THE SENSUOUS IN THE COUNTER-REFORMATION CHURCH

This book examines the promotion of the sensuous as part of religious experience in the Roman Catholic Church of the early modern period. During the Counter-Reformation, every aspect of religious and devotional practice, including the role of art and architecture, was reviewed and the invocation of the five senses to incite devotion became a hotly contested topic. Protestants condemned the material cult of veneration of relics and images, rejecting the importance of emotion and the senses and instead promoting the power of reason in receiving the Word of God. After much debate, the Church concluded that the senses are necessary to appreciate the sublime and that they derive from the Holy Spirit. As part of its attempt to win back the faithful, the Church embraced the sensuous and promoted the use of images, relics, liturgy, processions, music, and theater as important parts of religious experience.

Marcia B. Hall is The Carnell Professor of Renaissance Art History and Director of Graduate Studies at Tyler School of Art, Temple University. She is the author and editor of several books, including *The Sacred Image in the Age of Art: Titian, Tintoretto, Barocci, El Greco, Caravaggio*; *After Raphael*; and *Renovation and Counter Reformation: Vasari and Duke Cosimo in Santa Maria Novella and Santa Croce, 1564–77*.

Tracy E. Cooper is Professor of Art History at Tyler School of Art, Temple University. She is the author of *Renaissance*, and her book *Palladio's Venice: Architecture and Society in a Renaissance Republic* received the Phyllis Goodhart Gordan Prize from the Renaissance Society of America as well as a Special Mention for the Premio Salimbeni. She is the recipient of numerous fellowships, including, most recently, ones from the Renaissance Society of America and the Gladys Krieble Delmas Foundation.

THE SENSUOUS IN THE COUNTER-REFORMATION CHURCH

EDITED BY

MARCIA B. HALL

Temple University

TRACY E. COOPER

Temple University

CAMBRIDGE UNIVERSITY PRESS

CAMBRIDGE
UNIVERSITY PRESS

University Printing House, Cambridge CB2 8BS, United Kingdom

One Liberty Plaza, 20th Floor, New York, NY 10006, USA

477 Williamstown Road, Port Melbourne, VIC 3207, Australia

314–321, 3rd Floor, Plot 3, Splendor Forum, Jasola District Centre, New Delhi - 110025, India

79 Anson Road, #06-04/06, Singapore 079906

Cambridge University Press is part of the University of Cambridge.

It furthers the University's mission by disseminating knowledge in the pursuit of education, learning and research at the highest international levels of excellence.

www.cambridge.org
Information on this title: www.cambridge.org/9781107013230

First published 2013
Reprinted 2016

A catalogue record for this publication is available from the British Library

Library of Congress Cataloging in Publication data
The sensuous in the Counter-Reformation church / [edited by] Marcia B. Hall, Tracy E. Cooper.
p. cm.
Includes bibliographical references and index.
ISBN 978-1-107-01323-0 (hardback)
1. Counter-Reformation in art. 2. Senses and sensation – Religious aspects – Christianity. 3. Counter-Reformation. I. Hall, Marcia B. II. Cooper, Tracy Elizabeth.
N7862.S467 2012
704.9′482088282–dc23 2011047851

ISBN 978-1-107-01323-0 Hardback

CONTENTS

ILLUSTRATIONS

CONTRIBUTORS

Costanza Barbieri received her Ph.D. from Rutgers University. She is currently Assistant Professor of Art History at the Accademia di Belle Arti of Rome. She is the curator of the exhibition *Notturno Sublime. Sebastiano e Michelangelo nella* Pietà *di Viterbo* (Viterbo, Museo Civico, 2004), author of *Specchio di virtù. Il consorzio della Vergine e gli affreschi di Lorenzo Lotto in San Michele al Pozzo Bianco* (Lubrina, 2000), and coauthor of *Santa Maria in Vallicella. Chiesa Nuova* (Fratelli Palombi, 1995). Her field of interest is primarily sixteenth-century iconography. She recently published several articles on Sebastiano del Piombo and is preparing a book on the Loggia della Galatea.

Tracy E. Cooper is Professor of Art History at Temple University. Her book, *Palladio's Venice: Architecture and Society in a Renaissance Republic* (Yale University Press, 2006), received the Phyllis Goodhart Gordan Prize from the Renaissance Society of America. Other relevant publications include "Paolo Veronese – fa un *modo* per 'la riforma cattolica'?" *Crisi e rinnovamenti nell'autunno del rinascimento* (Leo S. Olschki Editore, 1991); "Locus meditandi et orandi: Architecture and Liturgy at San Giorgio Maggiore," *Musica, scienza e idee nella Serenissima del Seicento* (Edizioni Fondazione Levi, 1996); and "Singers and Setting: Choir and Furnishing in an Age of Reform," *Architettura e musica nella Venezia del rinascimento* (Bruno Mondadori Editore, 2006).

Robert W. Gaston, Ph.D., Warburg Institute, is Principal Fellow in Art History at the University of Melbourne. He taught art history at Bryn Mawr College, the University of Melbourne, Boston University, and La Trobe University. He was Visiting Professor at Villa I Tatti, the Harvard University Center for Italian Renaissance Studies, Florence, and Senior Research Fellow at CASVA, the National Gallery of Art, Washington, DC. He has written extensively on decorum, including an article in

Macmillan's renowned 1996 *Grove Dictionary of Art*. His latest major publication is a critical edition of Pirro Ligorio's Naples manuscript on waters in the forthcoming Edizione Nazionale. He is currently editing (with Louis Waldman) I Tatti's San Lorenzo monograph project.

Meredith J. Gill is Professor of Italian Renaissance Art at the University of Maryland, College Park. Her scholarly interests include art and spirituality in Italy from the late medieval era through the sixteenth century. She is the author of *Augustine in the Italian Renaissance: Art and Philosophy from Petrarch to Michelangelo* (Cambridge University Press, 2005), and she has contributed to *Rome* in the series Artistic Centers of the Italian Renaissance (ed. Marcia Hall, Cambridge University Press, 2005) and *The Renaissance World* (ed. John Jeffries Martin, Routledge, 2007). Among other projects, she has coedited, with Karla Pollmann, *Augustine Beyond the Book* (Brill, 2012), a collection of interdisciplinary studies on Augustine's reception.

Marcia B. Hall is The Carnell Professor of Renaissance Art and Director of Graduate Studies at Temple University. She has been writing about the Counter-Reformation since her first book, *Renovation and Counter-Reformation: Vasari and Duke Cosimo in Santa Maria Novella and Santa Croce, 1564–1577* (Cambridge University Press, 1979), in *After Raphael* (Cambridge University Press, 1999) and most recently in *The Sacred Image in the Age of Art: Titian, Tintoretto, Barocci, El Greco, Caravaggio* (Yale University Press, 2011). These are concerned with the relationship of midcentury *maniera* to the art of the subsequent Counter-Reformation. She contributed to and edited the volume *Rome* in the Cambridge series Artistic Centers of the Italian Renaissance, of which she is also series editor.

Stuart Lingo is Associate Professor of Renaissance Art at the University of Washington. He received his Ph.D. from Harvard University (1998) and has been a Fellow at Villa I Tatti, the Harvard University Center for Italian Renaissance Studies, and a Visiting Senior Fellow at the Center for Advanced Study in the Visual Arts at the National Gallery of Art. In *Federico Barocci: Allure and Devotion in Late Renaissance Painting* (Yale University Press, 2008), he explores the fertile tensions between artistic ambition and religious devotion in mid- to late-sixteenth-century Italy. His current work focuses on the shifting fortunes of the ideal nude in the period.

Maria H. Loh is Lecturer in the history of early modern Italian art and theory at University College London. She is the author of *Titian Remade: Repetition and the Transformation of Early Modern Italian Art* (Getty Research Institute, 2007) and the editor of *Early Modern Horror*, a special issue of the *Oxford Art Journal* (2011). She has also written on repetition and desire; sensation, special affects, and the moving image; and portraiture and loss.

She is currently working on *Past Perfect: On the Construction of Old Master Narratives*, which looks at pathos, process, and performance in the representation of early modern artists.

Peter M. Lukehart is Associate Dean at the Center for Advanced Study in the Visual Arts, National Gallery of Art. From 1992 until 2001, he was director of the Trout Gallery and Professor at Dickinson College, where he organized the exhibition and Web site *Writing on Hands: Memory and Knowledge in Early Modern Europe* (2000). His publications include contributions to *Taddeo and Federico Zuccaro: Artist-Brothers in Renaissance Rome* (J. Paul Getty Museum, 2007) and to *The Artist's Workshop* (National Gallery of Art, 1993) and the *Accademia Seminars* (Yale University Press, 2009), both published under his editorship. He is project director of "The History of the Accademia di San Luca, c. 1590–1635: Documents from the Archivio di Stato di Roma" (www.nga.gov/casva/accademia).

Opher Mansour is Assistant Professor, University of Hong Kong. His research focuses on attempts to reform or suppress art in the Catholic Reformation and on responses and resistance to such projects. He has published essays on the depiction of martyrs and martyrdom in Counter-Reformation prints, on the papal state portrait, and on the Camerino Farnese, and he is currently writing a book on the changing status of the body in Italian art and art theory, from the debates over Michelangelo's *Last Judgment*, to the renewed prominence given to the nude and to the human figure in the work of Annibale Carracci and Caravaggio.

John W. O'Malley, a specialist in the religious culture of early modern Europe, is currently University Professor in the Theology Department of Georgetown University. Among his seven monographs, *The First Jesuits* (Harvard University Press, 1995), winner of two best-book prizes and translated into ten languages, is perhaps the best known. He has received lifetime achievement awards from the Renaissance Society of America and the Society for Italian Historical Studies. He is a Fellow of the American Academy of Arts and Sciences and of the Accademia di San Carlo, Ambrosian Library, Milan.

Amy Powell, who received her Ph.D. from Harvard University, is Assistant Professor in the Department of Art History and the Graduate Program in Visual Studies at the University of California, Irvine. She is the author of *Perpetual Motifs: Scenes from the Late Medieval Church and the Modern Museum* (Zone Books, 2012) and is currently working on a project called *The Whitewashed Image: Iconoclasm and Seventeenth-Century Dutch Landscapes*.

Richard Schofield studied classics (Oxford, 1968–72), then art history (Courtauld Institute, Ph.D., 1979). He worked at Nottingham University and is now Professor of Architectural History at Istituto Universitario di Architettura di Venezia, Venice. He has written numerous articles on Lombard Renaissance architecture and sculpture and five books with co-workers: on Amadeo (1989), on Pellegrino Tibaldi (1994), translations of Palladio (with Robert Tavernor, MIT Press, 1997) and of Vitruvius (Penguin, 2009), and *Architettura e controriforma. I dibattiti per la facciata del Duomo di Milano, 1582–1682* (with Francesco Repishti, Electa Editore, 2004), in which he proposed an explanation of the doctrinal justification for splendor in post-Tridentine architecture.

Jeffrey Chipps Smith, Kay Fortson Chair in European Art at the University of Texas, Austin, specializes in German and Netherlandish art, 1400–1700. His publications include *Nuremberg: A Renaissance City, 1500–1618* (University of Texas Press, 1983); *German Sculpture of the Later Renaissance, c. 1520–1580* (Princeton University Press, 1994); *Sensuous Worship: The Jesuits and the Art of the Early Catholic Reformation in Germany* (Princeton University Press, 2002); *The Northern Renaissance* (Phaidon Press, 2004); *The Art of the Goldsmith in Late Fifteenth Century Germany: The Kimbell Virgin and Her Bishop* (Kimbell Art Museum, 2006); *Dürer* (forthcoming, Phaidon Press); editor, *New Perspectives on the Art of Renaissance Nuremberg: Five Essays* (Arthur M. Huntington Art Gallery, 1985); and coeditor (with Larry Silver), *The Essential Dürer* (University of Pennsylvania Press, 2010).

Bette Talvacchia is Board of Trustees Distinguished Professor Emerita of Art History at the University of Connecticut. She edited and contributed to *Sexuality in the Renaissance (1450–1650)*, volume 3 in the series The Cultural History of Sexuality (Berg Publishers, 2010). She has written a monograph on Raphael (Phaidon Press, 2007) and is the author of *Taking Positions: On the Erotic in Renaissance Culture* (Princeton University Press, 1999). Her most recent article in the area of gender studies is "The Double Life of Saint Sebastian in Renaissance Painting," in *The Body in Early Modern Italy*, ed. Julia Hairston and Walter Stephens (Johns Hopkins University Press, 2010).

ACKNOWLEDGMENTS

The idea for this volume grew out of several sessions that we organized for the annual meeting of the Renaissance Society of America held in March 2007 in Miami, Florida. The editors would like to thank all the participants in those stimulating sessions, many of whom are represented in this volume. Those contributors who subsequently joined the project have rounded out the topic and added additional perspectives. We would particularly like to thank John W. O'Malley, who began as the commentator on the sessions in Miami and has now, drawing on his incomparable knowledge of the subject, contributed a historical review of how the decree on the veneration of images of the Council of Trent came to be. It is an indispensable introduction to our topic and a touchstone for the authors of this volume.

We are most grateful to our acquisitions editor, Beatrice Rehl, Publishing Director of Humanities & Social Sciences for Cambridge University Press, and the publications team, in particular book designer Holly Johnson and copy editor Mary Becker, for their dedicated work on this complex volume.

Marcia B. Hall and Tracy E. Cooper

INTRODUCTION

Marcia B. Hall

THE THEME OF THIS volume is the promotion of the sensuous as a part of religious experience in the Roman Catholic Church of the early modern period. Here "sensuous" refers to the dictionary definition of the term: of, related to, or derived from the senses, usually the senses involved in aesthetic enjoyment. "Sensual" usually applies to the physical senses or appetites, particularly those associated with sexual pleasure. We have not excluded the sensual – indeed, Bette Talvacchia's essay deals explicitly with this area and others refer to it – but it is not our primary focus.

The origin of this book is two sessions at the 2007 meeting of the Renaissance Society of America, entitled "The Counter-Reformation Re-encountered."[1] By design, the sessions offered a range of perspectives: the presenters included historians and art historians, and the commentator, John O'Malley, is the leading historian today working on religion in the Renaissance. We all noted that the papers had, as a common thread, the role of the senses. It was apparent that classic formulations were being questioned by each of the authors, and this indicated that the time is right for a reassessment of the Counter-Reformation.[2]

Erasmus initiated the debate that developed between Protestants and Catholics over the role of the senses at the beginning of the sixteenth century, when he called for reform from within the Church. He described, and roundly condemned, the material cult of the veneration of relics and images that he saw all around him: lavish ceremonies displaying the wealth of the Church and superstitious practices, such as prostrating oneself before the statues of saints. Erasmus influenced Martin Luther in his formulation of *sola scriptura* and his rejection of good works as a means of salvation, including the patronage of churches, chapels, and monasteries. Reformed churches were whitewashed, stripped of images and of ornament. Although Luther eventually permitted didactic altarpieces, Calvin sternly prohibited them and eliminated all pomp and ceremony from the liturgy, with the intent that worshippers would have nothing to distract them from receiving the Word of God and pondering it with their mental faculties. Appeal to the senses was to be avoided because it created an emotional dependency on the Church, which Protestants regarded as an illegitimate hold over the faithful.

The definitive response from the Catholic side came from Alberto Pio, who bundled Erasmus together with the Protestant Reformers and proclaimed that joy must accompany every form of the divine cult.[3] The senses are necessary, according to Pio, to ascend to sublime things, and they derive from the Holy Spirit. The lines were drawn. In the thirteenth session of the Council of Trent (1551) the doctrine of Transubstantiation of the Eucharistic elements, rejected by most Protestants, was reaffirmed, together with the practice of carrying the Host in procession. When the Council finally pronounced the Church's position on sacred images (1563), it endorsed them, saying that "great benefits flowed from all sacred images" and that by them "the faithful should be aroused to adore and love God and to practice devotion."[4]

The role of the senses had always been recognized in the writings of the Church, and that written tradition played an important part in the arguments put forward against the Protestant Reformers.[5] The apologists for images in fact argued for the superiority of the senses over reason in promoting devotion. Alberto Pio, responding to Erasmus, had declared that all spiritual reality is transmitted to the mind by the senses, and Ambrogio Caterino echoed him.[6] Catholics recognized that emotion was a tool that Protestants had renounced and that it could therefore be used effectively to woo the lapsed back to the Catholic fold.[7] Images were an important part of the whole arsenal that included relics, liturgy, processions, music, and theater. Protestants held that reason, not emotion, should be the basis of religious experience. Both sides recognized the unconscious power images wield over thought and behavior, but for Catholics this was an indispensable bond that strengthened believers' relationship to God and tied them to the Church. The reassertion of this tradition of honoring the appeal to the emotions vitalized the reform after Trent, as the essays in this volume will show. In this introduction, some of the revisions and trends in current scholarship of both historians and art historians of the post-Tridentine era will be discussed, in particular with regard to the role of the senses.

The view of the Counter-Reformation held by historians until the past quarter-century has been summarized powerfully by John O'Malley:

> Serious historians of Christianity of the early modern period had until recently little interest in Catholicism as a subject of research. The Renaissance, they believed, was theologically vacuous, only superficially Christian, and the so-called Counter-Reformation was a restoration of the worst aspects of the Middle Ages, interesting only insofar as it threw light on the Protestant Reformation. The Reformation was modern, the

Catholic Church remained medieval. To such historians even religious art of the latter period reflected the monolithic uniformity of Catholicism at large. It adhered slavishly to the dictates of ecclesiastical authority, which acted on the well known lines on sacred art from the Council of Trent, and it was programmed as a reaction to Protestantism.[8]

O'Malley goes on to point out, however, that since about 1985–90 Catholicism has held a new allure: the stepsister, though not yet Cinderella, has attracted the unbiased attention of a young generation of scholars, particularly in North America, who often do not have a Catholic background.[9]

What I see as the single most important revision in this recent scholarship is the recognition that reform after Trent was not simply mandated by ecclesiastical authorities, then obediently and mindlessly implemented. Certainly there were efforts to impose conformity, but they collapsed, as for example in Carlo Borromeo's Archbishopric of Milan[10] – where they met with resistance from the civic authorities and barely survived beyond his death – or in the early days of the Jesuits. In 1558 the first General Congregation of the Order issued a ruling regarding the erection of houses (residences),[11] which was confirmed and enlarged on at the next meeting in 1565: "Jesuit structures should be neither lavish nor overly decorated, but should awaken the contemplation of poverty and built in the form and manner of our buildings." This is an unambiguous reference to an accepted Jesuit standard. All projects had to be examined by the Jesuit general and approved by him, after which no changes were permitted.[12] In the event, as the Society of Jesus spread geographically, it became impossible to exercise tight control and latitude was permitted.[13] It should be noted that the prohibition on decoration was not applied to churches. Jeffrey Chipps Smith shows in his essay just how lavish a Jesuit church might become by the seventeenth century.

In contrast to these efforts by Church authorities to dictate, a more typical procedure was exemplified by the project to renovate the churches in Florence.[14] In 1564, the year following the close of the Council of Trent, Duke Cosimo, on his own initiative, instituted reforms that transformed the Dominican and Franciscan churches, S. Maria Novella and S. Croce, into structures that privileged the laity as never before. The duke ordered that the rood screens, which blocked the view of the high altar from the laity's space, be removed and the friars' choirs be transferred from their elite position immediately in front of the high altar to the chancel behind it. Altars were constructed in each of the bays of the nave, and in S. Croce the subjects of the altarpieces were designed to follow a sequence of Christ's Passion, providing the laity with the opportunity to meditate on the narrative. The churches were thereby transformed: virtually all traces of the medieval hierarchical arrangement were eradicated,[15] and in accordance with the spirit of Trent, the churches were reoriented to the laywomen and laymen. What is noteworthy is that there is no evidence that the ecclesiastical authorities were even consulted, to say nothing of their having dictated or directed the project, and that the artists enthusiastically endorsed it. This is in sharp contrast with the way Carlo Borromeo proceeded with church-building reform in Milan,[16] but the contrast highlights the error of regarding post-Tridentine reform as a monolithic, top-down movement imposed by the Church on arts and architecture.

Scholars are recognizing increasingly, then, that the process of reform after Trent was not in the main one of enforcement or of issuing directives from above; rather it was catalyzed by the initiative of patrons and artists who sought new solutions addressing concerns that had been raised. Of particular interest is the development in recent Counter-Reformation scholarship of the concept of "negotiation." It is a kind of "counter-category," as O'Malley has dubbed it, to "social discipline," by which historians meant the imposition of standards of social behavior from above.[17] "Negotiation" points to responses of resistance and compromise to those efforts to impose standards. Such negotiating has been shown to take place at all levels: "between bishops and Rome, between pastors and bishops on the one hand and their flocks on the other, and between accused and inquisitors."[18] From the vantage point of art history, negotiation is proving to be an important key to interpretation. In fact, it can enable us to see through to what was really going on behind the official documents. A case in point is the infamous encounter between Paolo Veronese and the Venetian Inquisition over his decoration for the refectory of SS. Giovanni e Paolo. The study of it has normally been interpreted to fall in the category of social disciplining rather than negotiation: it is traditionally cited as the most egregious instance of the ecclesiastical authorities intervening between the artist and his church patrons. The case has been useful to scholars trying to understand the new norms for painting in the post-Tridentine period, because the court records of Veronese's interrogation have survived and show specifically what the concerns of the Inquisition were.[19] However, the compromise that concluded the case is not documented and is therefore generally overlooked by scholars. The painting was not destroyed; the painter was not punished. We can deduce from the present state of the painting, to which an inscription identifying the scriptural passage on which it is based was added, that all parties reached an agreement simply to change the subject from the Last Supper to the sacramentally neutral Feast in the House of Levi. The alternative view of this notorious case, informed by the new interpretive tool, is that when the Inquisition flexed its muscle to demonstrate that it could and would exercise oversight, both the patrons and the painter were able to negotiate a compromise. It is significant that this is the only recorded case of such intervention by the Venetian Inquisition that we know of.

Another example of negotiation was the system that evolved in the 1580s whereby the painter was required to present a drawing to the church

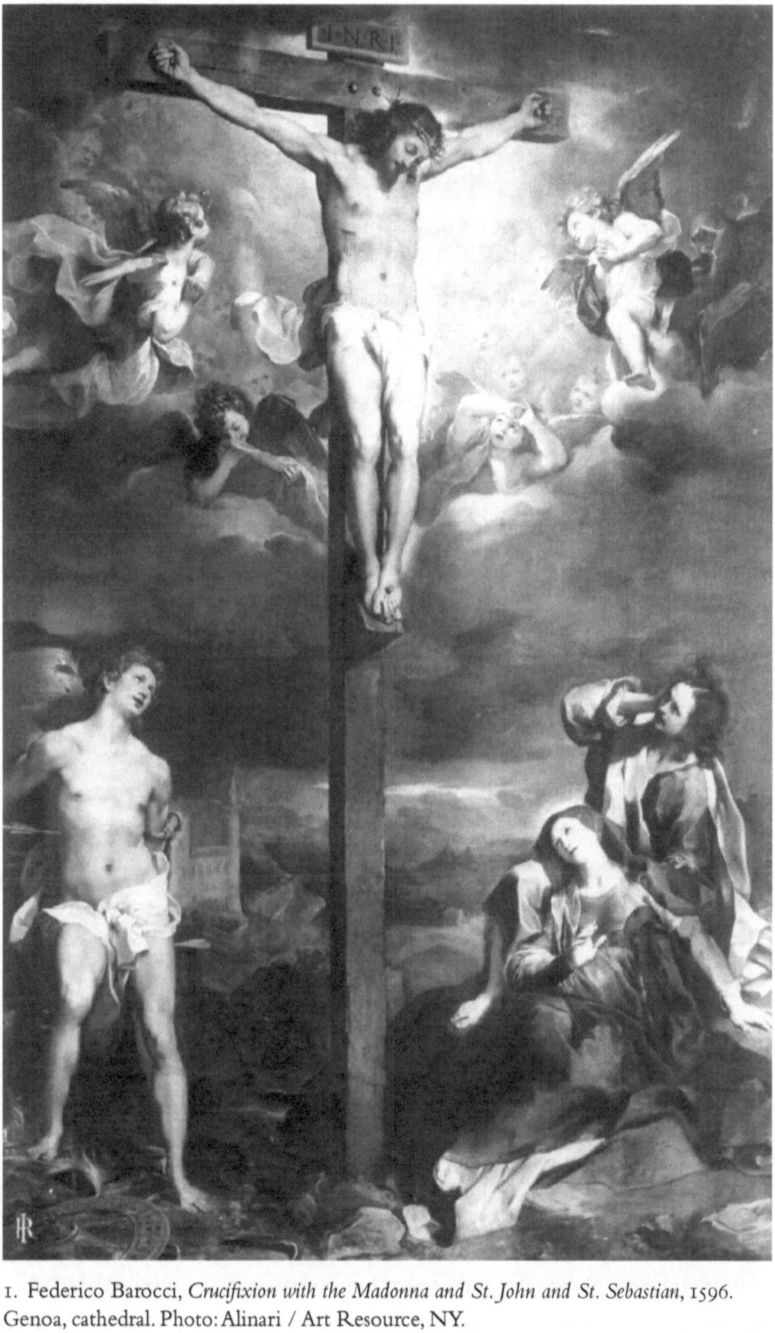

1. Federico Barocci, *Crucifixion with the Madonna and St. John and St. Sebastian*, 1596. Genoa, cathedral. Photo: Alinari / Art Resource, NY.

before executing an altarpiece. A documented early instance is that of the Oratorians requiring Scipione Pulzone to send a *cartone* of his *Crucifixion* to allow the fathers to assess it in situ.[20] This became required practice in 1593 when Cardinal Vicario Girolamo Rusticucci issued an edict that artists should submit a *bozzetto* for prior approval by ecclesiastical authorities.[21] Although an undeniable aspect of social disciplining is implied, the mechanism set up a situation in which negotiation between artist and patron could take place in advance to avoid any need for censure or rejection of the finished altarpiece.

In fact, enforcement of the decree was local, sporadic, and underfunded. Studies show that concern in the parishes centered more on the leaking roof than on the questionable decorum of the pictures.[22] Opher Mansour's essay on Clement VIII's visitation of the churches in his Diocese of Rome shows that although the pope had the power to effect reform, his efforts were often ineffective. Both patrons and artists sought new solutions for the sacred image, recognizing that the *maniera* paintings of the pre-Trent period did not provide satisfactory images to stir the worshipper's devotion.[23] The appeal to the emotions of the new sacred images that artists like Federico Barocci were striving for clearly struck a chord with patrons, if one can judge from the letter from Doge Senarega praising the *Crucifixion with the Madonna and St. John and St. Sebastian* that Barocci had executed for the Genoa cathedral (1596, Illustration 1).[24] He calls it "something divine," "beyond the reach of human praise." Senarega makes clear that it evoked in him deep emotions. "The Virgin arouses pity and consoles, and it seems precisely that her divine spirit, penetrating the wounds of Christ, enter into them to discover whether she is to be transfixed by the death of her beloved son or rather regenerated by the redemption of humankind." In attempting to describe its affect, he says that "it enraptures, tears asunder, and gently transforms us." Though the rhetoric may seem over the top to us, and therefore suspect, it signals a level of emotional involvement with the image that was desired and that would not have been possible with pre-Trent *maniera* sacred images.

LITERATURE ON ART OF THE POST-TRIDENTINE ERA

The literature on art of the post-Tridentine era has its own history. There is a noticeable lack of attention to the effects of the Tridentine decree in the seventeenth, eighteenth, and early nineteenth centuries, although the controversy surrounding the Jesuits had an impact on the way art was regarded, as we shall see. A few treatises continued to appear after the flurry culminating in Gabrielle Paleotti's *Discorso* in 1582,[25] most notably that of Giovan Domenico Ottonelli and Pietro da Cortona,[26] examined here in Maria H. Loh's essay, but writers about art, like Baldinucci, Malvasia, Bellori, and less well known local historians, followed the model of Vasari's biographies. Even Luigi Lanzi, who was trained as a Jesuit priest, wrote his *Storia Pittorica dell'Italia* without giving special attention to the genre of sacred images (1792–96). Although Lanzi depended heavily on Raffaello Borghini (1584)[27] in describing the altarpieces in Florentine churches, he largely ignored Borghini's critique from the point of view of Trent, mildly objecting in passing to Bronzino's *Christ in Limbo* (see Illustration 18) because the naked figure was better suited to an academy of design than to a church, a paraphrase of Borghini.[28] Stuart Lingo's essay in our volume examines Borghini's treatise in the light of the Florentine context.

The term "Counter-Reformation," which originated in 1776 in the plural usage of Johann Stephan Pütter (*Gegenreformations*), had been used by the historian Leopold von Ranke (1843), but he did not discuss art. The subject did not reenter the literature until Charles Dejob published *De l'influence du Concile de Trente sur la littérature et les beaux-arts chez les peuples catholiques: essai d'introductionà l'histoire littéraire du siècle de Louis XIV* in 1884.[29] Even after its publication, post-Tridentine sacred art was not separated out in the literature and would be discussed under the rubric of mannerism or late Renaissance art, that is, categorized by style rather than subject.

Certainly the appearance of Emile Mâle, *L'art religieux après le Concile de Trente, étude sur l'iconographie de la fin du XVIe, du XVIIe et du XVIIIe siècles en Italie, en France, en Espagne et en Flandre* (1932), drew attention to new iconography, although most of Mâle's examples were drawn from the seventeenth century.[30] His choices were no doubt circumscribed by the scarcity of photographs of works from the late sixteenth century – a situation that has not been fully remedied to this day – so that he did not adequately discuss the last third of the sixteenth century. Nevertheless, Mâle opened up the topic of Catholic ideology, showing how Trent's endorsement of the didactic function of sacred images came to be interpreted as a mandate to defend doctrines attacked by Protestants. Thus, we find, for example, the Virgin Mary the subject of increased devotion, and the cult of saints, especially martyrdoms, represented with a new fervor. Iconography that promoted the position of the Church is territory that continues to be mined to great effect in scholarship, for example, the colossal exhibition on art at the time of Sixtus V[31] and recent studies of iconographical programs of the Church. Not only iconographical innovation in individual images or programs, but entire genres, such as landscape and still life, emerged as new objects for devotional consideration after Trent and have received recent study by scholars such as Pamela M. Jones, whose *Federico Borromeo and the Ambrosiana: Art Patronage and Reform in Seventeenth-Century Milan* has provided a firm foundation for contextualizing preferences in patronage and collecting.[32]

The first book to focus on the *style* of Counter-Reformation painting in Italy was Federico Zeri's *Pittura e Controriforma. "L'arte senza tempo" di Scipione da Gaeta* (1957).[33] He characterized Scipione Pulzone as the quintessential painter of post-Tridentine sacred art, finding in his work a manner that removed the image from the immediacy of setting or moment, creating what Zeri called a timeless quality. For Zeri, the period was the beginning of the drying up of religious art that has continued to our own time. Although he showed insight in recognizing that Trent inaugurated a new era, he had no sympathy for it; the painters he selected to epitomize it gave Counter-Reformation art a bad name among connoisseurs. In fact, contrary to Zeri's premise, it is difficult to pick out any artist who is exemplary of this period. Gauvin Bailey has pointed out that "[i]n the decades before 1600 a greater variety of styles was being used than ever before in the history of Central Italian painting, as each artist went in his own direction to reformulate the rules of *arte sacra*."[34] In the English-speaking world, Zeri's first impact was on Sydney Freedberg, who applied his term "Counter-Maniera" to painting in relevant cases across the Italian peninsula.[35] In the 1980s, perhaps inspired by the reprinting of Paolo Prodi's important essay from 1962, "Ricerca sulla teorica delle arti figurative nella Riforma Cattolica,"[36] Italian scholars Alessandro Zuccaro and Claudio Strinati, among others, began turning their attention to the problem of style in post-Tridentine painters.[37]

A different approach proved more fertile. In 1940 Rensselaer Lee turned attention to the contemporary sources and the ways they addressed style in "*Ut pictura poesis*: The Humanistic Theory of Painting."[38] His study, particularly of Gilio, would sire a series of investigations of the application of the classical rhetorical principle of decorum in post-Tridentine art. Following Lee, Charles Dempsey recognized that decorum was a key to understanding how artists translated the decree into art and, conversely, how their art would be judged.[39] Robert W. Gaston's essay in our volume shows that the interpretation of decorum was as varied as the artists themselves, and thus contributes to our understanding of the diversity of the period.

Around 1960, publications of the sources began to appear, most notably that by Paola Barocchi, *Trattati d'arte del Cinquecento fra Manierismo e Controriforma*. The translation and analysis of *Charles Borromeo's "Instructiones fabricae et supellectilis ecclesiaticae," 1577*, by Evelyn Carole Voelker, added significantly to our understanding of the social-disciplining side of the reform.[40] Especially valuable are Giuseppe Scavizzi's analyses of sources in his various publications, first in Italian and culminating in *The Controversy on Images from Calvin to Baronius* (1992).[41]

Two decades previously, Anthony Blunt's influential summary of sources, *Artistic Theory in Italy, 1450–1660* (1940), first appeared, but it is misleading in its characterization of the spirit of the reform after Trent. Blunt's book has been a principal source disseminating the view of the Counter-Reformation as a top-down organization. He characterized the Counter-Reformers as diametrically opposed to the humanists: "It was their aim to undo all that the Renaissance had achieved, and to get back to a feudal and medieval state of affairs.... One of the first objects of the Counter-Reformers was to abolish the right of the individual to settle all the problems of thought or conscience according to the judgement of his own personal reason. They wished instead to set up the acceptance of authority, which was exactly the principle the Humanists had succeeded in destroying."[42]

Francis Haskell laid the broad foundation for studying systems of patronage in his book *Patrons and Painters* (1963), which was revised and enlarged in 1980, indicating its ongoing impact. It has spawned a large number of useful studies of papal and cardinalate patronage, including those on collections and collectors, and programs of architectural renovation and decoration.[43] Christian Adolf Isermeyer did some early work in this latter area, followed by Hall's study of the Florentine Mendicant Church renovations already mentioned.[44] Enlarging the field of Mâle's original investigation of persuasive imagery was the influential work of Joseph Connors, *Borromini and the Roman Oratory: Style and Society*.[45] Beginning in the 1990s, students of Connors and Irving Lavin began the systematic study of iconographical programs of the late Renaissance and baroque – for example, Jack Freiberg, *The Lateran in 1600: Christian Concord in Counter-Reformation Rome* (1995). The Cambridge series Monuments of Papal Rome, edited by Connors and Lavin, included Steven Ostrow, *Art and Spirituality in Counter-Reformation Rome: The Sistine and Pauline Chapels in S. Maria Maggiore* (1996); Louise Rice, *The Altars and Altarpieces of New St. Peter's: Outfitting the Basilica, 1621–1666* (1997); and Nicola Courtright, *The Papacy and the Art of Reform in Sixteenth-Century Rome: Gregory XIII's Tower of the Winds* (2004). In each case the author has shown how the subject matter of the decorative program and architectural decisions were shaped by the concerns of the Church. Taking the opposite viewpoint, that of the laity, Pamela Jones, who has authored several important studies of Counter-Reformation art and culture, offered in 2008 a study of the reception of altarpieces in Rome by contemporaries, providing us with a multivalent perspective on the outcome of such programs.[46]

THE SOCIETY OF JESUS

The association of Counter-Reformation art with "propaganda," that is, missionizing, however, reinforced a mistrust of it born of suspicion of the Jesuits.[47] The historiography of the Society of Jesus is an important chapter in the story of how the art of the post-Tridentine era has been regarded and deserves closer attention here. Because the Jesuits, unlike the other Orders, vowed to go on missions when ordered by the pope, which has been interpreted as an oath of loyalty to the pope, and because they grew rapidly and spread their mission not only across Europe but also around the world, their power made them increasingly an object of hostility. When the Jesuits fell into disfavor, culminating in the suppression of the Society in 1773, two aspects of their method came under suspicion. The first was their centralized and uniform approach, which suggested that all orders came from the top down. To the extent that the Jesuits and the Counter-Reformation were regarded as synonymous, the perception grew that the ecclesiastical authorities dictated initiatives for reform after Trent, which we have seen is a view only now receding. The second aspect was the Society's endorsement of the appeal to the senses as an especially effective way to stimulate devotion in the faithful; this fostered the suspicion that the Jesuits intended to subvert reason, to conquer the mind and the spirit "through visual intoxication" (phrase borrowed from Galassi Paluzzi).[48] In the age of the Enlightenment and its aftermath, this was a deeply sinister threat. It is in this context that one of the tasks of scholars interpreting the Counter-Reformation today is to reconstruct accurately and without prejudice the role of the senses and the emotions.

From the very start, the Society promoted the use of sacred images in devotion and encouraged an appeal to the senses. Ignatius of Loyola's *Spiritual Exercises* provided a model for the way the senses can be invoked to draw the participant into meditation.[49] Ignatius instructs the exercitant to concentrate all his senses and focus his imagination on the subject selected for the day's meditation, for example, hell. He is then instructed to see in his mind's eye the "composition," the place; then to feel it – the heat of hell's fire; then to hear it – the shrieks of the tortured damned, and so on through the senses.[50] A similar direct appeal to the senses characterized the worship experience in a Jesuit church.

It is useful to take a look at the Jesuits' adaptation of theater in order to gain insight into their methods because theater works the way liturgy does, appealing to the emotions through the senses. Professional theater was developing simultaneously with the founding and early years of the Society in the mid-Cinquecento. Recognizing the power of theater to change people, the Jesuits recognized as well the competition professional theater offered in the education and care of souls.[51] Theater educates, either for bad or for good, so they developed their own theater, making use of all the devices and techniques of professionals, but instead of educating their audiences in the vices – teaching how to lust after potential lovers, how to cuckold husbands, how to undermine the authority of masters, how to indulge the basest longings of the flesh – they taught them how to live virtuously in a world created and ordered by God.[52] The reason they were successful is that they in no way avoided sensuousness. Their spectacle competed with, and even surpassed, anything secular professionals had to offer.[53] "Jesuit dramaturgy operates in a thoroughly incarnational way: transcendence is achieved through the physical, through the word-made-flesh," in Michael Zampelli's words.[54]

Contrast this with Carlo Borromeo, who with puritanical zeal forbade comedy and dance in his Diocese of Milan. He objected to performances that competed with liturgical celebrations, disrupted holy days, indulged the imagination to no useful – that is, religious – purpose, and literally wasted time.[55] Although he temporarily persuaded Gregory XIII to his position, his victory was short-lived. Immediately following both their deaths, Gregory's successor, Sixtus V, permitted theatrical performances, though he banned women from acting.[56] By the seventeenth century, cardinals, conspicuous in purple, regularly attended the opera and theater.

Yet the anxiety in the Church over secular performance was never far beneath the surface. There is a substantial antitheater literature even among the Jesuits.[57] Gian Domenico Ottonelli, a Jesuit, first published a tract condemning immodest spectacles (*Memoriale agli spettatori delle teatrali oscenità*, 1640), then moderated his view in 1652 (*Della cristiana moderatione del teatro*). Two popes at the end of the Seicento, Innocent XI (r. 1676–89) and Innocent XII (r. 1691–1700), showed animosity to theatrical performance.[58] Nevertheless, the Jesuits' practicality and openness to modernity kept them at the cutting edge, borrowing from the secular world to devise every means to work with the laity for the good of their souls without requiring them to retreat into priggish renunciation of the pleasures of the world. In their theater, as in their approach to prayer and meditation, the Jesuits invested themselves in the human imagination, seeing it as critical to the formation of conscience.[59] The appeal to the imagination, activated by the senses, was also the hallmark of Jesuit devotional art.

The Tridentine decree on sacred images, which was intentionally left vague, called for images that moved the emotions of the devout, so the challenge for artists and patrons was how to implement it. In the wake of the decree, it was the treatise writers who spelled out how sacred images should be reformed. Though they were imprecise when they discussed style, they pointed to a fundamental fault in the devotional art of the previous generation, the lack of appeal to the emotions, or appeal that was problematic. Gilio's attack on Michelangelo's *Last Judgment*, which appeared a few months after the master's death, set the tone for much of what followed.[60] Gilio faulted Michelangelo for putting artistic effect above devotional efficacy and for relying on sophisticated artistic devices and iconography, which would not be understood by the ordinary worshipper. Although it was an ironic choice to single out as the scapegoat Michelangelo, who was as pious an artist as there was, there was justice in the complaint that the sacred images of Michelangelo's contemporaries were not successful when judged from the point of view of the Church.

THE FAILURE OF *MANIERA* SACRED IMAGES

The treatise writers who preceded and followed Gilio pointed to particular failures in *maniera* devotional art.[61] The cleric Ambrogio Caterino, writing before Gilio and the Tridentine decree, complained about the excessive artifice in paintings, saying, "Some images are so extravagant that you can hardly recognize the human figure in them,"[62] and Paleotti likewise objected to painters who "amass a multitude of figures and actions, which confuse your sight and intellect."[63] The *maniera* painters valued precisely this kind of artifice and copiousness, as we can see in Perino del

Vaga's drawings for the now dismantled Massimi Chapel in Trinità dei Monti (Illustration 2).[64] Scenes from the life of Christ were embedded in the richest possible framework, emulating the vaults of the pagan emperor Nero's palace, the Domus Aurea. Compartments were filled with gilded stucco ornaments and *grotteschi*, caryatids, masks – the entire repertory of antique decoration. The ornaments overwhelm the Christian narrative, in the same way that the musical *intermedi* had become the principal focus of a theatrical performance, overwhelming the comedy. What had begun in the Quattrocento as a musical interlude, an *entre'acte* to facilitate the transition between scenes, had become sumptuous pageants of costuming, set design, and cutting-edge stagecraft. This kind of inversion of priorities, this delight in surfeit, was an aesthetic that was not unique to the mid-Cinquecento, anticipated as it was by Nero. It characterized the taste of the elite who were the intended audiences: copiousness and *varietà* are the terms of praise one reads in Vasari and his contemporaries. For the painter of religious images, it is as if the multiplication of *bellezze* would serve as a substitute for the evocation of emotion.

The artifice Caterino denounced was precisely what the *maniera* painter sought. Take Domenico Beccafumi's decoration for the Pisa cathedral, for example (Illustration 3). Moses, descended from the mountain with the tablet of the law, finds the people worshipping a golden calf. Beccafumi is a master of dramatic lighting, here effectively dividing the righteous Moses in a band of light from the idolaters in the murky shadow. The dark, threatening sky suggests Moses' anger; however, the prophet's dance-like pose seems more concerned to model the perfect *figura serpentinata*[65] than to express plausible emotion. The river god reclining in the foreground shows off the painter's skill at foreshortening and chiaroscuro, but his nudity and his posture are difficult to explain in the context of the narrative. The woman placed frontally scarcely alters her choreographed pose to respond to Moses, lest we lose sight of her alluring body revealed through diaphanous drapery. When Gilio declared the painters more concerned with "the allure of art" (*la vaghezza de l'arte*)[66] than with inciting devotion, one has to admit he had a point.

Trent explicitly decreed that "all lasciviousness be avoided; in such wise that figures shall not be painted or adorned with a beauty exciting to lust." Figures like Beccafumi's woman are susceptible to the charge of a beauty "exciting to lust." Parmigianino's figures in the *Madonna and Child with Saints and an Angel* (Illustration 4) are not nude or even scantily draped, and yet there is an aura of the erotic about them. The angel who seeks our eye is lovely in excess. As Bette Talvacchia points out in her essay, the defenders of *maniera* would have argued that he is the embodiment of ideal beauty, which signals the divine, as is the Madonna herself. The intimate gesture and exchange of glance between the Christ Child and St. Margaret should be interpreted as divine love, yet there is a valence of carnality that cannot be denied. It was, to be sure, a short step from the ideality of Raphael to his

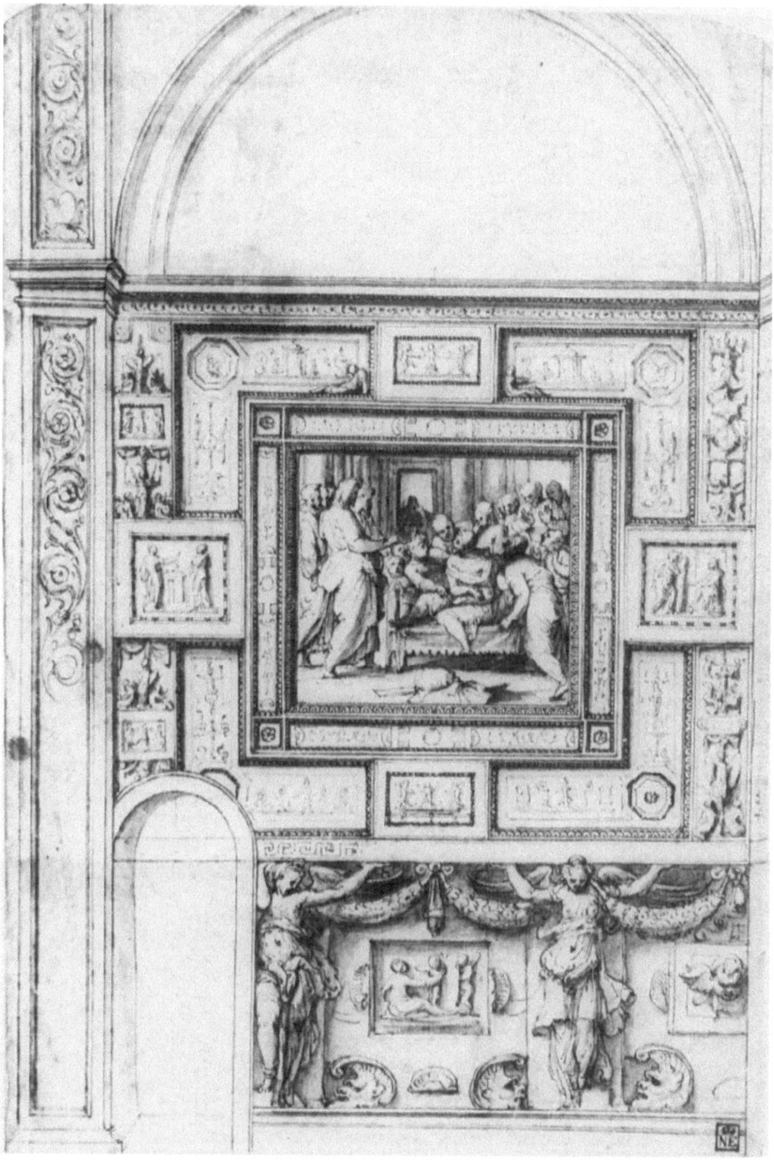

2. Perino del Vaga, Drawing for the side wall, Massimi Chapel in Trinità dei Monti, Rome, c. 1537–38. Budapest, National Gallery. Photo: Szépmüvészeti Museum, Budapest.

emulator Parmigianino, and yet some may feel that a line has been crossed; certainly the critics of the Counter-Reformation thought so.

An objection was voiced by Paleotti, and raised by many of the critics, to the "obscurity and intricacy" that made these paintings incomprehensible "without the help of a skilled professional philosopher or theologian."[67] The appeal of these pictures was more cerebral than emotional. That the obscurity was intentional is clear when one examines an altarpiece such as Bronzino's *Christ in Limbo* (Illustration 18). Vasari noted that it contained

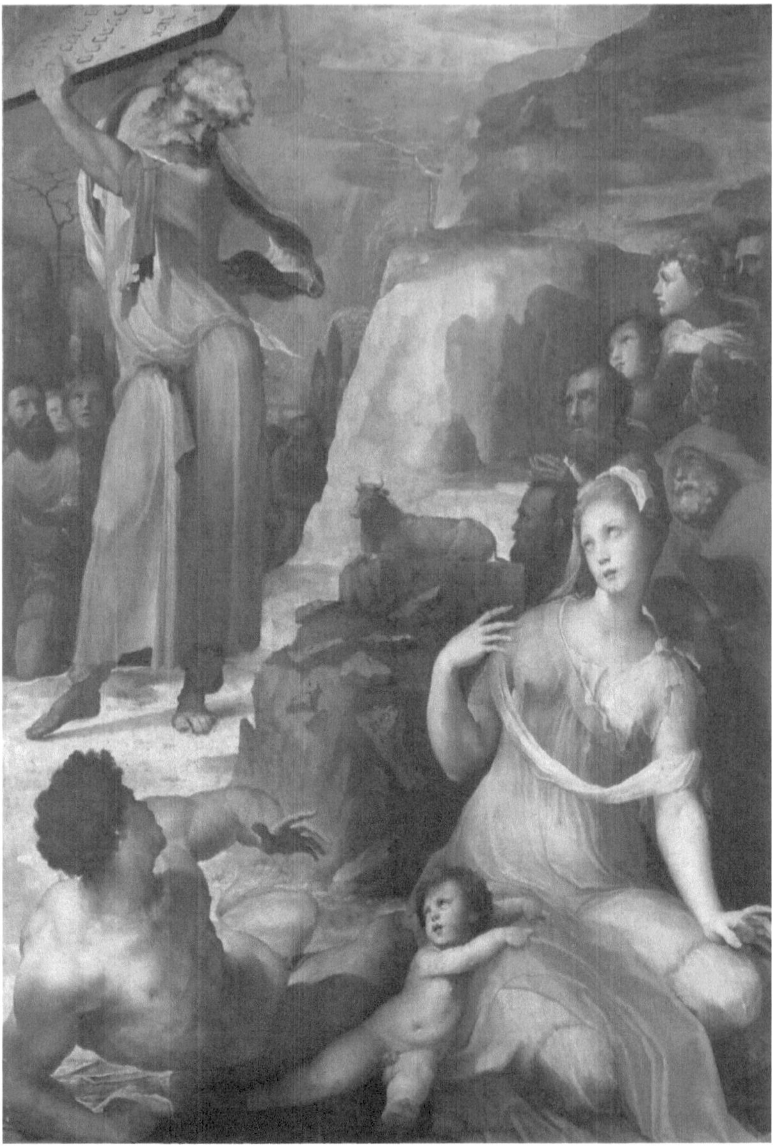

3. Domenico Beccafumi, *Moses Breaking the Tablets of the Law*, 1539. Pisa, cathedral. Photo: Scala / Art Resource, NY.

portraits of contemporary Florentines,[68] which is evident at a glance, and one can imagine the frisson that a member of the elite circle would have felt in recognizing his friends, but those outside the privileged circle would have been mystified and distracted by the apparent doubling of faces, as in the two arresting women who look out at us at the level of Christ's feet and the bearded twins behind his right shoulder. In Raffaello Borghini's dialogue, Vecchietti sternly rebuked Michelozzo for his "pleasure in gazing at the delicate parts of those beautiful women," saying, "We have already discussed how badly done are sacred figures made so lascivious. Now I tell you once more they are inappropriate, not only in churches but in every public place. They give a bad example and induce vain thoughts in the mind."[69] It is hard to avoid the impression that the painter was concerned mainly with addressing an insider group of cognoscenti and displaying his skill. The sheer aesthetic appeal of the coloring and these cold, marble-fleshed nudes is a substitute for the compassion we might expect

4. Parmigianino, *Madonna and Child with Saints and an Angel*, c. 1529. Bologna, Pinacoteca. Photo: Scala / Ministero per i Beni e le Attività culturali / Art Resource, NY.

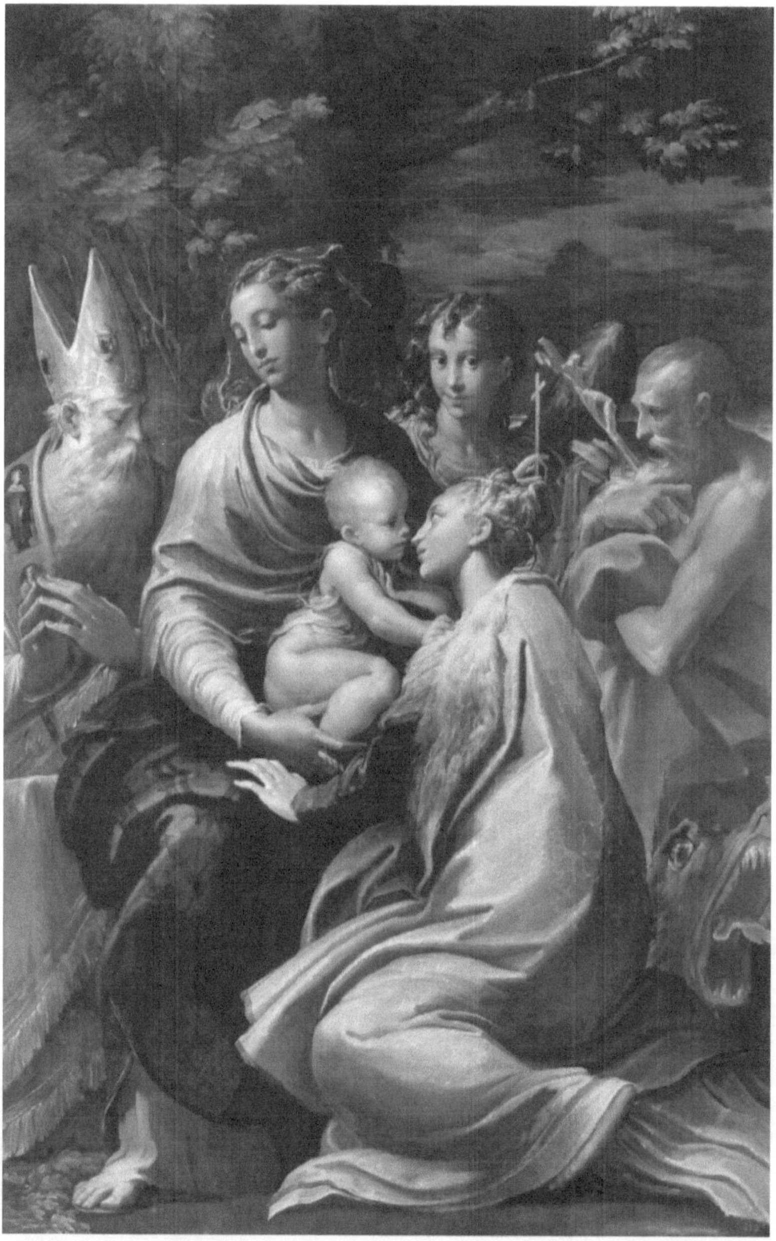

to feel for these men and women who have been hoping for release from limbo, to which they are condemned for eternity. It was the anesthetizing of emotion (as John Shearman called it) that was the principal and fundamental fault of *maniera* sacred images.

It was clear that ornament was not acceptable when used – as the *maniera* artist did – as a substitution for meaning and content, but there was a long tradition of adorning churches with rich materials to glorify God, traditionally supported by citing the instructions God had given to the Jews in building the Temple of Solomon.[70] There are competing views in the post-Tridentine era on lavish ornament and precious materials: Do they contribute to the sense of the presence of God, or do they distract the worshipper and violate the spirit of simplicity sought in the revival of early Christian religion? This issue remained unresolved in the last decades of the Cinquecento and early Seicento, as illustrated in this example of the Jesuits. They, like the other Orders, took a vow of poverty, so they were presented with a problem when donors insisted on adorning the gifts they made. Members of the Polish nobility made such a gift to the novitiate chapel of S. Andrea al Quirinale in the form of a tomb for a fellow countryman and former novice, Stanislas Kostka. Louis Richeôme was invited to Rome in 1608 by the father general of the Society, Claudio Acquavita, to write a handbook that would take the young novice on a spiritual journey through the images in S. Andrea. In his manual (1610), Richeôme, addressing remarks to the novices, says about the alabaster and gilding and precious materials with which the patrons had adorned the tomb: "All this work is a present of the devout affection and liberality of the Polish nobility made in memory of their compatriot; but none of this touches an atom of your devotion or of mine, which beholds a much higher design."[71] In other words, the novices do not need the precious materials for their devotion, but they are disciplined enough that they will not allow the materials to distract them.

Paleotti, as stern as he often was, made it clear from the outline of the unwritten chapters of his treatise that he was in favor of ornament in *pittura sacra* to enhance veneration. He intended a chapter in which he would discuss how the early Christians ornamented churches with sacred images of painting, sculpture, mosaics, and other precious materials.[72]

Notes

1 We are aware of the controversy surrounding the term "Counter-Reformation"; see O'Malley (2000). Our decision to use "Counter-Reformation" is deliberately based on its established usage as a period designation and our interest in revisiting associated issues in the immediate post-Tridentine climate.

2 According to the *Oxford English Dictionary*, 2d ed. (1989), "sensuous" was first used in 1741 by John Milton (*Reform*, I.3), in a context that linked it to religion: "The Soule ... finding the ease she had from her visible, and sensuous

collegue the body in performance of Religious duties ... shifted off from her selfe the labour of high soaring any more."

3 On the polemical exchanges between Erasmus and Alberto Pio, see Gilmore (1969); Minnich (1988).

4 Tanner (1990), 775.

5 See Scavizzi (1974), 171–213, esp. 186.

6 Cited by Scavizzi (1974), 183.

7 See the account by Fehleison (2005) of how the Jesuits staged a show within earshot of Calvin's Geneva.

8 O'Malley (1999a), 19. Cochrane (1981), esp. 477–80, 591 n. 1, provides a historical explanation of the Renaissance split between humanist historiography and *historia sacra*, the latter becoming a product of the Catholic Church and subject to its censorship (therefore suspect to anticlerical eyes). Alternatively, in the twentieth century, the study of heresy using the documents of the Inquisition radically reframed the relationship of the institution and its history, awakening the interest of new and successive generations of scholars both outside and within Italy from the 1960s to the 1970s: Carlo Ginzburg, of *Cheese and Worms* fame (Ginsberg [1976]), cites the importance of Delio Cantimori (1992), which has become more broadly associated with the study of Catholic Reform as a pluralistic series of reform movements ante- and post-dating Trent and coexisting, sometimes in tension, with its objectives. A cogent historiographical analysis of this dynamic situation can be found in Martin (2004); see esp. 5–8 on Cantimori and Federico Chabod.

9 O'Malley (1999a), 20.

10 Alexander (2007); Repishti and Schofield (2004); de Boer (2001).

11 The distinction here between Jesuit houses and churches is made clear in Padberg, O'Keefe, and McCarthy (1994), 98. I thank John O'Malley for this reference.

12 Bailey (1999b), 44–45, has discussed the degree of supervision intended and achieved; see also Bailey (2003), 6, 31.

13 Wittkower and Jaffe (1972) noted that by 1580 the efforts at centralization and the procedure put in place to ensure it were collapsing. The success of the Gesù plan meant that it was copied by the Jesuits and other Orders, and the peripatetic lives of Jesuit artists and architects resulted in a certain degree of stylistic conformity, but it was not imposed by fiat; rather it resulted from success.

14 Hall (1979). I return to this case in the present instance because I appreciate to a greater degree now than when I first studied it that this Florentine project illustrates an initiative taken at the local level and not dictated from above by the Church. Nothing in the documentation suggests that the Orders even had a say in the renovations.

15 They did not attempt to remove the steps that separated the upper and lower churches in S. Maria Novella, which had symbolically designated the friars' church closer to the altar as higher than the lay (lower) church.

16 See Borromeo's (1577) very precise instructions for how to built or renovate a church. As Scavizzi (1992), 124, remarked, "Borromeo's *Instructiones* cover absolutely every aspect of the church and contain a description of every utensil needed for the administration or for other liturgical purposes."

17 Paolo Prodi in particular has used the term "social discipline" in studying the Italian situation; see Prodi and Möller-Luckner (1993); Prodi and Penuti

(1994). The concept of "negotiation" has been influentially articulated by Greenblatt (1988), vii: "This book argues that works of art, however intensely marked by the creative intelligence and private obsessions of individuals, are the products of collective negotiation and exchange." Greenblatt's conception has been discussed by Pieters (2001); see particularly "Theories of Culture: Bakhtin, Gramsci, and Williams," for some background in "language and/as ideology."

18 O'Malley (1999a), 21.

19 See Cooper (1991) on Veronese and Catholic Reform. The text of the interrogation is available online in English translation by Charles Yriarte at several sites, including www.efn.org/~acd/Veronese.html, and translated in Chambers and Pullan (1992), 232–36. See also Fehl (1961), 325–54. Martin (2004), 166, described this as a process of mediating boundaries between sacred and profane, clerical and lay; see also Marinelli (1974), 302–64.

20 Verstegen (2003b), 59–60.

21 Zuccari (1984), 16–19. Varriano (1999), 206, cites Beggiao (1978).

22 See Hall (2011), ch. 5.

23 *Maniera* is employed here and in relation to "Counter-Reformation" in the manner described in Hall (1999), xii–xv; this is discussed further later in the chapter.

24 Bury (1987), 327–56.

25 Paleotti (1582). On Paleotti, see also P. Jones (1995).

26 Ottonelli and Cortona (1652).

27 Borghini (1584). Stuart Lingo in his essay in this volume examines Borghini's treatise in the light of the particular Florentine context.

28 Lanzi (1809), 1: 191.

29 Dejob (1884).

30 Mâle (1932).

31 Madonna (1993).

32 P. Jones (1993). Jones (2006), 153–65, has cogently summarized the new place of Counter-Reformation art.

33 Zeri (1957).

34 Bailey (2003), 16. Attendant problems with identifying a Counter-Reformation style of patronage are discussed by Robertson (1992), esp. 206–207.

35 S. J. Freedberg (1993).

36 Prodi (1962). Prodi's theories of a Counter-Reformation style were quickly taken up in a substantial review by Jedin (1963), 321–39. See the account by Courtright (2006), 135–52.

37 See, e.g., Strinati (1980), 15–48; Zuccari (1984, 1992).

38 Lee (1967).

39 Dempsey (1982); see also Dempsey (2006), 388–402.

40 C. Borromeo (1577). See a number of these treatises now in digital form on Paola Barocchi's Web site, Fondazione Memofonte, under "Trattati d'Arte," www.memofonte.it/index.php?option=com_content&task=view&id=45&Itemid=38.

41 Scavizzi (1974, 1981, 1987, 1992).

42 Blunt (1978), 105; also in paperback (1962) and now in its fourteenth printing.

43 Robertson (1992). See Hallman (1985) for a skeptical view of motives; the influence of the direction of this research is reflected in the recent essays

in Hollingsworth and Richardson (2010), esp. ch. 10, Pamela Jones, "The Court of Humility: Carlo Borromeo and the Ritual of Reform."

44 Hall (1979), with references to Isermeyer, notably on Vasari. Isermeyer's work on monastic patrons and reform led him to Palladio, on which see Cooper (1990; 2006). The notion of such "programs" of decoration and architectural renovation for sacred buildings has been studied more broadly than the brief indications given here, where our concentration is on Counter-Reformation rather than Catholic Reform concerns. Indeed, the category of buildings affected by concerns of reform can be expanded to include charitable institutions, such as *scuole*, *ospedale*, and confraternities; see also Cooper (2005), pt. VI.

45 Connors (1980).

46 P. Jones (2008).

47 The Sacred Congregation *de Propaganda Fide* was founded in 1622 to foster the spread of Catholicism and to oversee the operation of the missions in non-Catholic countries. It was renamed in 1982 the Congregation for the Evangelization of Peoples.

48 Galassi Paluzzi (1951), as used by Y. Levy (2004), 32. The author offers a provocative account of the reception of Jesuit art in the twentieth century in the light of the coloration given to ideological art by Nazism and Stalinism.

49 For a detailed discussion of the *Spiritual Exercises* and bibliography, see Bailey (2003), 7–10 n. 19.

50 On Ignatius and the *Spiritual Exercises*, see Ganss (1991).

51 Bjurström (1972), 99–110, outlined the development of Jesuit theater from the mid-1560s. Baroque Rome as a "theatre state" has been explored by Rietbergen (2006), 11; on the post-Tridentine culture, 377–78.

52 Zampelli (2006), 563.

53 Zampelli (2006), 562.

54 Zampelli (2006), 563.

55 Zampelli (2006), 552; see also Taviani (1969), esp. 10, 22–23.

56 Dejob (1884), 217.

57 See Taviani (1969).

58 Dejob (1884), 219–20.

59 Zampelli (2006), 564.

60 Gilio (1961). On Gilio's critique, see Dempsey (1982) and Hall (2005a), 35–38.

61 The literature on mannerism is vast, but the modern debate has centered on the writings of Friedlaender (1957); Smyth (1992); Shearman (1967); and S. J. Freedberg (1961, 1965, 1993).

62 Caterino (1552), 130–40, quoted by Scavizzi (1992), 251.

63 Paleotti (1582), 411, quoted by Scavizzi (1992), 134.

64 Several of Perino's drawings for the chapel survive, including the highly finished project for the side wall in Budapest, reproduced in Hall (1999), fig. 96. On the chapel and its drawings, see Parma Armani (1986), 284–86, figs. 214–20.

65 On the *figura serpentinata* as a quintessential maniera device, see D. Summers (1972).

66 Gilio (1961), 80, the term and the passage cited by Stuart Lingo in his essay in this volume.

67 Paleotti (1582), 452, quoted by Scavizzi (1992), 135.

68 Vasari (1881), 109. Vasari mentioned Pontormo, Giovambatista Gelli, the painter Bacchiacca, Camilla Tebaldi del Corno, and Costanza da Sommaia, but he made no suggestion as to why these particular portraits were included.

69 Borghini (1584), 109–10.

70 See Scavizzi (1992), 122, discussing Pietro Cataneo, *I quatro libri d'architettura* (1554) and Onofrio Panvinio, *Le sette chiese romane* (1570).

71 Richeôme (1611), 48–49, quoted in Bailey (2003), 58.

72 I thank Anne Muraoka for this reference.

ON THE SENSUOUS

RECENT COUNTER-REFORMATION RESEARCH

Tracy E. Cooper

WHERE DOES OUR particular attention to the *sensuous* in the Counter-Reformation take us? This volume participates in what we recognize as a much wider phenomenon, recently characterized as a "turn to the sensuous" by Patrizia Di Bello and Gabriel Koureas, who propose that "[g]oing back to the senses might be a way to rediscover the artworks we are supposed to be concerned with historicizing."[1] They characterize "aesthetic intuition as sensitive knowledge" conjoining philosophical and art historical inquiry, what David Summers termed "the judgement of sense."[2] Interest in the senses as both a method and subject of study has been in the forefront of a number of disciplines since the mid-1980s; sensuous anthropology constitutes an entire subdiscipline in which it is possible to discern a range of approaches. One of its early innovators, David Howes, has collected influential contributors in *Empire of the Senses: The Sensual Culture Reader*, Marshall McCluhan – one of Howes's teachers – among others.[3] In his introduction to the volume, Howes performs an analysis of a seventeenth-century painting known as *The Yarmouth Collection*, describing it as "a portrait of a particular sensory order – or rather, of a number of sensory orders, which interact and challenge each other." In calling our attention to the notion of sense taxonomies, he further notes that "[w]hile the arrangement of the collection in the painting might appear to be haphazard or dictated only by aesthetic concerns, the different objects and beings are in fact entwined through powerful bonds of sensuous and moral significance."[4] Indeed, among the objects one might see depicted, a mirror without reflection is not only a *vanitas* symbol, but a stand-in for the project of elevating our attention to senses other than that which we accord to sight – as the blind must do.

Howes and his colleagues put senses in relationship to each other, an "intersensoriality," and to our understanding of them as cultural systems, an approach that has been taken up by other disciplines, including history – for example, Mark M. Smith in his *Sensing the Past: Seeing, Hearing, Smelling,*

Tasting, and Touching in History.[5] According to historian Robert Jütte, "There can be no such thing as a natural history of the senses, only a social history of human sense perception."[6] Other disciplines also have explored enough of the sensuous to engage in the process of self-reflection, notably geography (on which see Paul Rodaway)[7] and sociology (on which see Phillip Vannini, Dennis Waskul, and Simon Gottschalk).[8] With relevance to the subject of our volume, Richard Newhauser has asked, "What can the historical disciplines that focus on the Middle Ages and the Renaissance bring to the study of the senses?" He insists on the now "essential place of the sensorium in any intellectual histories of the Middle Ages and the Renaissance."[9]

There is, however, a multifocal historical dimension to be considered in the construction of a sensuous description of the past. "We 'other Victorians,'" as Michel Foucault's influential *History of Sexuality* reminds us, have inherited different codes about the body from those historical peoples whom we study, as have contemporary histories of the body acknowledged this differentiation of practices.[10] Indispensable to the study of the senses in the Renaissance is François Rabelais, who was deliberately provocative in his aggressive adoption of a sensory mode, no doubt a provocation made by eliding a medieval sense of decorum with that of his contemporary early modern world, as we learn from Mikhail Bakhtin's description of Rabelaisian festive culture; for the Renaissance his "grotesque realism" overturned tenets of classical literature: "To be understood he requires an essential reconstruction of our entire artistic and ideological perception, the renunciation of many deeply rooted demands of literary taste, and the revision of many concepts." The reader must be prepared for the sensory assault of the marketplace and the banquet table, for with "[t]he awareness of a purely human material bodily power.... [a]ll mystical fears are dissipated." Thus, a popular culture equivalent of the classical symposium or the Christian Last Supper becomes a liberating experience through the metaphysical and sensory level of shared bodily functions in the imagination of the reader.[11] But today's reader now takes these sensations as representing historical artifacts of experience rather than recognizing their perception as a process of translation filtered through our relatively sanitized world: Would the Renaissance reader have been equally distanced from the popular excesses to have the flavors, smells, and noises register in an analogous way? The modernist conception of the cultures of classicism (including the Renaissance) has transmitted to us codes of purity that did not admit a messy physicality in our aesthetic consideration of the past, although if we go by the multisensory descriptions of social experience, the long continuum of daily life suggests it was otherwise.[12] As Mark Smith writes in his explanation of the preeminence of context for a study of the historical world of the senses, "Most sensory historians do not assume that what smelled foul to a medieval English nose is the same thing as what modern English noses would deem stinky." He goes on to posit a post-Enlightenment privileging of the visual, with hearing also granted a continuous intellectual and social status, while smell, taste, and touch were given lower value.[13] It is not very surprising, therefore, to find the study of multiple senses well advanced in scholarship of the medieval period, where such biases have been less pronounced, for which see the volume edited by Stephen G. Nichols, Andreas Kablitz, and Alison Calhoun, *Rethinking the Medieval Senses: Heritage/Fascinations/Frames*.[14]

Privileging the visual, however, can be moved earlier than Smith posits it as both a historical and historiographical phenomenon. In literary and media studies, another student of McCluhan, Walter J. Ong, S.J., characterized the technological revolution of printing, as the spoken word gave way to typographical space, as one that would privilege "visiles" over "audiles."[15] The reception of the new media transformed thought processes and communication through the increased use of "the spatial model as key to the mental world." Margaret Miles wrote on visual history being associated with the intellectual, civilizing process of the Renaissance but also cautioned that it, too, meant something quite different from the way we experience it now in a hypermediated society, removed from context and function, and aestheticized. For religious art, "[t]he individual viewer confronted the image as a member of an interpreting community, and the image itself was also part of the architectural and liturgical presentation of an ordered cosmos of being, reality, and value.... In addition, religious images were interpreted verbally and reinforced by the liturgy of the churches in which they appeared." Also, theories of vision then and now have been fundamentally altered, from the classical notions of emission and intromission (rays emanating from the eyes or being received by the eyes) that permeated the early modern characterization of sight, replaced by nineteenth-century optics of the visual system (light entering the eye and processed by the brain). She further described the emotional and spiritual implications of the interaction between the person's eye and object of sight as inflected by such influential interpretations of vision as Augustine's, in which what was seen would actively affect (or infect) the person: "This heightened, even exaggerated, respect for the power, for good or evil, of visual experience is very far from modern understandings of what occurs in vision."[16] Robert Nelson also has effectively argued against "normative" theories of vision in the introduction to his edited volume *Visuality Before and Beyond the Renaissance: Seeing as Others Saw*.[17]

If Miles was making a plea for the importance of visual history as a constructed practice to text-based historians, David Freedberg in his 1989 *Power of Images: Studies in the History and Theory of Response* was making a case for the inclusion of reception and perception by art historians as a means to account for the visceral period responses to the image in Reformation iconoclasm and censorship.[18] Current work on the parallel "crisis" of the image in the Italian Renaissance and Counter-Reformation includes Hall's *Sacred Image* and Alexander Nagel's *The Controversy of*

Renaissance Art.[19] It has been persuasively argued that an emphasis on the visual in the Counter-Reformation also could be justified by its inclusion in meditative tracts on spiritual development, notably the influential *Spiritual Exercises* of Ignatius of Loyola, as Jeffrey Chipps Smith shows regarding the deployment of images (*Bildung*) in *Sensuous Worship: Jesuits and the Art of the Early Catholic Reformation.*[20] Yet for Robert Jütte it was the even more complete "exploitation" of *all* the senses that the Counter-Reformation was able to achieve through such texts, recognizing that the duality of sensuous association with both virtue and vice could be remediated through a program of education.[21] The prevalence and widespread diffusion of meditative practices were thus not limited to affecting the experience of a beholder of a work of art, but acted as well to inform its maker, as has been posited for artists employing naturalism in Counter-Reformation religious subjects. Caravaggio's work has long been promoted as the "pictorial equivalent" of the meditative process in which the religious subject was meant to be imagined as if taking place and experienced by sensory means.[22] In this volume and elsewhere, Stuart Lingo has investigated such strategies as those used by Agnolo Bronzino and Federico Barrocci to engage multiple senses through the visual image in order to heighten the spiritual impact and the translation of that experience into a new, more *sensitive* language.[23]

The persuasive capacity of a more fully embodied response has attracted attention to the operation of the senses in the Counter-Reformation. Bette Talvacchia identifies the Council of Trent as having made the concept of the body more explicit.[24] And even more sweeping is the claim that "Western religion is the main reason why sensation is important for Western art."[25] This receptive condition has been explained influentially as "incarnational theology" by John O'Malley, S.J., and invoked by Leo Steinberg to underpin his theory of the sexuality of Christ as "an ostensive act, a palpable proof."[26] The close relation between the sensuous and the sexual is treated in the introduction to this volume, but it is worth revisiting the problem of corporeality as it is implicated in both the beholder's experience and that of the representation – thus the strictures of Carlo Borromeo against the dangerous body, the gendered body, as well as circumscription of the suffering body, the ecstatic body. If "[f]or medieval people, the experience of seeing and imagining a body that was ravaged and bleeding from tortures inflicted upon it lay at the centre of a constellation of religious doctrines, beliefs and devotional practices," then in the era of "art" (*pace* Hans Belting) the sensuous map of the spectacular body was reformed and controlled to meet the new expectations.[27] The study of the intensity ascribed to sensuous experience and the mechanics of its invocation forms part of a new wave of sensuous art history as it relates to various trends in somatic studies. An important direction has been the return to emotion, now based on a new alliance between art history and cognitive science, as in the neuroaesthetic research program of David Freedberg: "Even the ancients knew that sight could activate the other senses, but now we have a much clearer idea of how this happens. Thanks to the polymodal consequences of sight, viewing a work of art also restores some of what is truly lost – the vitality of body and hand – and endows movement with the possibilities of emotion."[28]

Such studies incorporate more than the five external senses; they acknowledge the participation of senses often described as internal, operating together as an "ecology of sensual relations."[29] Oscillation between early modern individual and societal sensory experience has been previously explored in the phenomenology of place. In 1971 Christian Norberg-Schulz wrote, "The character of Baroque art brought forth a 'phenomenization' of experience, which made man more conscious of his own existence." In his reading, the baroque was characterized by *persuasion*, a means of enactment common to both the Catholic and Protestant churches, whether by visual images' stimulation of imagination and empathy in the former, or the appeal of sermons in common language and sacred music in the latter, to achieve *participation*. His notion of a lived perspective saw architectural developments, such as Carlo Maderno's longitudinal axis for St. Peter's, as the corollary "of the Counter-Reformatory epoch to make the church become an active participant in its spatial environment, thereby expressing the role of the Church in the world."[30]

In conclusion, early modern sensuous art history has been devoted largely to its perception (phenomenology, cognitive), aesthetics (philosophy, neuroaesthetics), and representation (imagery, iconography, iconology). The study of literal representation also has caught the attention of sensuous anthropologists, as the earlier discussion of *The Yarmouth Collection* indicates, and has been identified as a distinctly secular phenomenon until the Renaissance. Carl Nordenfalk's 1976 survey of the iconography of the five senses showed the distrustful attitude of the Church: "Given the popularity of the theme of these secular iconographic traditions, it is remarkable that ecclesiastical art, which after all was predominant in the Middle Ages, so seldom included the theme of the Five Senses in its pictorial teaching. This is all the more surprising as the Five Senses occur quite frequently in Christian texts – in commentaries on the Bible, in sermons and other educational material – mostly with a moralizing cast, as dangerous gateways to the Vices." These medieval secular traditions of symbolic representation employed mostly allegorical series of animals, men with attributes, or the sensing organs. Nordenfalk noted several meaningful breaks in those traditions around 1500, whose effects were expanded by printing and dissemination. Changes included a switch from male to female personifications, which he identified as reinforcing an association with the "instruments of sin," as well as the introduction of models from classical culture and the study of anatomy, leading to the depictions of the senses in emblem books, broadsheets, programs of decoration, and a new genre of images combining narrative subjects from the life of Christ with the five senses.

The potential of allegory as a paratactic strategy for the proscribed religious image, with its pedagogical tone and moral instruction, distanced from cultic devotional practice, would find a receptive audience in the Reformation and Counter-Reformation.[31] The authors in this volume investigate in various ways just what was at stake with the representation of the sensuous in the early modern period.

Notes

1 Introduction to Di Bello and Koureas (2010), 14; on the "sensual turn," 15, n. 19.
2 Summers (1987), 8, in the framework "of Western tradition of psychological speculation and its relation to the language of art" (14), associated with the emergence of naturalism in the early modern period. Another example is Osborne (2000). See also various essays in Sanger and Walker (2012); over a broader period see Bacci and Melcher (2011); for our period see the essay by Geraldine A. Johnson, "The Art of Touch in Early Modern Italy." The latter reflects a trend often remarked upon in the study of *individual* senses in various disciplines; for example, Harvey (2003); more broadly Paterson (2007). Haptic/optic has been a long-standing discourse in art history since Alois Riegl.
3 Notably Alain Corbin, Constance Classen, Steven Connor (on Michel Serre's 1985 *Le cinq sens*, trans. 2009), as part of the publisher's influential Sensory Formations series: Howes (2005); his full bibliography and an excerpted version of the Introduction can be found at www.david-howes.com/DH-research-sampler-TheSensesCollected.htm.
4 The painting is also known as *The Paston Treasures* (Norfolk, Norwich Castle Museum and Art Gallery(www.culturalmodes.norfolk.gov.uk/projects/nmaspub5.asp?page=item&itemId=NWHCM%20:%201947.170%20:%20F), with former attributions to Dutch artists working in England, Franciscus Gysbrechts and Peter Gerritz van Roestraten, dated in the 1660s; see the *National Inventory for Continental European Paintings* online at VADS: the online resource for visual arts, www.vads.ac.uk/large.php?uid=85377. In addition to the citations given in Howes (2005), for an interesting analysis of the genre, see Honig (1998), 166–83, esp. 177; also Kemp (1995), 177–96. Another way to look at this work might be ontologically, as creating "a bloc of sensation, that is to say, a compound of percepts and affects," proposed as the function of art by Deleuze and Guattari (1994), 164.
5 M. Smith (2008), esp. 1–18, for a survey of approaches, on which see Howes (2008), 442–51.
6 Jütte (2005), 9, and see ch. 4, esp. 81–82, on the Counter-Reformation.
7 Rodaway (1994).
8 Vannini, Waskul, and Gottschalk (2011).
9 Newhauser (2010), 5–9, another Berg publication.
10 Foucault (1980), 1–14. The phrase "other Victorians" was taken from Steven Marcus and was used in his part 1 title.
11 Bakhtin (1984), 3.
12 For a formative figure of the "Modernist Sensorium," see C. Jones (2006).
13 M. Smith (2010), 860–63, who optimistically claims that we can "recover the meanings of taste in a pre-refrigerator age." For such an example, see Wheeler (2007), 25–38.

14 Nichols, Kablitz, and Calhoun (2008); also Woolgar (2006). There is something of an analogy to the concept of primitive culture as being more sensorial, e.g., animal, but operating in reverse and stripping our sensitivity to it.

15 Ong (2004), 314.

16 Miles (1985), 7–9.

17 Nelson (2000), 1–21, which provides an overview of the now expansive literature on visuality, to which add Summers (2007). Also see Clark (2009); Melion and Wandel (2009).

18 D. Freedberg (1989). See his updated preface to the second Italian edition (*Il potere delle immagini*, 2009), available on his faculty Web site in English: www.columbia.edu/cu/arthistory/faculty/Freedberg/Power-Images-Italian-Preface.pdf.

19 Hall (2011); Nagel (2011). Behind these stand Belting's (1994) influential inquiry into the icon.

20 Jeffrey Chipps Smith (2002); and see his essay in this volume. A new book promises the examination of pre- and post-Reformation practices across the channel: Millner (2011) (not available at the time of writing). Of interest is a future publication: Göttler, de Boer, and Roodenburg (forthcoming).

21 Jütte (2005), 157–59.

22 Chorpenning (1987), 149–58, in which he presents a summary of views for and against Caravaggio's understanding of meditation directly through his patrons or as more generally understood as a popular practice.

23 Lingo (2008).

24 See her essay in this volume and Talvacchia (2010), ix, arising from a 2002 conference.

25 Quiviger (2010); on the Counter-Reformation, see 66–69.

26 O'Malley (1979), 138–39; and see his essay in this volume. L. Steinberg (1983), 8, 10; L. Steinberg (1997). "The Incarnation changes everything," as famously stated by Merleau-Ponty (1964), 174.

27 Merbeck (1999), 19. Karant-Nunn (2010), in a sensitive discussion of gender, states that the notion that women were considered to be inescapably physical and easily moved to emotion was implicated in relation to the 'crisis'; she notes that "the physicality of early modern piety underwent reduction" (67). See the essay in this volume by Richard Schofield on Borromeo and that by Robert Gaston on decorum.

28 D. Freedberg (2011), 352. Onians (2007) gives a historical perspective on art history and cognitive science.

29 Vannini, Waskul, and Gottschalk (2011), 7, 9, explicitly decry a "dualist ontology" (mind/body) and instead see the "*senses as interaction*" (10). They give the usually cited exteroceptive senses as sight, hearing, taste, smell, and touch; the most common interoceptive senses as pain, thirst, hunger, proprioception (often cited as a third category, an internal sense of the parts of the body communicated through the nervous system), balance, movement, temperature, time, and orgasm. Howes (2009) has contributed another sense, as illustrated by the title of his edited volume, *The Sixth Sense Reader*, in the Sensory Formations series.

30 Norberg-Schulz (1971), 12–13, 108. The phenomenological context of the proprioceptive (haptic, touch) is covered in Paterson (2007).

31 Nordenfalk (1985b), 1–22; for the quote see 2. Also see Nodenfalk (1985a), 135–54, and Quiviger (2010), on allegories, 88–95.

TRENT, SACRED IMAGES, AND CATHOLICS' SENSES OF THE SENSUOUS

John W. O'Malley

THROUGH THE CENTURIES Christians have had a wide spectrum of attitudes toward the arts, a fact the studies in this volume confirm even for a quite specific period.[1] Within that spectrum the Catholic Church as an institution steered a virtually hands-off course in stated policy. It pronounced on the matter in official and universally binding declarations on only two significant occasions – at the Second Council of Nicaea, 787, and at the Council of Trent, 1563.[2] In both these instances not a desire to regulate the quality or decorum of the art in question but serious outbursts of iconoclasm occasioned the decree. In essence these declarations affirmed two things: first, iconoclasm was wrong, and, second, images of sacred subjects were legitimate and helpful. Trent added a third: such images should be appropriate to their setting and subject.

After the Council of Trent, despite the debate and controversy that swirled among Catholics about what was appropriate for art in religious settings, the Church *as such* issued no pronouncements and pursued no consistent or broadly enforced policy regarding music, painting, sculpture, or architecture. In 1571 Pope Pius V established the Congregation of the Index, which was the equivalent of a department of state. Its function was to censor and if necessary suppress dangerous books. Gabriele Paleotti, archbishop of Bologna (1527–97), advocated creating an official and detailed list of criteria for detecting and correcting in religious art deviations from Trent's directive, in imitation of the norms the Index provided for books. Yet no such handbook or index was ever created.[3]

In those same decades after the Council and, indeed, for the next two centuries, popes, cardinals, and bishops continued to be among the most important patrons of the arts, manifesting in their patronage a great diversity of taste and a similarly great diversity of attitudes about what was appropriate, what was not, and what should be done to correct any problems. For that reason extreme caution must be exercised in speaking of "the Church" in relationship to the arts in this period. It is much safer to specify Pope X, Bishop Y, Theologian Z, or Synod ZZZ. It is at the same time important to realize that even popes, bishops, and inquisitors were rarely able to impose their will on offending parties without meeting resistance. They often had to enter into some form of negotiation, which resulted in a compromise or a blunted impact.

During the latter half of the sixteenth century, a wave of moralizing reform swept over parts of Europe, most notably in those where Calvinist – but to some degree also Catholic – influence was strong. This "severe morality," as it is sometimes called, had an impact, of course, on the appreciation of art. Whence did it come? Many factors, surely, were responsible for it, but not to be underestimated is the moral imperative at the heart of the humanist tradition as revived in the Renaissance.[4] Early in the century no one propounded a strict public morality more insistently than Erasmus, Europe's most esteemed and widely read author.

An inveterate moralizer, Erasmus espoused a prudish attitude toward art, as Erwin Panofsky showed many years ago. His strictures on the subject in his treatise, "The Institution of Christian Matrimony," for Queen Catherine of England (Aragon), 1526, are characteristic:

> What shall I say about the licence so often found in statues and pictures? We see depicted and exposed to the eyes what would be disgraceful even to mention.... Why is it necessary to depict any old story in the churches? A young man and a girl lying in bed? David looking from a window at Bathsheba and luring her into adultery? Or the daughter of Herodias dancing? These subjects, it is true, are taken from the Scriptures, but when it comes to depictions of women how much naughtiness is admixed by the artist![5]

By its disciplinary decrees, most of which dealt with the proper behavior of bishops and pastors of parishes, Trent added to the force of the moralistic wave. More pointedly, as our volume makes clear, Trent's decree on sacred images had an impact on artists, patrons, and other interested persons to the point that it is legitimate, though perilous, to speak of Tridentine art. For that reason, it may be useful, before reviewing the origins of the decree, to place it in the larger framework of the Council.

The Council of Trent met over the course of eighteen years, from 1545 to 1563, in three distinct periods: 1545–47, 1551–52, and 1562–63. It had an extraordinarily troubled history. Popes, kings and queens, the emperor, bishops, and Protestants threw obstacles of all kinds in its way, including war. One result of these problems was the relatively small number of bishops who participated. The Council opened in December 1545 with only some 30, and at its peak in 1563 the number reached only about 225.

None of the three popes under whom the three periods unfolded attended the Council, a condition insisted on by Emperor Charles V in the negotiations for its convocation. They therefore appointed legates to preside over it. An efficient courier service allowed communication back and forth between Rome and Trent, but of course with a delay of some ten days between message and response. Through the legates, the popes had considerable, but imperfect control over the Council's course.

It was a political miracle that the Council was able to meet at all – then meet again, and after an interval of ten difficult years meet yet again, but this last time with an almost entirely new cast of bishops and theologians. Nonetheless, due largely to the skill of Cardinal Giovanni Morone, the leader of the papal legates directing the final phase of the Council's third period, Trent was finally concluded on 4 December 1563.

Given the bad press the Council often receives, it is important to observe in interpreting it the distinction Giuseppe Alberigo made between Trent and *tridentinismo*, that is, between what the Council enacted and how its enactments were later interpreted and implemented – especially when the interpretation and implementation exaggerated or distorted the Council's intent.[6] It is equally important to take account of how careful and, in the context of the times, even moderate the Council was in its decisions. Many of the bishops attending the Council, while they may have had a meager theological education, were experts in canon law, trained to frame official statements in cautiously precise terms.[7] The theologians who assisted them and who by their direct interventions on the floor of the Council provided the first framework for the decrees were professionals drawn from prestigious universities or equivalent institutions. As Hubert Jedin, the great historian of the Council of Trent, observed for the first period, 1545–47, the caliber of the theologians was extraordinarily high.[8] A similarly high caliber prevailed in the other two periods. For all the limitations in the Scholastic theology of the period, its practitioners were trained in the art of examining evidence and facing it squarely.[9]

True, the bishops and theologians for the most part simply assumed that Luther and other Reformers were guilty of heresy in their teaching about justification and the sacraments. Nonetheless, they did not respond in knee-jerk fashion or assume the Reformers were wrong in every detail. They took extremely seriously the problems Luther raised about justification and spent seven months elaborating the decree on it. They sifted through the pertinent sources with great care before arriving at their position. After they approved the final form of the decree in April 1547, they moved to the sacraments, which became the almost exclusive doctrinal issue occupying them for what remained of the first period and for the entirety of the second and third.

They were in sympathy with much of what the Reformers were saying about reform of the Church. They shared many of the same grievances, which was a common heritage of the cries for Church reform, especially reform of the papacy, that resounded in Europe for a century from the time of the Council of Constance, 1414–18, to the outbreak of the Reformation. Luther's "Appeal to the German Nobility," 1520, in large part echoed these grievances, even as it proposed them in particularly inflammatory language and went beyond them.

Within a short time, Luther and then other Protestants began calling not for a reform of the papacy but for its abolition altogether, to which of course the Council could not subscribe. Nonetheless, criticism of the institution was virulent at Trent and a radical reform of it high on the agenda of many bishops, especially those from outside Italy. In the winter and spring, 1562–63, conflict over papal authority brought the Council virtually to a standstill for ten months. Only the extraordinary diplomatic skill of Morone saved Trent at this point from utter disaster.[10]

On three concrete and explosive issues that seemed almost designed to provoke a strong reaction from the Council, Trent either refused to commit itself or took a notably moderate stand. It refused, for instance, to assert the necessity or usefulness of clerical celibacy.[11] It passed onto the papacy whether or not the Eucharistic cup could be allowed to the laity.[12] Finally, contrary to what is often said, Trent did not decree that the mass must be celebrated in Latin. It, rather, forbade the opinion that the only legitimate form was the vernacular: "Although the mass is full of instruction for the faithful people, the council fathers did not think it advantageous that it should everywhere be celebrated in the vernacular."[13] Latin, therefore, was legitimate but not prescribed.

Trent did not undertake a general review of the state of Catholicism, as for instance did Vatican Council II in the twentieth century. Few phenomena of the sixteenth century, for instance, had a greater long-range impact on the future of Catholicism or were more characteristic of the Church in that century than the great waves of missionaries sent by the religious orders to Latin America and Asia. About such missions, however, Trent uttered not a word. They did not enter the Council's purview.

The Council had a narrowly focused agenda that it pursued under two large and traditional headings: doctrine and reform.[14] Under "doctrine," the Council meant to treat only Protestant teaching that was seen to conflict with Catholic teaching. Thus, Trent made no pronouncements about the Trinity, the Incarnation, or other doctrines that Protestants accepted. In this regard Trent had Luther principally in mind, with only scant attention to Zwingli, the Anabaptists, and even Calvin. However, during the last period of the Council, 1562–63, the threat of Calvinism in France was much on the mind of the prelates at Trent and gave impetus in fact to the decree on images.

Reform for the most part had a similarly precise focus. For the bishops at Trent, "reform of the clergy and Christian people" – or, as it was at the time more commonly expressed, "reform of the Church" – meant essentially reform of three offices in the Church, namely the papacy, the episcopacy, and the pastorate. This focus was traditional but had become urgent after Constance and especially after Luther.

Because of the popes' adamant refusal to allow the Council to deal with reform of the papacy, the Council made practically no headway on the issue. In its reform of bishops and pastors, Trent was successful in passing strong legislation. Radically improving the pastoral functioning of these two offices was the epicenter of the Council's reform. Trent set its eyes on the canonical traditions regarding those offices and determined to put teeth in them to make sure they were observed.

In particular, the Council tried to correct two related and notorious abuses of canon law: bishops' absences from their dioceses and their holding more than one diocese at the same time. With legislation firmly in place on those problems, Trent set about providing job descriptions for bishops once they set up residence in their diocese. Although the prelates at Trent made correlative provisions for pastors of parishes, they applied the most consistently stringent discipline and penalties for nonobservance to themselves.

This focus helps explain why, despite all the time and effort the Council spent on reform, it dealt with indulgences, relics, the cult of the saints, and the veneration of images at the last moment, even though they were explosive issues "out in the trenches," especially in northern Europe. These issues did not neatly fit into the template the fathers at Trent had adopted for themselves. Contrary to what art historical literature sometimes suggests, the issue of sacred images was not only not a major issue at the Council, but until the very last minute not an issue at all. As Hubert Jedin correctly observed many years ago, there is about it "virtually nothing in the official records of the council."[15]

During that third period the largest number of bishops by far came from Italy, more than two-thirds of the total. Spain provided the next largest number, followed at considerable distance by Portugal. In these countries iconoclasm was virtually unknown. The same was not true for France, where iconoclasm had broken out as early as the 1520s. The iconoclasm was little more than a symptom of the more general infiltration of "Lutheran" ideas into France and especially into the capital. In response to the infiltration, Antoine Duprat, cardinal-archbishop of Sens, convoked in 1527 the most important local synod (or council) of the sixteenth century before Trent. An irrefutable confirmation of its importance is the fact that at Trent Italian and Spanish prelates invoked its decrees when it served their purpose.[16]

Held in Paris, the Council of Sens, as it is known, issued a large number of decrees on a wide range of subjects. Two of the decrees pertained to sacred images. The first was a relatively long but traditional justification of them. The second, much shorter, dealt with their quality:

> So that nothing improper take place in the church of God, it seemed right and reasonable [to decree] that, because of the sensuality of some images [*lascivas*] and their deviation from the truth of Scripture, in the future none be placed in the churches unless the bishop or his vicar approve beforehand and visit the church.[17]

This was the first time in the period that this issue was raised in an influential way in an official, though local, ecclesiastical document.

Despite the religious unrest in the kingdom, the French tried to prevent the convocation of Trent and boycotted it once it finally opened in 1545. King Francis I saw the Council as strengthening the hand of his enemy, Emperor Charles V. But in November 1562, after the death of Francis's successor, his son Henry II, and after the third period of the Council had already been under way for ten months, a relatively small but important delegation led by Cardinal Charles de Guise finally arrived at Trent. The religious situation in the kingdom had become desperate, and even Henry II's widow, the regent, Queen Catherine de' Medici, realized that recourse to the Council was unavoidable.[18] Iconoclasm had meanwhile broken out once again as the Huguenots grew stronger.

The veneration of images was a concern, but marginal, for others at Trent besides the French. Because of their direct experience of iconoclasm, the French bishops felt a keener urgency in the matter and assigned it a high priority. Even in the rapidly deteriorating religious and political situation in France, the regent had earlier unrealistically hoped to calm the waters by bringing leaders of the Huguenot and Catholic parties together so that through conversation they might resolve their differences. At the Colloquy of Poissy, 9 September to 9 October 9 1561, Theodore Beza was the leading Huguenot spokesman and Charles de Guise the Catholic. Among many other issues, image veneration was hotly debated. The Colloquy resolved nothing. In desperation Catherine called another colloquy, which met in the queen's own quarters at the Château-de-Saint-Germain-en-Laye, 27 January to 11 February 1562. The proceedings broke down on the first item on the agenda, the veneration of images.

After the colloquy at the Château, a new rash of iconoclasm broke out. Catholics were outraged. Claude de Sainctes, abbot of Lunéville and future member of the French delegation to the Council, published his *Discours sur le saccagement des églises catholiques* and dedicated it to Cardinal Charles de Guise. The situation was rapidly deteriorating. On 1 March Duke François de Guise, the cardinal's brother, discovered a congregation of Huguenots holding a service in Vassy, a small town on his lands. An altercation ensued, which resulted in the death of sixty Huguenots, the famous "massacre of Vassy" that set off thirty years of religious wars in France. The outbreak of what amounted to civil war, plus the impossibility at Saint-Germain of reaching an agreement over image veneration, which the queen regent had considered among the easiest issues to resolve, convinced her that she now had no alternative but to support French participation in the Council.[19]

On 13 November 1562, the "cardinal of Lorraine," Charles de Guise, arrived at Trent with twelve bishops, three abbots, and eighteen theologians. This relatively small delegation, which was later somewhat enlarged, proved itself extremely influential, due largely to the forceful personality of de Guise, who from this point forward played a role at the Council second in importance only to that of the papal legates.[20] On 3 January, little more than six weeks after the French arrived, they presented the Council with a memorandum of thirty-four articles on reform, one of which (number 29) dealt, not surprisingly, with images:

> 29. Because iconoclasts have arisen in our times, men who believe images must be destroyed, which has resulted in grave public disturbances in many places, the council must take measures to assure that the faithful are properly instructed in church teaching regarding the veneration of images. The council should likewise take measures to eliminate the abuses and superstitious practices that have grown up in that regard. Similar provisions should be made for indulgences, pilgrimages, the relics of the saints and the so-called brotherhoods [confraternities].[21]

The legates took the French proposals extremely seriously and in early February sent to Rome three reports that were article-by-article reactions to them – one by Tommaso Campeggio, bishop of Feltre, a seasoned and highly respected canonist; another by Giovanni Antonio Facchinetti, bishop of Nicastro; and a third that was a report from an eleven-person committee, made up principally of canonists, that the legates had created to provide their own considered response.[22] On number 29, the committee said simply, "Let the matter be treated in the catechism."[23] Facchinetti, a member of the committee who filed a separate report, did not even mention article 29. Campeggio recommended following the decree of Nicaea II, where, he maintained, the issue was adequately handled. He said, further, that the Council should ensure that "abuses and superstition be removed."[24]

When the legates sent these materials to Rome, they pleaded for a speedy response. It was a delicate moment at the Council because, while the legates and Pope Pius IV were eager to keep the French there after their sixteen-year boycott, they were wary of them and especially of Charles de Guise. They recognized in de Guise a powerful personality, who had the potential for swaying the Council on crucial issues. They were suspicious of his Gallican leanings in ecclesiology and, more immediately, of the conversations on the Augsburg Confession that he on his own had initiated only a few months earlier with the Lutheran Duke Christopher of Württemberg.

When the materials arrived in Rome, the pope asked the opinion of his trusted and prudent confidant, Cardinal Morone, not yet appointed legate to the Council. As to article 29 Morone said only, "Regarding images let there be a declaration [from the Council] to observe what the seventh synod [Council of Nicaea II] prescribed."[25] Pius responded to the legates as swiftly as they could have desired. On 13 February the papal reply came in a letter from Carlo Borromeo, secretary of state to his uncle, the pope. The comment on number 29 – "The most reverend legates responded well" –seemed to mean either that the matter should be relegated to the catechism or that, if deemed necessary, the decree of Nicaea II should be reissued.[26] To reissue Nicaea II would have meant, as mentioned, a simple condemnation of iconoclasm and an affirmation of the legitimacy and usefulness of images for Christian devotion and instruction.

This correspondence between Trent and Rome about the French proposals was published only in 2001 in the final volume of the critical edition of the acts of the Council of Trent under way since 1910. It was not, therefore, available to Jedin when he wrote in 1935 that there was "virtually nothing" in the official documentation on the decree. Nonetheless, even this new material does not substantially alter Jedin's assessment, because in February 1563 the decree was a thing of the distant future. It does, however, make clear that neither with the legates at Trent nor with the pope in Rome were "images" a particular concern.

The French proposals, like similar documents from the Spanish bishops and from Emperor Ferdinand I, never made it to the floor of the Council, nor were they distributed to the bishops. Images, therefore, were still not on the agenda of the Council. Other matters, including the crisis over the authority of bishops in relationship to the pope that, as mentioned, brought the Council almost to a halt, took precedence through the rest of the year. As the months passed, Pius IV pressed the legates to bring the Council swiftly to conclusion. Despite strong Spanish resistance to the idea, in the middle of November the legates succeeded in setting 9 December as the terminal date. Not until then did they begin to set in motion procedures for dealing with relics, indulgences, purgatory, the invocation and veneration of saints, and the veneration of images. One of the many ironies of the Council of Trent is that indulgences, which were the spark setting off the Reformation, got such late and such cursory attention.

Although the circumstances in which the decree on images was formulated are well known since Hubert Jedin's reconstruction of them, they bear repeating.[27] As time ran out, Morone was able on 15 November to push through a plan to have documents on these matters prepared by special committees or deputations and to consider them as dealing with reform rather than doctrine, which much simplified and speeded up procedures. The deputations went to work, but whatever they accomplished seems to have had little effect on the final decree.[28]

The plan ran into difficulties, which led to its refashioning on the morning of 29 November. A new deputation went to work immediately that afternoon and met in the quarters of Cardinal de Guise. But when late in the evening of the next day news arrived at Trent from Rome that Pope Pius IV was so seriously ill that his life was in question, the legates insisted that the Council be concluded immediately. If the pope died before the Council officially declared its business finished, it would automatically be suspended. Not only would it suffer the delay occasioned by a possibly long conclave, but its very existence would be in jeopardy because there was no guarantee that the new pope would reconvene it.[29] On 1 December the legates were able to gain approval from the Council that the next day would be the last working day of the Council and that the solemnities ending it would be held on 3 and 4 December, known as Session 25. ("Session" designated a day or, in this case, days, principally ceremonial, when documents already debated, amended, and in principle approved were formally accepted.)

Jedin convincingly argued that in dealing with image veneration the deputation had to have had a prior document that provided them with a pattern for a decree they needed to formulate in such haste. Otherwise, they could hardly have produced their text in such short order. Charles de Guise in fact had such a text in his possession, the *Sententia* (opinion or position paper) on the matter formulated by theologians from the Sorbonne for the colloquy at Saint-Germain, a fact he had made known in the Council weeks earlier. Five theologians from the Sorbonne who had constructed the *Sententia* formed part of the French delegation to the Council. Even if Guise had not carried the text with him, the theologians were surely able to supply him with it.[30] Almost from the moment of his arrival at Trent, the French cardinal became the most powerful and insistent voice there demanding that the Council issue a decree on images.

By a careful comparison of the *Sententia* with the Tridentine text, Jedin showed the latter's dependency on the former. The latter text, though considerably shorter, follows the sequence in which the *Sententia* developed its position. It occasionally quotes the *Sententia* verbatim, more often paraphrases it. The *lascivia* in the Tridentine text, a word much discussed in the studies in this volume, is a simple reworking of *impudica et lasciva* in the Saint-Germain text, which itself may have been an echo of Sens.[31] Although, as already mentioned, the veneration of images was by no means exclusively a French concern, Jedin goes so far as to state that the matter was at the last minute taken up by the Council "so as to provide the French Catholics with a shield against the iconoclast fury" that had broken out.[32]

The decree as we know it was presented to the Council, along with many other documents, in the General Congregation in the afternoon of 2 December, the Council's last working day. Although two bishops took the occasion to suggest minor changes, the decree was not debated. Then at Session 25 it was solemnly approved. It was, as we have seen, never submitted to theologians for vetting and never discussed on the Council floor. No record of the deliberations of the deputation that formulated it has survived. Thus, all we know about the construction of a text that had such influence on artists and patrons and that in the past hundred years has generated so much scholarly comment is that Charles de Guise was a principal player in its evolution, that it was in a general way based on the *Sententia* of Saint-Germain, and that it was put together with almost desperate haste.

After 4 December the bishops left Trent for home with the self-imposed mandate to implement the Council's decrees. The bishop of Rome, though he never set foot in Trent, felt himself under the same mandate, of course, but perhaps in an even more urgent way because of the preeminence of his bishopric and because of the need he must have felt to reassure the world that the harsh criticism the papacy had received at the Council for being the major obstacle to reform was no longer justified. In consistory on 30 December 1563, Pius IV, now fully recovered from his illness, declared to the cardinals, with self-serving exaggeration, that the Council's reform decrees were milder than if he had done them himself. He would see to it that the decrees were implemented.[33]

In the same consistory, accordingly, the pope created a deputation of cardinals to review the decrees to see what could and should be put immediately into action in Rome and to lay the groundwork for his bull ratifying the Council's decisions. The membership consisted of Giovanni Morone and Ludovico Simonetta, both of whom had been legates to the Council, plus Carlo Borromeo, Giovanni Battista Cicala, and Vitellazzo Vitelli. To the deputation were added three canonists: Gabriele Paleotti and Ugo Boncompagni, both of whom had been at Trent, and Francesco Alciati. The deputation met three times between 18 and 21 January and dealt with a wide spectrum of issues.

The final meeting of the deputation, 21 January, dealt, for instance, with questions about benefices, marriage dispensations, the diocesan and provincial synods the Council had mandated, and similar matters.[34] Among those matters was the implementation of the decree on images: "The pictures in the Apostolic Chapel are to be covered, as [is to be done] in other churches if they display anything obscene or obviously false, according to decree 2 in Session 9 [25] under Pius."[35]

In the literature about the relationship between Michelangelo's *Last Judgment* and the Council, there has been considerable confusion. Some scholars have mistakenly identified the action of the Roman deputation as a decision of the Council itself.[36] Romeo De Maio in his influential book on Michelangelo made essentially the same mistake by asserting that the *Judgment* was discussed by name at the Council. He cited Jedin's article on the origins of the decree to validate his claim, but in the article Jedin never once mentioned either Michelangelo or the painting.[37] Mistakes like these unfortunately became established and unquestionable verities in scholarship about the painting.

As best as I have been able to ascertain, no one has discovered a mention of the painter or the painting in the acts of the Council. It is plausible that in the discussions of the deputation that at Trent met in de Guise's quarters, the *Judgment* was adduced by some members as an example of a deplorable *lascivia*. That is, however, pure speculation. There is no textual basis for asserting that it or any other specific work of art gave impetus to the stipulation in the decree that in sacred images "all sexual allurement must be avoided, so that images are not painted or adorned with seductive charm."[38]

We can reasonably infer that the corresponding passage in the *Sententia* of Saint-Germaine sufficiently explains the origins of the stipulation. That text reads, "It is also by no means a small abuse if images are painted and shaped in an indecent and sexually alluring form and one at odds with the chastity and upright character of the holy men and women the images represent."[39]

The notoriety of the *Judgment* easily accounts for the Roman deputation's action. As is well known, from the moment of its unveiling twenty-two years earlier, it had been harshly criticized for its nude figures and been the object of public controversy at least since the publication of Pietro Aretino's letter of 1545 deploring the indecency of the images "in the most sacred chapel upon the earth."[40] The offending painting was the *Judgment*, even though there were, of course, other *ignudi* in the Sistine Chapel.

Not until 21 January, therefore, do we have a document that relates the decree to the *Judgment*. That is the moment, moreover, when the more general application of the decree to the Diocese of Rome was officially set into motion. At about the same time, other conscientious bishops set to work implementing the new duties the Council imposed upon them. But if we are to believe Paleotti and others, most bishops in Italy did not prove themselves particularly diligent in pursuing this one. Nonetheless, as our volume makes clear, the decree by no means remained a dead letter.

I have dealt at some length with Trent's decree because of the important role its *Nachleben* played in Catholics' relationship to "the sensuous," but our volume ranges more broadly over attitudes related to the body, the senses, the sensuous, and even the sensual. I will conclude, therefore, with some very general comments about Catholic attitudes in those regards. In some cases I will not do much more than confirm (or implicitly challenge) points the other contributions have made.

Passages from the New Testament suggest a conflict between flesh and spirit, and Platonic or Neoplatonic philosophies, which almost from earliest times infiltrated Christian theologies and spiritualities, promoted the idea that sloughing off the material, the physical, and the fleshly as much as possible was prerequisite to rising to a more spiritual state. In the early fifteenth century, the little collection of axioms about the devout life, *The Imitation of Christ*, quickly gained popularity throughout Europe. The call it issued in the very first chapter "to withdraw thy heart from the love of visible things and turn thyself to things invisible," traditional though it was, achieved through the *Imitation* and similar works wider appropriation as a spiritual ideal, especially once the book appeared in print.

What the *Imitation* proposed was mild in comparison with what some other Christians texts proposed. From at least the late second century, an ascetic tradition appeared in which "despising the flesh" was almost the central tenet, a tradition that implied a sharp body–soul dichotomy. Some Christians – Montanists, for instance, and Cathars – took hatred of the body to such an extreme that they were condemned as heretics. In the sixteenth-century Catholic context, nobody better exemplified, within the bounds of orthodoxy, this tradition than San Carlo Borromeo, the "Counter-Reformation saint" par excellence. He seemed intent on punishing his body to the limit, which surely contributed to his death at the early age of forty-six.

Even in this period of "severe morality," however, only an infinitesimally small minority of Christians followed such a drastic course, and even other saints of the era exemplified and promoted a different ideal. Among them was San Filippo Neri in the joyous, music-filled spirituality he inculcated for his Oratory. Neri's older contemporary, the founder of the Society of Jesus, Ignatius of Loyola, moved from the draconian asceticism he imposed on himself immediately after his religious conversion to advocacy of a spirituality of ascetic moderation. In the *Constitutions* he drew up for the Jesuits, he laid down that care of the body was praiseworthy and should be observed by all members of the order.[41]

Correlative of these two broad ascetic traditions were two broad theological traditions. The one placed an emphasis, more or less great, on the dire consequences of the Fall and the implications of Christ's redemptive death on the cross. It antedates St. Augustine but with good reason is attributed to him. Luther and Calvin belong to this tradition, in which Original Sin had rendered the human soul corrupt.

The other tradition tended to focus more on humankind's creation in God's "image and likeness" and on the implications of the "Word becoming flesh" in the Incarnation. As the axiom put it, "God became man that man might become God." The idea can be traced back to St. Irenaeus in the second century and was especially developed by the Greek fathers of the Church, but the axiom that became so popular occurs in a sermon of Pseudo-Augustine. Thinkers as diverse as Aquinas and Petrarch quote or paraphrase it.

When this latter tradition was fully articulated, as it was by some important Italian thinkers in the Renaissance, it resulted in a much more positive attitude toward a range of issues that correlated with one another, such as the relationship between "reason and revelation," between "nature and grace," and between "body (or flesh) and spirit."[42] This theological tradition may have suffered an eclipse in the later sixteenth century, but it was too deeply ingrained in too many authors to have lost all force.

It correlated with principles endemic to Scholasticism. The great turning point in the history of Christian theology occurred in the late twelfth and early thirteenth centuries as a result of two developments. The first was the founding of the universities and the founding within many of them of theological faculties. The second was the translation into Latin of a large corpus of works from Greek antiquity.[43] These two developments radically transformed the theological enterprise, effecting a momentous paradigm shift. The new paradigm brought with it important consequences for "the sensuous."

To a degree never experienced before, the most urgent and fundamental task facing theology was how to reconcile the Bible with philosophy. In practice philosophy was synonymous with Aristotle – and Aristotle became virtually synonymous with "reason." (Although Platonic and Neoplatonic influence was strong in the Middle Ages, Plato's works were not translated until the fifteenth century.) Long before the twelfth century theologians had, of course, dealt with aspects of the problem but in fragmentary ways and generally only in passing. Now the problem framed the theological enterprise and was addressed in an incomparably more professed, systematic, and clearly articulated fashion.

Theologians espoused a range of opinions on the degree the reconciliation between "reason and revelation," as it came to be known, was possible, but the role Aristotle, as well as a few other pagan thinkers, played in university learning almost forced them to admit some correlation. Aquinas was among those who went furthest in pursuing compatibility between the two. "Grace perfects nature" (it therefore does not destroy or oppose nature) was for him a fundamental axiom guiding his theological synthesis.[44]

What this meant was intense reflection on the potential of the intellect, even unaided by grace, in the pursuit of truth. With that specific reflection came a consequent reflection on human nature as such. This reconciliation process that defined the theological enterprise for many of the major Scholastic thinkers led them to a new emphasis or more closely argued emphasis on the goodness of all that was natural (i.e., not supernatural), including the human body. Theologians, of course, had to reckon with the consequences of Adam's sin, but they shied away from the drastic Augustinian position of the total corruption of human nature, which implied a sharp nature–grace, body–soul, flesh–spirit dichotomy. This emphasis on the goodness of "the natural" was especially true of the scholars working in the traditions of Thomas Aquinas, the leading Scholastic from the Dominican Order, and of Duns Scotus, the most influential Franciscan. These were the two Scholastic traditions strong in Italy at the time of Trent.[45] The substance of the Renaissance theme of human dignity, which through classical rhetoric was in Renaissance Italy often orchestrated into a paean, is found in most of the mainline Scholastic theologians from the thirteenth century into the seventeenth.

This state of affairs was ensured by the application of Aristotle's metaphysical theory of matter and form to the body–soul relationship. This application moved Aquinas and others toward postulating an integrated union of the two and moved them away from theories that conceived of the soul as an entity dwelling in the body – or even a prisoner of the body and at enmity with it. The soul, instead, was the "form" of the body, that which to a large extent made it what it was. It was inexorably destined to rejoin the body "on the Last Day" after the unnatural separation that occurred with death. When the Scholastics replaced with Aristotle the Neoplatonism that for centuries had implicitly undergirded Christian theology in the West, a new anthropology (if I may use the word) resulted.

This anthropology had epistemological consequences and correlated perfectly with Aristotle's theory about the process of human cognition. Fundamental to Aristotle was the postulate that cognition originated in the senses, which was altogether different from theories generically dependent on Plato in which ideas somehow descended from above. Aquinas and other Scholastics put the matter clearly: "Nihil in intellectu quod non prius in sensibus" – there is nothing in the intellect that is not ultimately dependent on sense knowledge. Within the parameters of that dictum, the Scholastics subscribed to a range of opinions, but that does not alter the fact that the adoption of Aristotle's epistemology promoted and validated "the sensuous" in the terms the editors of this volume defined it: "of, related to, or derived from the senses."

Contrary to what is often said, the Council of Trent did not recommend or impose Scholastic theology, even though the theologians who advised the bishops were Scholastics. Once again, the matter fell outside the purview the Council set for itself. Moreover, the Council did not have to make such a move because, despite humanists' attacks, Scholastic theology, especially in its Thomist forms, had been experiencing a revival in Italy, Spain, and elsewhere for decades before the Council.[46] After the Council, Thomist theology received a boost in 1567 when Pius V declared him a "doctor of the Church," putting him on the same level as the four traditional doctors – Ambrose, Augustine, Jerome, and Gregory the Great. Aquinas was the first saint in history to be thus elevated.

Where there was Catholicism after Trent, there almost certainly was Scholasticism. Where there was Scholasticism, especially in its Thomist form, there was at least a theoretical acceptance of a close and positive body–soul relationship and a recognition of the integral role that the senses play in one of the most spiritual, noncorporeal realities of which we have direct experience, abstract thought or concepts.

I must be clear: Augustinian influences remained strong, sometimes very strong, in Catholic theology and religious thought in the early modern period. They were to be found even in mainline Scholastics. With the appearance of Jansenism in the seventeenth century, moreover, the Augustinian tradition experienced in Catholicism a coherent and powerful revival. Nonetheless, the tradition more widely favored among professional theologians was that of Aquinas, Scotus, and others whose principles were similar to theirs.

So much for the rarefied atmosphere of academic philosophy and theology. The Church was engaged, however, in battles over more pressing matters and, therefore, so was the Council of Trent. Although one of the battles was against iconoclasm, there was another, related to it but far more threatening and more central to the very heart of traditional worship. This was the battle over "ceremonies." Under attack were not only images, but also the traditional rites and rituals of worship itself, which included the vessels, vestments, and furnishings that were an integral part of them. As Edward Muir has pointed out, the sixteenth-century crisis was a crisis in "communal, performative signs."[47]

Outside the universities, the Neoplatonic tradition continued strong. Throughout his life, Erasmus advocated simplicity and intelligibility in worship and campaigned relentlessly against what he considered the superstitions and excesses of medieval piety. In so doing he minimized the visible and material aspects of worship in favor of a more interiorized religion. In one of his earliest and eventually most popular works, *The Handbook of the Christian Soldier*, he wittingly or unwittingly echoed *The Imitation of Christ* when he pronounced that you can establish perfect piety only when you "progress from visible things ... to the invisible."[48]

In the sixteenth century, largely through the influence of Erasmus, the very word *ceremoniae* acquired in some circles the pejorative meaning of "petty little rituals." Erasmus criticized and satirized aspects of worship he thought superfluous, superstitious, or too elaborate and sumptuous: "What is the use of so many baptistries, candelabra, gold statues? What is the good of the vastly expensive organs, as they call them? What is the good of that costly musical neighing when meanwhile our brothers and sisters, Christ's living temples, waste away in hunger and thirst?"[49]

Erasmus was certainly no enemy of the traditional mass or the sacraments as such. One of his lesser-known works, in fact, is a full mass liturgy he constructed – that is, he wrote the prayers for the mass, selected the appropriate readings from Scripture, and composed a homily.[50] He was shocked at the iconoclast fury and at the attacks on the mass and the sacraments. But there can be no doubt that radical Reformers and even iconoclasts like Andreas Karlstadt could find comfort in his words.

In Wittenberg as early as 1521, Karlstadt was arguing for the destruction of images in the churches, but his war against "idolatry" was also a war against "ceremonies" – two aspects of the same onslaught. According to him, if images were idolatrous, so was the mass. On 3 December 1521, a mob, Karlstadt-inspired, forced its way into a church, destroyed the liturgical books, and drove the priest from the altar. Such attacks were ultimately attacks on the sacramental principle of the invisible being mediated through visible objects and performance. More specifically, the attack on the mass was an attack on the Real Presence of Christ in the Eucharist. The mass, nothing more in this perspective than an adoration of bread and wine, was thus as idolatrous as adoration of a painted canvas. Karlstadt represented an extreme in this regard, but there was a direct correlation between how present or absent the Reformers considered Christ to be in the Eucharist and how moderately or radically they changed the mass from its medieval form.

The up-front controversy over whether Christ instituted seven sacraments or fewer, important though it was in itself, sometimes acted as a red herring, as a distraction from the radical attack on traditional understanding of the very meaning of religious ritual. The attack sprang from a mentality that saw ritual observance, especially when embellished with rich furnishings, as a diversion from the truly spiritual or, worse, as a manipulative fraud.

The massive attention the Council of Trent devoted to the sacraments and to the mass was explicitly directed to the doctrinal deviations of the Protestants. Nonetheless, in expending so much time on the matter, the Council implicitly reaffirmed the sacramental principle of the invisible being mediated through the visual, of the spiritual through the corporeal. It thus implicitly reaffirmed the validity and even the necessity of the appeal to the senses. At one point it directly addressed the question of "ceremonies" and their embellishment:

> Since human nature is such that it cannot easily raise itself up to the meditation of divine realities without external aids, holy mother church has for that reason duly established certain rites, so that for instance some parts of the mass are to be said in quieter tones and others in louder. It has established ceremonies and in them makes use of symbolic blessings, lights, incense, vestments and other things of this sort in accordance with apostolic usage and tradition. By such means the majesty of the great sacrifice [of the mass] is enhanced, and the minds of the faithful are aroused by these visible signs of religious devotion to rise to contemplation of the high mysteries hidden in them.[51]

By the time the Council of Trent concluded, besides liturgy another form of performance with sometimes spectacular appeal to the senses was already on its way to becoming a characteristic of post-Tridentine Catholicism – Jesuit theater. Within a decade of opening their first school, the Jesuits began exploiting theater for its educational and propagandistic value, in which they became famous, or notorious, for their elaborate costumes, stage sets, music, dance, and "special effects." These were features that later brought down on them scathing and unrelenting criticism from the Jansenists and others influenced by the Augustinian tradition. These same features characterized the elaborate spectacles they created for municipalities to celebrate important civic events.[52]

By the early decades of the seventeenth century, the Jesuits had become the most important producers of religious emblem books, which were aids to meditation and reflection, intended for an educated readership, that combined image with poetry. It was a genre characteristically baroque in its literary and visual conceits, and although it was important in its own era, study of it has until relatively recently been minimal.[53] In these pursuits as well as others, the Jesuits wrote theoretical justifications for what they were doing, which resulted in their creating, according to Ralph Dekoninck, a veritable "theology of the visible."[54]

Regarding the "sensuous," no mention of the Jesuits would be complete without calling attention to the *Spiritual Exercises* and their recommendation, as an aid to focusing one's attention at the beginning of a meditation, to conjure up "a mental representation of the place ... for example, when we contemplate Christ, our Lord, the representation will consist in seeing in the imagination the material place where the object is that we wish to contemplate" (n. 47). The book also recommends a form of contemplation that consists entirely in "the application of the senses." It enjoins, in the first place, seeing the persons and their circumstances and "then draw[ing] some fruit from what has been seen;" second, "hear[ing] what they are saying;" third, "smell[ing] the infinite fragrance and tast[ing] the infinite sweetness of the divinity;" finally, "apply[ing] the sense of touch, for example, by embracing and kissing the place where the persons stand or are seated, always taking care to draw some fruit from this" (nn. 121–26).[55] In such a context Jerónimo Nadal's *Adnotationes et Meditationes in Evangelia*, with its magnificent series of 153 copperplate illustrations of scenes from the New Testament, was an easy, almost logical step to take. Ignatius of Loyola himself seems to have sown the seed for the idea in Nadal's mind.[56]

Rubens was the major artist with whom the Jesuits had the longest and closest relationship.[57] As early as 1605 he painted *Circumcision of Christ* for the high altar of their church in Genoa, and he, devout Catholic and member of the Jesuits' Marian Congregation in Antwerp, from that point forward collaborated with them on numerous projects until his death in 1640. The "severe morality" of the immediate post-Trent decades had by then begun to fade. In the work Rubens produced for the Jesuits he observed the niceties of religious decorum. But few masters of the baroque painted more flesh than he, for which he seems never to have suffered reprimand.

I conclude these comments, therefore, as I began. In the early modern period after Trent, the Church in its official capacity continued to maintain its tradition of condemning iconoclasm and defending the legitimacy and usefulness of images even in sacred places. To a degree unknown before, however, controversies swirled in elite circles over what in images was religiously and morally acceptable. In play in the controversies were diverse theological and philosophical assumptions about the senses and, in particular, about the relationship of body and soul, flesh and spirit. On these controversies the Church made no pronouncement. Individual popes, bishops, theologians, and other religious leaders, as this volume makes abundantly clear, evinced great variety in their attitudes about such matters – and they acted in accordance with those attitudes.

Notes

1 O'Malley (2004a), 179–233.

2 For the decrees in the original Greek and Latin, with English translation, see Tanner (1990), 1: 135–37, 2: 775–76. Constantinople IV, 869–70, repeated the substance of the decree of Nicaea II (1: 168). In passing, other councils have mentioned images, e.g., Lyons II, 1274; see Tanner (1990), 1: 323. The Trullian Synod, 692, an assembly whose disciplinary decrees were not recognized by the Western Church, forbade licentious or obscene images, as noted by Loh in her essay in this volume. As Hubert Jedin showed, with the outbreak of iconoclasm as the Reformation gained force, a number of local synods took up the problem of images, but none of these measures were binding beyond the local level; see Jedin (1963), 326–27.

3 See, e.g., Prodi (1959–67), 2: 557. As Prodi reports Paleotti's proposal, as in a *memoriale* he circulated to friends in 1596: "Nella sesta risposta è proposto il rimedio ritenuto fondamentale: fare comporre un'opera, un commentario che particolareggiatamente insegni a riconoscere gli abusi ed a correggerli." See also Jedin (1963), 333. Jedin, quoting from Paleotti's *Tractatus*, reports the same idea: "Dunque, essendosi dal sacro Concilio Tridentino con l'Indice dei libri data buona regola per discernere quali siano i libri permissi e quali i proibiti, potrà la istessa servire per norma al conoscere quali siano le pitture da essere seguite o fuggite dal cristiano."

4 See, e.g., Kallendorf (2002).

5 As quoted by Panofsky (1969), 209–10; see also Eire (1986) and Minnich (1988).

6 See Alberigo (1981) and Alberigo (1988), esp. 219–23.

7 See, e.g., Helmholz (1996), esp. 394–99.

8 See Jedin (1957–61), 2: 59–61.

9 See, e.g., O'Malley (2004a), 103–15.

10 See Jedin 1967, 80–120.

11 See, e.g., O'Malley (2006a), 102–105.

12 See Tanner (1990), 2: 741, 728.

13 See Tanner (1990), 2: 735; also 736: "If anyone says ... that mass should be celebrated only in the vernacular ..., let him be anathema."

14 See, e.g., Alberigo (1988), n. 6, and O'Malley (2002). The history of the Council by Hubert Jedin (1948–75) is, of course, indispensable.

15 See Jedin (1966), 460: "Man kann getrost sagen: Über die Entstehung des Bilderdekretes nihil fere in actis."

16 On the French relationship to the Council, see Tallon (1997), 448, 450–51.

17 See Mansi (1960–62), 32: 1200: "Et ut nihil sine discretione in ecclesia Dei fiat, expediens et rationabile visum est, propter lascivas imagines et veritati scripturae non convenientes, si in posterum, praecendente episcopi aut commissi ejus judicio et visitatione, imagines in ecclesiis collocentur" (my translation); for the longer decree, see 1175–76.

18 See Tallon (1997).

19 See Tallon (1997), 326–27, and Nugent (1974), esp. 190–203.

20 On him, still basic is Evennett (1930). See also Tallon (1997) and Carroll (2003).

21 See *Concilium Tridentinum* (1901–2001), 13/2: 108, my translation. See also Tallon (1997), 842–67.

22 For the pertinent documents, see *Concilium Tridentinum* (1901–2001), 13/2: 114–40.

23 *Concilium Tridentinum* (1901–2001), 13/2: 120. In the Biblioteca Nazionale of Naples there is a long but anonymous reaction to the French proposals. Whether it was ever circulated at the Council or in Rome is not known. What it adds to the others is a request that the Council add to its decree on the matter a brief teaching about veneration of images and about the mind-set with which one should approach it (13/2: 138).
24 *Concilium Tridentinum* (1901–2001), 13/2: 117: "Ad XXIX. Placet, quod tollantur abusus et superstitiones, et quod observentur decreta septimae synodus generalis, quibus plene provisum fuit contra censentes sacras imagines evertendas."
25 *Concilium Tridentinum* (1901–2001), 13/2: 115: "Quoad imagines servetur septima synodus et fiat declaratio."
26 *Concilium Tridentinum* (1901–2001) 13/2: 125: "Ad 29. Bene responsum est per reverendissimos legatos."
27 See Jedin (1963, 1966b).
28 See Jedin (1966b), 488–93. On procedures at Trent, and specifically on the role of theologians, see Beumer (1971); Jedin (1966a), 2: 577–88; and Minnich (1998), 431–34. The primary basis for reconstructing the procedures is the authoritative summary of them prepared after the Council by its diligent and talented secretary, Angelo Massarelli, in *Concilium Tridentinum* (1901–2001), 13/2: 680–96.
29 See Jedin (1948–75), 4/2: 164–89, and Jedin (1967), 121–58.
30 See Jedin (1966b), 488.
31 For a side-by-side comparison of the texts, see Jedin (1966b), 482.
32 See Jedin (1963), 324: "[D]as auf Verlangen des Kardinals Karl von Guise dem Konzil in letzter Stunde vorgelegt wurde, um den französischen Katholiken einen Schild gegen die aufflammenden Bilderstürme in die Hand zu geben."
33 See the summary of the address in *Concilium Tridentinum* (1901–2001), 9: 1143–44. See also Jedin (1948–75), 4/2: 225–27.
34 Stefan Ehses, the editor of the ninth volume of *Concilium Tridentinum* (1901–2001), transcribed the full list of items from all three meetings of the deputation (9: 1144–49).
35 See *Concilium Tridentinum* (1901–2001), 9: 1149: "Picturae in capella Apostolica cooperiantur, similiter in aliis ecclesiis, si aliquid obscoenum aut evidenter falsum ostendant, juxta decretum 2. in sess. 9 [25] sub Pio" (my translation). For the meeting on 21 January, Ehses, in *Concilium Tridentinum* (1901–2001), vol. 9, drew on three manuscripts in the Archivio Segreto Vaticano, Conc. 9, ff. 7r, 84r ("e scriptis Paleotti"), and 80r. There is, however, a manuscript in the Vatican Library that contains a notable variation from Ehses's text. As cited by Melinda Schlitt, for instance, and checked by her against Vatican manuscript Borg. Lat. 61, ff. 318–21, at 318v, the text reads: "Picturae in capella Apostolica cooperiantur, in aliis autem ecclesiis deleantur, si quae aliquid obscenum aut evidenter falsum ostendant, iuxta decretum secundum in sess. 9 sub Pio." See Schlitt (2005), 145, n. 10. The *deleantur* ("let them be effaced," or even "let be destroyed") in the second version is, obviously, a significant alternative reading. Unless the discrepancy can be resolved through certification of a reliable urtext, which, given the extensive research of the past hundred years on documents related to Trent, seems unlikely, there are reasons for preferring the reading in the *Concilium Tridentinum*. First, why would the deputation establish a double standard for the implementation of the

decree – one standard for the Sistine and another for everyplace else in the diocese? Second, why would there be such a drastic measure for elsewhere? Third, whereas the provision of the minutes was literally and immediately carried out for the "Judgment," we have no evidence, as far as I know, of parts of other "pictures" in the city of Rome being "effaced" at the time. Finally, I find it unlikely that the members of the deputation, many of whom were present at Trent and knew well the anti-iconoclasm origins of the decree, would call for such drastic action against images in Rome. To do so would seem almost to play into the hands of the iconoclasts and give them grounds for saying, "See, you're doing it too!" Of course, the possibility that *deleantur* is the correct version cannot at this point be ruled out. As Peter Lukehart shows in his essay in this volume, the members of the Università dei Pittori in Rome were told in May 1563 that, unless they depicted sacred subjects "virtuously," their work would be "thrown out and destroyed." That was a warning or threat, however, not a directive meant for actual implementation, as was the case with the text we are considering.

36 See, e.g., De Vecchi (1986), 194.
37 See De Maio (1978), 39. On the same page, De Maio mistakenly identifies Morone as a Theatine and therefore a "reactionary" and inclined to prudish judgments about art. But Morone, a friend of Michelangelo's, not only was not a Theatine but had been persecuted by the Theatine pope Paul IV and, cardinal though he was, tried for heresy and thrown into prison by him.
38 See Tanner (1990), 2: 775–76: "[O]mnis denique lascivia vitetur, ita ut procaci venustate imagines non pingantur nec ornentur." I have slightly modified Tanner's translation.
39 Jedin (1966b), 482: "Non parvus quoque est abusus, si pingantur et effingantur imagines forma impudica et lasciva et quae non conveniat castitati et integritati sanctorum et sanctarum, quos repraesentant" (my translation).
40 See, e.g., Hall (1999), 189.
41 See Ignatius of Loyola (1970), 167–70, nn. 292–306; see also O'Malley (2006a), 10–14.
42 See, e.g, Trinkaus (1970); O'Malley (1979); and L. Steinberg (1996).
43 See, e.g., O'Malley (2004a), 87–103.
44 See, e.g., *Summa Theologiae*, 1.1.8, ad 2am: "Cum autem gratia non tollat naturam sed perficiat, ... "
45 See, e.g., Monfasani (1993).
46 See, e.g, Kristeller (1992) and O'Malley (1981).
47 See Muir (1997), 181.
48 Erasmus, "Handbook," in O'Malley (1988), 66: 65.
49 As quoted in Eire (1986), 44.
50 Erasmus, "Liturgy of the Virgin Mother Venerated at Loreto," in O'Malley (1999c), 69: 79–108.
51 Tanner (1990), 2: 734. I have made a few modifications of the translation.
52 See, e.g., Filippi (2006), 512–29, and more extensively Filippi (2001); Zanlonghi (2002); Hsia et al. (2005); Rocke (1996); W. Summers (1999); and Irving (2010). But Jesuits at the same time severely criticized secular theater; see Zampelli (2006).
53 In the middle of the last century Mario Praz (1964) produced a pioneering study that defined the genre and piqued scholarly interest in it. On the Jesuits see, e.g., Manning and Van Vaeck (1999); Höltgen (1999); Salviucci Insolera (2004); Dimler (2007); and, most recently, Campo and Daly (2010).

54 See Dekoninck (2005), esp. 19–30. See, more broadly, O'Malley and Bailey (2005) and Bailey (2003).

55 This feature of the *Exercises* is often commented on, but see especially Dekoninck (2005), 145–86, n. 54.

56 See the translation and reproduction of parts of the work in Nadal (2003–2007).

57 See, e.g., O'Malley and Bailey (2005: n. 54, passim); Knaap (2005); and O'Malley (2008), esp. 3–4.

THE WORD MADE FLESH

SPIRITUAL SUBJECTS AND CARNAL DEPICTIONS IN RENAISSANCE ART

Bette Talvacchia

Two things have always been considered marvelous about the art created in Italy during the Renaissance: the technical virtuosity attained by its masters and their enthrallment to the expressive beauty of the human form. These elements carried particular implications for the production of religious art. Do a style predicated on the perfection of an idealized naturalism and a cultural bias that privileges the concreteness of physical symbols and metaphors embody an inherent conflict with spiritual expression? My contention is that the mainstream of Italian religious art throughout the Renaissance period manifestly used sensuous corporeality as a vehicle for spiritual expression.

Beginning with the example of Giotto, and developed over the course of the fifteenth and sixteenth centuries, belief in the efficacy of carnality to express spiritual truths held sway in the visual arts. This practice was modified in response to the religious upheavals of the Protestant movements, codified in the decrees of the Council of Trent, and diffused after mid-century. However, even after the Reformers achieved ascendancy, change in the visual arts was never systematic. The transformation of styles and imagery took place by degrees and differed from city to city, decade to decade, and patron to patron. While censorship could be locally imposed, no universal decree or governing body was ever in command of cultural developments throughout the peninsula. Conventions in the visual arts were governed by centuries of traditions expressed through fierce local pride; individual artists were formed by professional genealogies transmitted through workshops and environment – formations that could not be erased by the pronouncements of a council, no matter how authoritative.

In tracing the tenacity of an approach to religious art commanded by the symbolic capacity of the perfected human form, it is important to begin with the founding mystery of Christianity as conceived by the Catholic Church: the doctrine of the Incarnation. From this belief of the deity's transformation into human form derived the ruling metaphor that the abstract Word was changed into the physicality of flesh. The immediacy of the Italian term *carne* is retained in our description of the "Word Incarnate"; it is a concept that was taken to heart by Italian culture and its artists. The consensus ruled that, following the central belief of the Incarnation, bodies reified spiritual mysteries. Renaissance art developed along lines that would literally embody that prescription, searching for techniques that fostered increasing naturalism tempered by idealization of the body, able to attract the viewer through its beauty and to convince by its tactility. The push toward these qualities quickly incorporated striking elements of sensual beauty that eroticized the bodies represented, and it is exactly this intersection that most demands exploration with "a period eye" that is markedly distant from our own culture's point of view.

Negative judgments about particularly striking Renaissance images usually assume that a conflict between carnality and spirituality was posited in contemporary values. However, such opinions often are the products of much later periods, or they use as a documentary basis the writings of Counter-Reformation critics from the late 1500s. This is a tactic that presupposes the answer to what is ostensibly being explored: the post-Tridentine treatise writers found fault with religious art that had elements of nudity, sensuousness, and distracting levels of artistic beauty. This is no surprise, since it expresses their particular ideological stand, formulated in opposition to a practice that permeated long-standing traditions. We would never have the enormous corpus of extant works featuring sensuous figures composed to express religious narratives if this were a transgressive practice. The volume and the quality of this type of art – some of it still in situ in the churches for which it was created – tell us that it was sought after by the wealthiest patrons, proudly displayed, and carefully preserved. If we discount the charge of subversion or inappropriateness, a more slippery and rewarding question to ask is how the nudity, sensuousness, and beauty functioned when employed in the service of religion.

If we agree that there could not have been an intended conflict between sensuous form and spiritual content in the mainstream of religious art, then we are able to explore how such art constituted spiritual messages that were instructive to the people who created it, commissioned it, and consumed it as devout believers. At the same time, it is crucial to take note of the contrary voices that were in circulation, quietly or more vociferously dissenting against this strategy, even during those moments when spiritualized carnality was most accepted. Just as is the case today, during the Renaissance opinions that were not in fashion were strongly stated, and although the culture was more homogeneous than our own, it was not monolithic.

In the Italian stylistic traditions, the personages in religious narratives and devotional images have a pronounced and commanding physical presence. The precise cultural impulses that gave rise to this convention would probably be impossible to trace, but they are easy enough to observe in the art. And every now and then the reasoning behind the images can be textually recovered. For example, in an imperious response to clerical patrons who complained about a depiction of the Creator carried out in their church, Giulio Romano, former student of Raphael and prestigious court painter to the Gonzaga dynasty in Mantua, declared:

> I understand that I have been maligned for painting God the Father, who is invisible. I respond that apart from Christ and the Madonna, who are in heaven with glorified bodies, all the rest of the saints and spirits and angels are invisible, and yet it is the custom to paint them. And it is no news to Your Lordships that paintings are the scripture of the unlettered and uneducated, and it is impossible to paint the invisible.[1]

This communication is interesting for its tactics. Essentially the painter declares that it is part of his profession to invent representations of the "unseeable"; he must find eloquent ways to embody abstract ideas. Giulio then supplies a bit of theological reasoning to impress the priests and to show that he understands the issues at stake. And finally he sententiously intones a truism about the function of religious art as a guide for the illiterate. This is a statement, however, for which we can be grateful, since it testifies to the general circulation in the Renaissance of the belief in art as a text available to all. These are the justifications that are repeatedly called upon when necessary: professional prerogative, theological reasoning, and the impact of visual communication.

In his letter Giulio Romano stated the need to clothe his figures in earthly bodies, but he did not mention anything about the physical qualities that would be adequate to represent divinity. However, we know that the diffusion of Neoplatonic concepts within general culture provided a source of ideas about the appropriate appearance of "glorified bodies" and spiritual entities. As popularly received from complex discussions in Neoplatonism, beauty was understood to be analogous to goodness, so that intensely beautiful bodies could be used as symbols of particular sanctity. Once more we can turn to a letter from the sixteenth century, in this instance written by an educated but not erudite woman, for an unselfconscious statement of this idea. Isabella Andreini was a famous actress, originally from Padua, who was also an accomplished writer. Her play, *Mirtilla*, published in 1588, was a great success. When she wrote to congratulate a friend on the birth of a daughter, her remarks (encouraging the father to be enthusiastic about his child's gender) included a prediction about the infant, "who, as she grows in beauty (as is to be expected), will be perfect in body and soul, since corporal beauty is a clear sign of the beauty of the soul."[2]

Physical beauty was considered a "sign" of spiritual goodness, and the artists reveled in their ability to perfect the signage. And it was not just in the realm of comeliness that artists sought to be convincing. All the elements of corporeality were called upon in the service of producing convincingly human renditions of the sacred stories. Starting with the naturalism established by Giotto's style in the Arena Chapel, religious narratives were presented with the accomplished storyteller's ability to highlight the eloquent detail. This can be strikingly observed in the two-handed shove that the high priest lands on Joachim as he expels him from the temple in the scene from the cycle dedicated to the life of Mary, which was painted at the start of the fourteenth century. The telling thrust was echoed by Jacopo della Quercia in his carving of the Expulsion on a panel for the portal of San Petronio in Bologna, dating to the 1430s. This time it is the irrevocable gesture of the avenging angel, making sure that Adam is physically banished from paradise, with a push in the direction of the gate, delivered just below the pelvis.

In contrast, the potent physical touch could be quite tender in an unexpected moment, as when a kinder angel discreetly takes Peter by the hand to reassure him while leading the saint out of prison, a detail in the rescue as Raphael imagined it for the Stanza of Heliodorus, painted in the Vatican's papal apartments in the early sixteenth century. Sanctified tenderness received insistent comment in the visual tradition, and it was a staple element in depictions of the Virgin and Child. From the fourteenth to the sixteenth century and beyond, artists communicated the love between the sinless mother and her divine son by envisioning the physical manifestations of their affection. Mary is shown nursing her baby, reciprocating his embrace, covering his nudity, and supporting his faltering first steps, in countless representations that make indelible impressions.

The potency of touching, in fact, was often used to great effect in devotional icons, conveying the bonds of love between two characters in unconventional ways, which surprise the viewer into reexperiencing a routine image. In a tragic vein, a stirring example of a very tangible expression of grief is Pietro Lorenzetti's motif of Mary clasping the hair of her dead son in the artist's *Deposition* from the 1330s, in Assisi (Illustration 5). The two heads are tightly pressed together so that the eyes meet, practically on the same axis, one pair closed in death, the other narrowed in pain. The arrangement is given increased visual interest by virtue of the upside-down juxtaposition of the faces of mother and son, and its pathos is palpable.

The Catholicism that was the shared religion of these artists and their audience encouraged such corporeal expressions of holy events by its structuring beliefs. Most central was the Incarnation of the second member of the Trinity, God who truly became man in the person of Jesus Christ; next was the equally crucial doctrine that after Christ's humanity had been extinguished, his glorified body rose from the dead and ascended to heaven; and the last was the doctrine that Christ gives his body and blood to his followers for spiritual nourishment while they remain on earth, through the sacrament of the Eucharist, the Real Presence of God under the species of consecrated bread and wine. The emphasis in all these doctrines is on the commingling of the divine with the human and on the physical body as a carrier of spiritual matter.

One strategy, therefore, for conveying these doctrines, which receives validity from the very nature of the beliefs represented, is to express them and stress their significance through graphic bodily metaphors. Explication

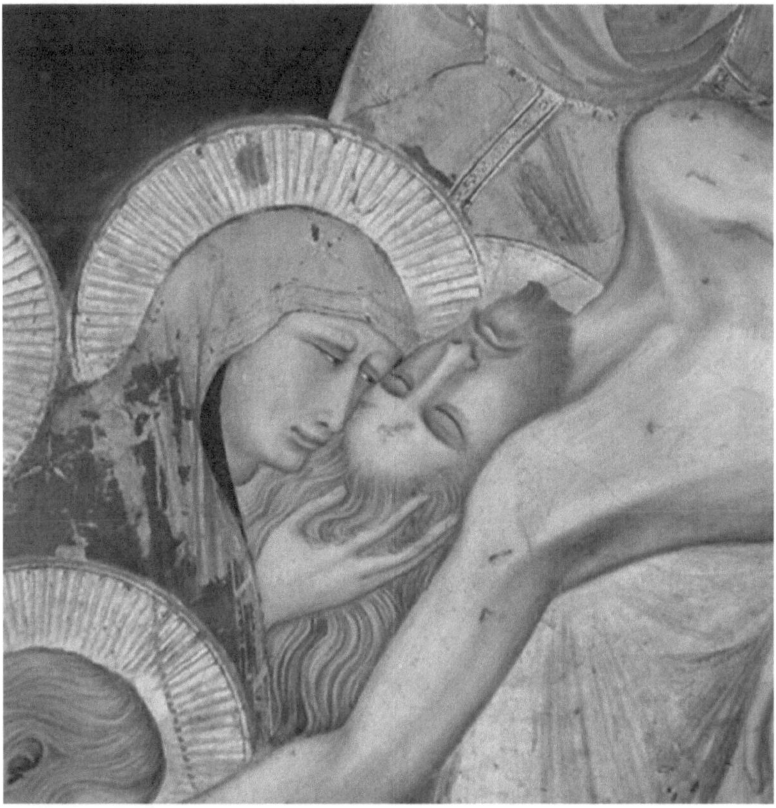

5. Pietro Lorenzetti, *Deposition*, 1330s. Assisi, Lower Basilica of S. Francesco. Photo courtesy of Sailko (license: CC-PD-Mark).

through carnal representation gives the faithful both a shared point of reference and an instant impact on which to anchor theology that could be quite abstract and often unfathomable. For example, the belief that the body and blood of Christ are truly, rather than symbolically, present in the consecrated Eucharist is irrational and comes down to a matter of faith. The crucial concept, however, could be expressed with power and immediacy through images of the Savior's corporeality, as shown by closely related versions of *The Blood of the Redeemer* by Carlo Crivelli (Illustration 6) and by Giovanni Bellini (National Gallery, London).

In both paintings the Eucharistic mystery is conveyed by the dark red blood that spurts from Christ's wound. Christ emphasizes the presence of his wound and applies pressure on it to make the blood freely discharge. This occurs quite dramatically in Crivelli's panel, where the gaping cut is trawled by Christ's thumb. The flow is caught in a chalice for direct distribution to the faithful by an angelic agent in Bellini's vision, while Crivelli portrays a saintly figure that is ready to ingest the divine blood. When taken seriously and literally, as they were by believers, these representations of the mystery of Christ's sacrifice can be powerful to the point of disturbance.

There is a further distinction about Crivelli's Christ: his short drapery is slung very low on his hips, low enough to expose a shadowy area of pubic hair (a trait that appears in many paintings of the dead Christ). This may ostensibly be an unseemly and unnecessary particular, until we further reflect on the doctrine of the Incarnation. An insistence on the true human nature of Christ and on his manhood in all of its physical minutiae becomes adherence to, and exposition of, sacred doctrine by visual means. Such detail provides an inescapable reminder, even by its ability to shock, that God became human. This is related to another path followed for imaging the sacred through the carnal, a strategy that has been exhaustively discussed after having been first mapped out by Leo Steinberg: the demonstration of the Incarnation by openly displaying the genitalia of the Christ Child.[3] Literally revealing the child's sex unequivocally attests to the double nature of Christ, simultaneously God and man. In some cases the nudity is emphasized by having the child squirm or wriggle in his mother's lap, which is appropriate (naturalistic) behavior for a baby, allowing him to twist around and raise up a leg for maximal "ostentatio genitalium" in the phrase favored by Steinberg. This particular convention was used extensively throughout the fifteenth and sixteenth centuries; in fact, it may be said to have been pervasive.

While I believe the Incarnation hypothesis to be a convincing interpretation of the practice, I do want to make an additional observation, which may be considered a slight emendation of the single-minded emphasis of Steinberg's thesis. It is clear that throughout the Italian Renaissance, early and late, north and south, the nudity of very small children was accepted as neutral. Genital display was never dishonorable or in the least offensive when it came to babies, and the infant Christ was not made an exception to this rule. It persists even in the rigid system of Giovanni Andrea Gilio, a conservative ecclesiastic, writing his treatise in 1564, the year following the Council of Trent's decree on images. Gilio allowed that the portrayal of nudity in very young children (*piccioli fanciulletti*) was harmless.[4] The acceptance of any type of nudity within Gilio's severe morality is notable; even more striking is that he sanctions such display on the basis of the "innocence and purity without evil and sin" of the subjects. The justification comes from the nature of the subject rather than the effect on the viewer. But this one instance is exceptional; nudity, according to Gilio, is never allowable in the representation of grown men or women. This provides textual evidence, from an unexpected source, for the acceptability of representations of the Incarnation that we have been considering. When, however, artists of particularly sensuous and elegant styles took up this theme, and added gloriously beautiful and very physically persuasive treatments of Mother and Son to the tradition, the line of acceptability for the overall image came close to being crossed, or at least the potential for indecorous effects on the viewer might be feared.

The paintings of Correggio, whose delicate figures with glowing skin have always been esteemed as the epitome of a particular strain of beauty, make no compromises with their sumptuous lyricism in the treatment of religious subjects. In fact, the humanistic culture that developed in the fifteenth century and flourished through the first half of the following century made beauty a central and a positive concern. As we have seen, beauty was linked conceptually to goodness and flawlessness, and was therefore

6. Carlo Crivelli, *Saint Francis with the Blood of Christ*, 1480s. Milan, Museo Poldi-Pezzoli. Photo courtesy of the Yorck Project (license: PD-Art-Yorck Project. GFDL).

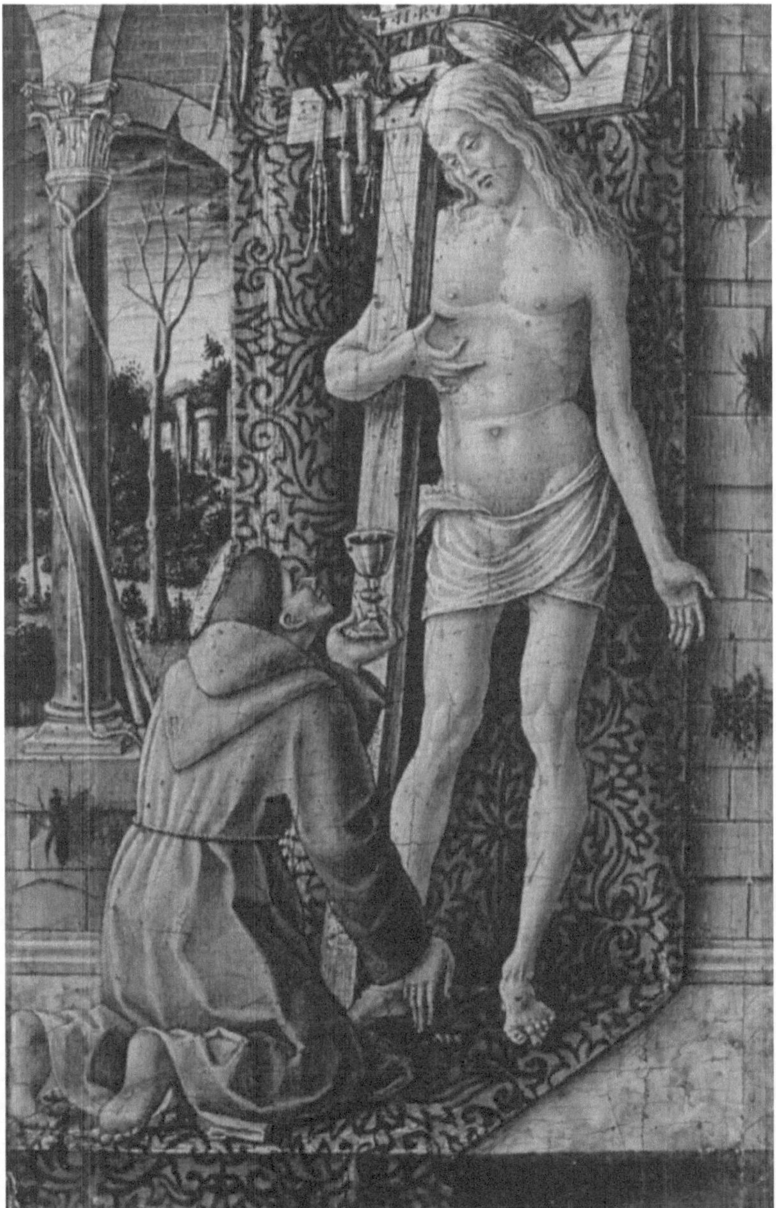

not only a legitimate but a most appropriate vehicle for the delineation of divinity. Linked especially with the sense of vision, beauty was believed to be a force of attraction that could lead the soul – through passage from the eyes – to the contemplation of goodness and ultimately to a higher sphere removed from the coarseness and imperfection of the earthly realm. But high-minded meditation on comeliness abuts a fragile boundary; if the postulate of beauty as a virtuous conduit toward a higher perfection is lost, only the force of humanity's lower appetites remains.

Therefore, outside of the immediate context of the highly idealizing Christian humanism from which these images took their validity, the seductive aspects appear to be purely carnal, with an allure that does not beckon beyond into purified spheres. When later viewers confront Correggio's religious images, often the perception of lasciviousness remains, while the spiritual element has evaporated. In the nineteenth century, at least one observer who was neither captivated nor ushered toward meditation by the transcendent beauty of Correggio's paintings left a strongly worded complaint about their effect. John Addington Symonds harangued against the inappropriateness of the characterizations he perceived in the holy personages. Symonds blustered that if Correggio's saints could walk out of their canvasses, "of what exemplary action would they be capable? That is the question which they irresistibly suggest; and we are forced to answer, 'None!' "[5]

As the sixteenth century progressed, the young Parmigianino would vie with the accomplishment of his immediate local predecessor. Working in the same stylistic tradition, Parmigianino redoubled insistence on virtuosity in constructing images of stunning elegance and overwhelming refinement and beauty. Did this virtuosity go too far and become indecorous for religious subjects? The fact that Parmigianino was extremely successful, attracting requests from both lay and clerical patrons for both private and public religious commissions, demands the acknowledgment that his output was sought after, valued, and supported by many of his contemporaries. Later his voluptuous style was criticized for detracting from the content of religious subjects, but his painting *Madonna of the Rose* (Illustration 7) had been copied at least fifty times by the mid–sixteenth century, according to Vasari's count.

The claim is often repeated that the *Madonna of the Rose* originally portrayed a Venus and Cupid. But that idea stems from a piece of eighteenth-century criticism, found in a monograph by Ireneo Affò. The author's supposition is that since the work was, on Vasari's authority, first intended for Pietro Aretino, "l'uomo più libertino de' giorni suoi," it must have had a licentious subject.[6] Affò's assessment of Aretino's character becomes his analysis of Parmigianino's painting. However, Parmigianino's evolving composition for the painting is documented by a wealth of drawings, in the words of David Ekserdjian, an "unparalleled number of drawings for a domestic painting."[7] The material evidence contradicts Affò's hypothesis and instead indicates that the subject ended up as it started out: a treatment of the traditional Madonna and Child theme with a long and venerable

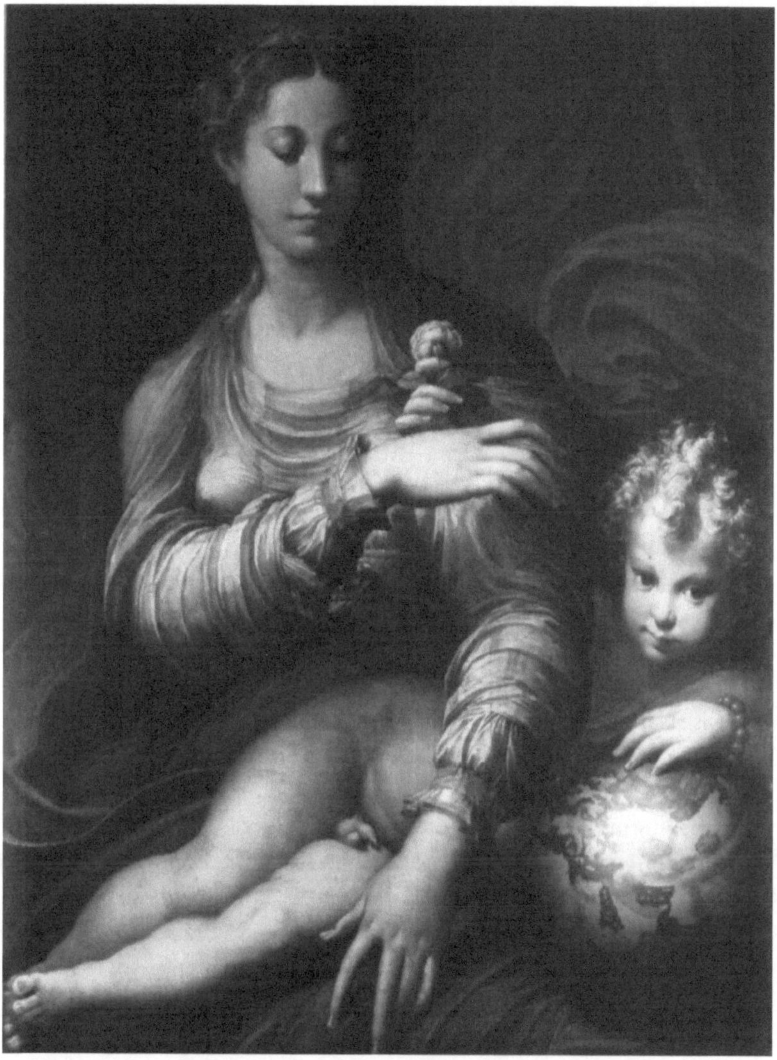

7. Parmigianino, *Madonna of the Rose*, 1528–30. Dresden, Gemäldegalerie. Photo courtesy of the Yorck Project (license: PD-Art-Yorck Project. GFDL).

history, which exploited the nudity of the infant for symbolic purposes. Parmigianino explored ways of making the subject new and vital, concentrating on the movement of the child out from Mary's lap where he usually sat and on the complex and graceful composition of intertwined hands and arms. The format and elongated shape of the stretching child recalls Raphael's *Bridgewater* Madonna. Parmigianino's love of the Urbinate's work and his extension of Raphael's graceful forms was a lasting heritage of the younger artist's Roman sojourn. Parmigianino's figures of Mary and Christ are as attenuated and sumptuous as possible, of course, but as we have seen, their beauty can be read in a positive light, and the child's nudity is practically demanded by tradition.

Another instructive detail in Parmigianino's work shows us the strategy of exploiting the attractiveness of childish innocence to full compositional effect in religious images. In his Prado *Holy Family with Angels* from the 1520s, the artist prominently places on the extreme right of the panel a vivacious cherub, whose golden curls in disarray indicate that he is rushing into the scene, at the same time that his figure closes the composition. The *putto*'s diaphanous garment, so revealing to begin with, pulls away from his body as he makes an apron of it to present his offering of gathered flowers, which Christ accepts. The action of the childish figure reveals his chubby thighs and buttocks, and swings them out toward the viewer. It is a teasing motif that enlivens the grouping, meant to delight the viewer on a visceral level, because it is frisky but completely ingenuous at the same time.

Putti often have this function, and religious art is full of them, frolicking in their nudity, beguiling in their corporeality, yet tempered by their angelic status and their childish stature. They can have an attractive presence even in the most solemn of subjects, where they often function as a chorus of mourners. In Giovanni Bellini's exquisite *Dead Christ Supported by Angels* (from Rimini), they support for our contemplation the heroic, wounded torso of the Redeemer, yet their short tunics, which fall open more or less discreetly, might prove a distraction along the way. For the devout, however, the seduction of the motif is enjoyable but concentration on it is fleeting. Having been drawn into the image, the viewer's gaze is moved along to the inescapable message. Once attention is engaged, prayer proceeds to its higher levels of contemplation. The strategy implies captivation, counting on the enthralled viewer to become enrapt in contemplating the figure of Christ, whose dead body represents the consequences of our sins. Perhaps first attracted by the *putto* on the right, with its shining hair falling into lowered eyes, the viewer's gaze might then caress the lovely bared shoulder of the child and wonder at the slippage of the fabric, probably caused by the weight of the gem on the slim strap. This path of scrutiny would then culminate in meditation on the hand of Christ held up by the attractive angel, its dark wound a visual counterpoint to the heavy broach previously inspected across the undraped shoulder. Thoughts and observations that might begin in profane matters (always the most easily accessible even to noble minds encased in weak human flesh) can lead, in the hands of a great artist, to supremely important issues of faith.

We can turn to Giorgio Vasari for a timely comment about these developments in the art of his contemporaries. His view is ardent and clear. He lodges a grievance against the ill-informed people who equate clumsy and inept figures in art with devoutness in life, and continues with an eloquent condemnation:

> Now I would not have any man deceive himself by considering the rude and inept as holy, and the beautiful and excellent as licentious, as some do, who, seeing figures of women or of youths adorned with loveliness and beauty beyond the ordinary, straightaway censure them and judge them to be licentious, not perceiving that they are very wrong to condemn the

> good judgment of the painter, who holds the Saints, both male and female, who are celestial, to be as much more beautiful to mortal man as Heaven is superior to earthly beauty and to the works of human hands; and what is worse, they reveal the unsoundness and corruption of their own minds by drawing evil and impure desires out of works from which, if they were lovers of purity, as they seek by their misguided zeal to prove themselves to be, they would gain a desire to attain to Heaven and to make themselves acceptable to the Creator of all things, in whom as most perfect and most beautiful, all perfection and all beauty have their source.[8]

Vasari's correlation of beauty with heavenly perfection is the underlying justification for acceptance of the sensuous figures, along with the technical proficiency of the artist. Significantly, as a practicing artist, Vasari exculpates his fellow professionals and places all blame for a potential fall from propriety onto others; the fault lies in the unseemly reaction of the viewer, not in the beauty of the representation. However, Vasari's text also shows that by midcentury such a defense had to be strongly voiced.

The tradition that Vasari upheld so staunchly was specifically that of Tuscan art and the humanism that helped to form it. In that milieu, a priority was always placed on attaining consummate skill in the representation of the human form and on developing a style that grew from the study of nature and the models of antiquity. Those values were elaborated by using the human figure as a basic means of expression, and its mastery was the proving ground of the artist. I believe that this concept was in place even before it had time to be fully developed in actual objects, as evidenced by two precocious and eloquent carved reliefs that symbolize the sculptor at work. Both reliefs were placed on highly visible public monuments in Florence, whose influential decorative programs were matters of both pride and instruction.

The earlier is the representation of the art of sculpture on the lower register of the Duomo's campanile, in the hexagonal panel of the series in praise and exhortation of human labor (Illustration 8). Designed by Giotto, the scene was executed in the 1330s in the circle of Andrea Pisano. The venerable figure of the sculptor, with a flowing beard and dressed in a long robe, works intently with hammer and chisel on his project, the execution of a nude male figure. Set on an incline to facilitate the carving, the angle of the sculpture-in-the-making also clearly reveals the anatomically detailed subject to the viewer's gaze. In this iconic scheme the sculptor's task is to create a true-to-life human form.

About eighty years later, the same idea is repeated but situated in a scene pertaining to workaday life rather than dwelling in the realm of symbol. The carved *predella* of Nanni di Banco's *Four Crowned Martyrs* (1410–14), set up in the niche devoted to the Guild of Stone and Wood Workers at Or San Michele in Florence, again addressed the theme of the sculptor practicing his profession. In this case we see four practitioners grouped in a working environment, performing the various skills overseen by the

Guild. On the far right of the relief, a bearded man bends down to carve a figure on an inclined panel – certainly paying homage to Giotto's relief, as well as to contemporary practitioners. In both cases the art of sculpture is characterized by the creation of the nude figure; in Nanni di Banco's updated version, the larger-scale sculpture now has the features of a *putto* in a pioneering *all'antica* style.

These reliefs were carried out at a time when the classicizing, free-standing nude was not common, although by the second decade of the fifteenth century the painting and sculpting of the nude were about to be reintroduced into mainstream practice. In addition to the interests of Neoplatonic humanism and antiquarian studies, it can be argued that the emerging acceptance of the display of the nude human body in art was linked to the conception of the artist's creative capacity as a mirror of divine creation. This idea had a continuous valence in Christian art, often expressed in images of God as the architect of the universe. The idea of the symbolic possibilities of human creation was a forceful one, with obvious appeal to artists. The preference for classical models (fundamental for the stylistic development of idealized naturalism in the visual arts), Neoplatonic theories of virtue and beauty, and artists endowed with and committed to technical expertise, all resulted in painting and sculpture of staggering impact. The artists' increasing ability to conceive and execute facsimiles of corporeal perfection, so much the apes of nature that concupiscence might naturally arise in encountering them, did cause problems for some segments of the original audience – especially those concerned more with religious import than with artistic statements.

Despite an account that Michelangelo's *David* was pelted with stones as it was moved from its work site to the Piazza della Signoria under the cover of darkness in May 1504, our culture admires this sculpture so much that we are unwilling to speculate on its lack of acceptance in the past. The problems attending its reception were certainly in part political, given its pronounced republican symbolism, and possibly in part a response to innovative art, with reference to its monumental nudity. Perhaps a political agenda was furthered by way of censorship. In a letter of 1545, Pietro Aretino alludes to a *ghirlanda* put in place to cover the statue's genitalia, testimony largely ignored by scholars, even after it was discussed by Renato Ristori in the 1980s.[9] The late date of Aretino's remarks had been invoked to dismiss the thought wholesale; now the further research of Francesco Caglioti puts forward uncontestable documentary evidence. Records stipulate that a certain "Raffaello di Giovanni" was paid to gild the garland after it had deteriorated from exposure to the elements, confirming the prolonged use of camouflage to minimize the impact of the colossal nude statue.[10]

Later, the more famous Raphael of Urbino included the girded statue in a slightly teasing detail in the border of one of the Vatican tapestries. Setting the entry of Leo X in the Piazza della Signoria in Florence, Raphael

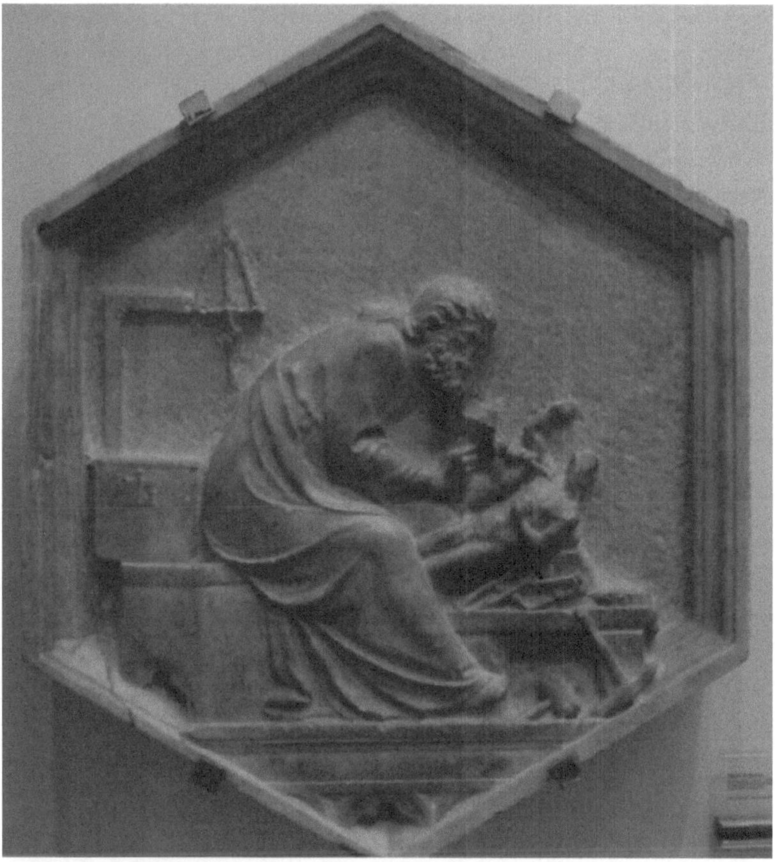

8. Andrea Pisano, *Art of Sculpture*, c. 1334–37. Florence, Museo dell'Opera del Duomo. Photo courtesy of Sailko (license: CC-BY-SA. GFDL).

incorporated the *David* into the scene. Not able to resist a jibe at his temperamental colleague, the younger artist employed a point of view that cut off the statue's head but featured its groin wreathed in leaves, accompanied by several figures that have clambered up the massive sculpture for a better view of the event. In Raphael's clever way, he has at one and the same time paid homage and disrespect to the venerable master and to the ambiguous success of Michelangelo's rendering an *all'antica* practice in contemporary terms. It was too close to the mark for some viewers. Our own resistance to the evidence that David's nudity – in monumental form and a public location – did provoke controversy stems from our penchant for imagining an essentially "pagan" High Renaissance culture, where Christianity hovered in the background but was pushed to one side when it came to art. This is mistaken; religious art was meant to be a legitimate expression of the Church's creed. But as artists pushed their styles in the direction of classical prototypes, virtuosity, *varietà*, and *ornato*, some of their audience found its comprehensive result problematic. During the period with which I am concerned, squeamishness regarding nudity in art was not the view of the majority, especially not in the powerful circles of wealthy, private patronage or the uppermost ranks of the clergy.

Representation of the nude figure, in all of its palpable sensuousness, followed rules of propriety in the Renaissance far removed from our own sense of appropriateness. A colossal nude in a civic context could threaten decorum, while full-scale figures in the nude found a certain level of acceptance within religious structures. The link to spiritual subjects is complex but crucial; for example, an expert on northern art of the same period has stated, "The nude in German art during the fifteenth century appeared exclusively in religious or moralizing themes and was in fact extremely rare."[11] In Italian art of the fifteenth century, where the nude figure was becoming the supreme artistic challenge and a staple of representation, it crossed the lines of both religious and secular subjects and situations.

For certain themes, nudity of even the adult Christ was permissible. Occasionally he was undraped during his baptism, although many examples of this scene finesse the matter by immersing the body of Christ in water that acts as a shield of modesty, rendering at times a murky rather than explicit depiction. Other Christological subjects, however, are unequivocal. Rosso Fiorentino's *Dead Christ* (in the Boston Museum of Fine Arts) shows his body in all of its unveiled, heroic humanity, strongly lit to give emphasis and clarity to the representation. Michelangelo's *Risen Christ* in S. Maria sopra Minerva, which was originally commissioned, conceived, and executed as a nude figure, unfortunately has appeared for some time with a garish loin cloth applied to its surface. The significance of its initial state is explained by Alexander Nagel as follows:

> Michelangelo offered ... a pristine and radiant dead Christ based on the models of antique sculpture. This was more than a stylistic preference. It was fundamentally a restoring of theological perspective, for it turned attention away from the immediate story of tragic suffering and death to the ultimate victory that resulted from Christ's sacrifice. This, too, was a preference shared by prominent advocates of reform.[12]

The virtuosity of such an exercise goes without saying; the emphatic sexuality of the figure goes without comment in the passage quoted, but it is justified by the symbolism that Nagel attributes to the presentation of the figure. The statement that such a characterization would find favor among the Catholic Reformers shows how difficult it is to draw the line about acceptability; various ideologies and convictions could easily make boundaries collapse, contingent on the valence of particular arguments.

Benvenuto Cellini's full-scale crucifix is another instance of a representation of Christ whose "pristine" nudity has been covered over to make it acceptable to modern standards (Illustration 9). The sculptor brags in his autobiography about how he set his own challenge to carve this piece, which was daunting to execute. The recitation helps us to understand the

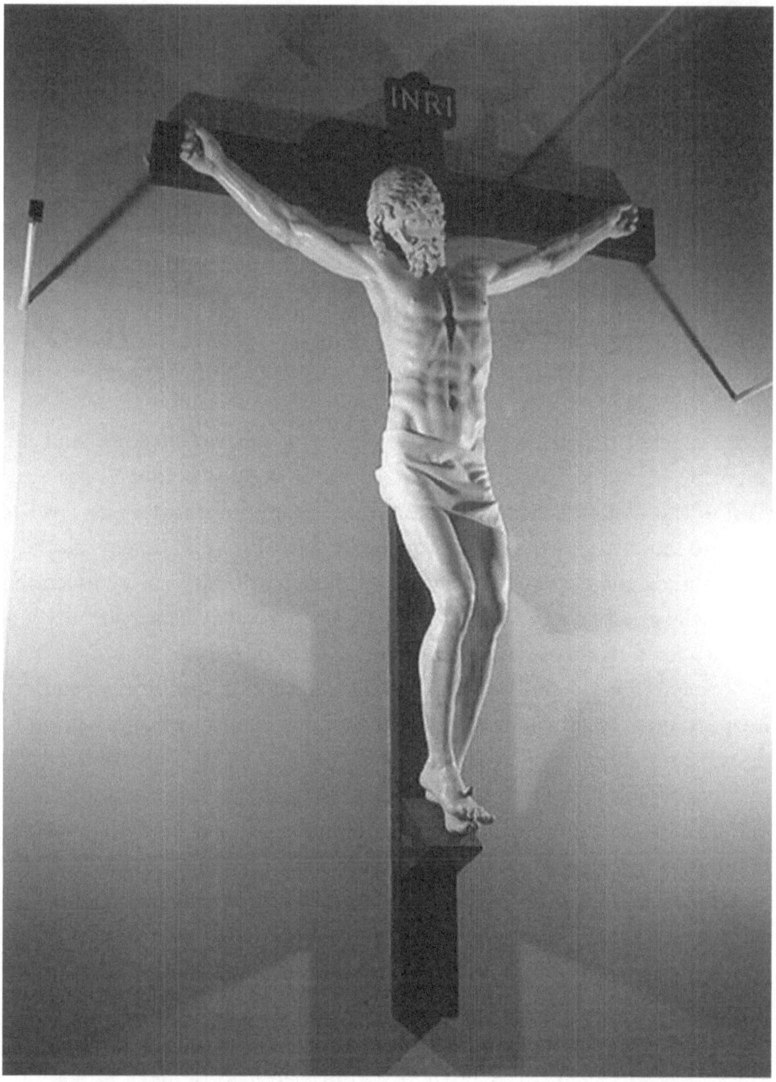

9. Benvenuto Cellini, *Crucifix*, 1556. San Lorenzo, El Escorial. Photo courtesy of AnTeMi (license: CC-BY-SA-3.0. GFDL).

crucial place that the demonstration of artistry had in the creation of such figures. I suggest that artists were given generous license when such "art figures" appeared in the context of religious subjects, because this professional training was tantamount to application for admission into the ranks of the virtuosi. The challenge taken up by Cellini in the creation of a life-size nude figure of the crucified Christ has one of the most noble traditions in the history of Renaissance art, starting with the competition that Vasari records between Brunelleschi and Donatello in the successful realization of the subject (and still available for our judgment in the Florentine churches of S. Maria Novella and S. Croce), followed by the young Michelangelo, whose result can be studied in the sacristy of S. Spirito.

If one category of creative license was virtuosity in the presentation of human figure, another was that of decoration. *Ornato* is the term that was used for this aspect of the creation of art, related to the English "ornament" and "ornamentation." It is a word of abundant meanings, as well as a category from classical theories of rhetoric, and it provided a rich source of analogies and guidance for systems of visual art. Leon Battista Alberti used terms linked to *ornato* in his treatise on painting, applying the concept of *ornamentum* to describe the ancillary area of the composition. Alberti encouraged the use of enrichment through variety in connection with the work's narrative component, the *istoria*, because it would "hold the eye" of all viewers, learned and unlearned, and it would do this through a sensation of pleasure.[13]

Passages of ornamentation in a religious *istoria* would command the attention of the viewer and rivet it, so that through prolonged contemplation the devout worshipper would pass from the initial entry level of profane sensation to the sphere of spiritual truths. This strategy placed a premium on the elements of artifice and skill, particularly in the invention of visually gratifying and complex motifs, and so became a particularly fertile area for displays of virtuosity. Defining this category of artistic creation as "ornament" was well founded in the context of specifically religious imagery, since *opus ornatus* is the term found in the exegetical tradition to describe the third phase of God's inceptive creative act. *Opus ornatus* refers to the formation of the stars and planets, plant and animal life, and human beings; we can, with justification, see this as the first instance of *varietà* and copiousness produced within the universe of forms.

Human imitation of the Divine Creator's *opus ornatus* was highly valued during the Renaissance, and it flourished as a driving stylistic force. An exquisite example of the striking use of *ornato* can be seen in the pages of Giulio Clovio's book of devotions known as the *Farnese Hours*, completed in 1546 for Cardinal Alessandro Farnese. Thirty-seven of the book's pages contain texts situated within elaborate borders, in addition to twenty-six full-page miniatures that are also surrounded by sumptuous framing devices. Embellishment was clearly a defining strategy of this luxury object, and the decoration followed its own rules, separate from the visual narratives and verbal texts. The patterns that emerge from the borders privilege *all'antica* decorative elements and feature the idealized nude figure, fictively represented as sculptures and reliefs. There is so much emphasis on the bordering devices that often the scale of the fictive sculptural figures outdoes that of the "live" figures populating the narrative scenes. Despite the elaborate, some might say "overblown," nature of the ostensibly ancillary elements, they were considered to be highly successful, indeed models of the genre.

Vasari fills about three pages of Clovio's biography with over-the-top praise for his accomplishment in the Farnese illuminations and ends by favorably commenting on the "variety of bizarre ornaments ...

appropriately placed at the border so as to enrich the work"[14] (my emphasis). Significantly, Vasari associates ornamentation with propriety, linking concepts of decoration to decorum, and in fact the words derive from the same root.[15] This semantic linkage has real potential for furthering our sensitivity to the period's understanding of *ornato*, because it is so often just this question that troubles our interpretation of many Renaissance works of religious subjects: Does the alluring decoration remain decorous? According to Vasari's comments, even "bizarre" elements are proper in a book of prayers, since they are used to embellish its appearance, taking their rightful place in the margins of the main subject.

The medium of the *Farnese Hours* puts it in the long tradition of medieval manuscript illumination, whose pages abound with marginalia. Visually commenting on the texts, sometimes in a polemic or a teasing manner, the drawings are literally "images on the edge" in the telling formulation of Michael Camille.[16] Camille analyzes the function of marginalia as a type of gloss that surrounds and amplifies the central text, at times with truly "edgy" intent. Two sheets from the *Rutland Psalter* (in the collection of the British Museum) transcribe Psalm 67 embellished with a simian-featured rider astride an ostrich-like bird, who advances with an arrow pointed across the page to the exposed buttocks of a nude youth who is bending over, with a gesture that can be read as either alarmed or obliging. It is not obvious what this has to do with Psalm 67, and luckily Camille has a smart suggestion. The vignette is a playful comment on the text, where the word *iuvencularum* sits above the bending youth: the drawing, we might say, "deconstructs" the text, embodying the *iuvenis* (youth) and *cul* (backside).[17]

We can consider these representations, which take advantage of a certain license in order to startle the reader back into serious consideration of the main text, as predecessors of Renaissance treatments of eye-catching devices. These extracurricular visual texts can operate as powerful contrasts along the spectrum of human experience, which abruptly jolt the heavenly sphere back toward the earthly venue for a moment of human, humorous contact, before demanding contemplation of the spiritual is renewed. Such interaction of carnal and spiritual indicates that these cultures saw the sacred and the profane as existing along a continuum with extreme reaches, not as binary opposites.

The freedom that medieval artists appropriated for themselves in marginalia can arguably be seen as a paradigm of the type of inventive liberty that Renaissance artists maintained in their relationship to the compositional framing and embellishing of their works. A creative use of this tradition appears in the arrangement of the Solomonic columns in Raphael's cartoon for the tapestry of the *Healing of the Lame Man*, where they bracket the main protagonists of the narrative from the crowd of observers (Illustration 10). The twisted columns are adorned with vines and with numerous *putti*. The inclusion of these decorative motifs within the composition has elicited the wrath of some spectators, and not just the usual suspects. Henry Fuseli referred to the columns as that "barbaric colonnade, loaded with profane ornament."[18] What Fuseli missed in the eighteenth century was the original justification for the motif, an impeccable model well known to Raphael in the sixteenth century. For the scene of miraculous curing set at the Temple of Jerusalem, Raphael manifested what has been called his "archaeological" interests by including versions of the twisted columns from St. Peter's, which survived the destruction of the old basilica and were believed to have been brought to Rome by Constantine. The naked *putti* were taken directly from the prototype. The graceful torsion of these columns was much admired by Renaissance artists, and those in Raphael's circle in particular included them often in their compositions. Parmigianino created a glorious set to frame his fresco of St. Cecilia in the Steccata, entwining the columns with rich drapery and arranging to great and sensuous effect the little figures within the coils.

But perhaps the most curious and startling use of *colonne tortilli* can be seen in an earlier work, an enthroned Madonna with saints in S. Maria Nuova, in Gubbio. As conceived by Ottaviano Nelli, an Umbrian artist whose known works were painted in the first quarter of the fifteenth century, the slender columns that frame the sacred grouping are filled with neither vinous motifs nor rollicking *putti*. Instead, the swirling spirals carry many energetic, nude figures of both sexes. A few of them are, without any doubt, engaged in intimate embraces, and perhaps copulation. The activity looks specific, indicating that it makes an iconographic contribution to the image as well as an adornment. The coiling progression of the different levels indicates that they might be representations conceived of as similar to the *bolge* from Dante's *Inferno*, the eternal theater of sins and their punishment. Such graphic imagery would be a legitimate – if disquieting – marginal commentary on the iconic image of salvation history embodied in the representation of the Madonna and Child, presenting the Savior in his humble, human form.

Consideration of the particular tradition and potential functions of sacred characters and narratives in frames provides new avenues of approach to figural series whose meanings remain elusive despite intense study. Michelangelo's *ignudi* from the Sistine ceiling are an illustrious case. Perhaps the sanction for their existence is caught up in the framing conventions that I have been describing, endowing their presence with more weight as ancillary commentary and less emphasis as conveyors of symbolic meaning. In his biography of the master, Condivi stresses the framing nature of the *ignudi*, outside the main stories of Genesis: "But no less marvelous ... is that part which does not appertain to the narrative. These are certain *ignudi* which, seated on bases above the aforesaid cornice, support at either side the medallions.... In all these things ... Michelangelo displayed consummate art."[19] In this passage Condivi describes skill and the function of framing but makes no mention of allegorical intent. The fanciful forms and exaggerated postures of the athletic figures designed by

Michelangelo fit comfortably into the liberties allowed and taken in marginal decoration that was approved by long tradition.

Within the ceiling's decorative framework, the apparent function of the *ignudi* is to support the flowing garlands, which are traditional bordering devices taken from the classical repertoire. Following the conventions connected to this motif, the *ignudi* become oversize, muscular variants of the more usual childish *putti* found in ancient decoration. As Charles Dempsey has shown, these captivating figures seduced Renaissance artists, starting with Donatello, who translated them into Tuscan *spiritelli*, introducing renewed interest in these figures.[20] The joyous, often rollicking figures abound in the decoration of sacred spaces throughout the Renaissance, whose unselfconscious nudity was legitimized by both their preadolescent innocence and their *all'antica* pedigree. The parade of garland-sustaining, nude *putti* can be followed in the Florentine tradition from the intarsia friezes in the sacristy of the Duomo, to Donatello's *spiritelli* placed above the cornice in his S. Croce *Annunciation*; they are transported to Rome by Michelangelo's monumental versions in the Sistine ceiling, which Bronzino then reclaims in the vault of Eleonora da Toledo's chapel in the Palazzo Vecchio, painted during the 1540s. Bronzino derived the postures of his small-scale *ignudi/putti* from their monumental prototypes, while shrinking them back to childish forms as they grab at the festoons that rise behind

10. Nicholas Dorigny, after Raphael, *Healing of the Lame Man* (tapestry cartoon, 1515–16, Hampton Court). From *Pinacotheca Hamptoniana*, late seventeenth century. Etching and engraving on paper. London, Victoria and Albert Museum (Dyce.2562). Photo courtesy of Victoria and Albert Museum, London. Bequeathed by Rev. Alexander Dyce.

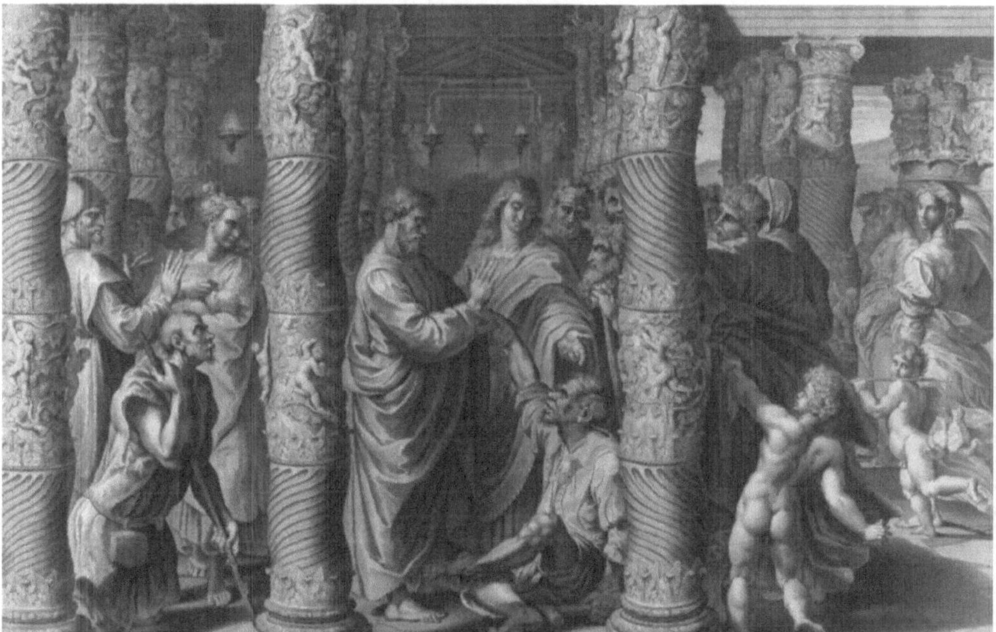

them. The continuous development of this motif, spanning the fifteenth and sixteenth centuries, enriched painted and sculpted decoration commissioned specifically for sites of worship, emphasizing the acceptability, if not the neutrality, of this type of nudity in decorative passages around sacred subjects, which at times could even encroach on the main narratives.

Bacchiacca'a *Flagellation*, in the National Gallery in Washington, DC, displays even more latitude taken with framing devices and the concept of *ornato*. The composition is patterned in strict symmetry, with Christ's body placed on axis at the *Santa Colonna*, located in the middle of an arch whose piers are bisected by two pilasters, resting between two other arches cut off in compositional space at their center point. Framing Christ are his two tormentors, one totally unclothed, the other garbed only in soft strips of a charming shade of rose, loosely knotted with a spiraling tie, defying gravity to hang together. The two flamboyant flagellators are, of course, "art figures," skillfully composed and painted, calculated to mirror each other in their motions and ready to deflect complaints made in the *paragone* about painting not being capable of showing a figure from more than one side at a time. The helmets are fantastic, truly displaying the *fantasia* of the artist. The panel is small in scale, a private devotional piece, made for a patron's individual delectation as well as devotions and honorable within the terms of Alberti's theory, which posits that elements pleasing to the eye lead the viewer to look longer and more closely. (The more conservative Alberti, however, might not have admired this later, ostentatious solution.)

Two images from Raphael's Vatican loggia can serve as a basis for further exploring how the concept of *ornato* could function in a complex decorative program. One of the narrative scenes in the loggia's vault depicts the Old Testament story of Isaac and Rebecca. The couple's legitimate sexual union, recorded in Genesis, is of crucial import within the Judeo-Christian tradition. Their progeny established a principal tribe of God's chosen people, which culminated for Christianity in the ancestry of Christ. The allusion to coupling, integral to the significance of the representation, is made in a decorous manner, conveyed by the "slung leg motif" that symbolizes sexual intercourse. After such discretion, it is surprising to find that in the nearby decorative areas stucco reliefs display less inhibited versions of the theme of sexual activity, this time without the validating factor of a biblical narration. Or perhaps the contrasting motif is not so surprising, since it follows the pattern that I have been suggesting, where the framing device comments on the main subject in a contrasting key.

A stucco relief in a highly classicizing style found on a *sottarco* shows two men facing each other and mutually displaying their sexual members. It is true that the typology of the loggia structure permits lighthearted decoration, but we might legitimately wonder if Giovanni da Udine pushed the limits with such explicit sexual content. The relatively private nature of the loggia and its function as a site of relaxation, even within the official Vatican residence of the pope, certainly allowed for less rigorous subjects, especially if they were discreetly placed in the upper reaches of the stuccowork. However, I believe that the real exculpating factors for the inclusion of this *osé* motif is its adherence to the tradition of decorative marginalia, given a level of prestige (if not respectability) by its classical pedigree. It may well have been copied from an ancient stucco relief, whose recipes and techniques Raphael encouraged Giovanni da Udine to imitate in the decoration or modeled on an intaglio carving found on a gem or cameo.

From the carnal display in reliefs surrounding Old Testament scenes, the discussion can move to passionate embraces displayed within a religious subject. Since it was unveiled in 1541, Michelangelo's *Last Judgment* has been the focus of much controversy around several issues connected to carnality in religious subject matter. The most notorious complaint centered on the nudity of the figures, but grievances were registered in other matters of content. One suspect iconographic detail shows several couples locked in embraces in the groupings of the elect.

When commented upon, these details are sometimes blurred over with discomfort, seen as indecorous and inexplicable manifestations of the artist's personal expression.[21] Personal and heartfelt they may be, as in the gentle motif found in the upper right of the fresco, where a young man engages an affectionate caress of a much older figure's beard. The artist's expression could also be emphatic, as displayed by the intensity with which another young man puckers up and pushes forward to kiss his companion. However, these expressions of love are not simply the self-indulgences of one idiosyncratic master; rather, they participate in a long-standing theme found in religious art, generated by visual precedent and sound theology.

As an example, the coupling of same-sex partners to symbolize spiritual bliss in paradise is present in the *Last Judgment* of Fra Angelico, housed in the Museum of San Marco in Florence. The artist, who was also a practicing member of the Dominican monastic community, has always been seen as a man of pious character and a propagator of authoritative spiritual imagery stemming from the established canon of institutional Catholicism. So far from being puzzling or transgressive, the segregation of men and women that was a fact of separate religious communities was most likely the basis for Fra Angelico's representation of intimate spiritual celebration symbolized by the affectionate exchanges among the elect included in his painting.

Similarly, Giovanni di Paolo's *Paradise* is conceived as a garden filled with hugging and kissing partners in all combinations, with a preponderance of same-sex twosomes in the fragmentary panels in the Metropolitan Museum (Illustration 11) and Siena's Pinacoteca. Many traditions converge in this interpretation of paradise: the prelapsarian Garden of Eden, the garden as a setting for lovers, and the usual division of the elect according to gender. In addition to mirroring the arrangement of religious communities, the distribution might also have been related to practices of worship that grouped males on one side and females on the other in places of worship. However, beyond the conspicuous interaction within the segregated assemblages of the faithful, it is the motif of the kiss that assumes an even more arresting impact in Christian ritual and symbolism, and in the art that records it.

The canonical (and mesmerizing) model of the carnal kiss that becomes a spiritual vehicle of expression is contained in the first line of the Song of Songs, whose literal transcription is: "O that he would kiss me with the kisses of his mouth, for lovemaking is better than wine."[22] The remarkably explicit imagery of the canticle, incorporated into the biblical canon, is one of the principal authorizations for the use of sexual metaphors in Judeo-Christian symbolic systems. In his commentary on the Song of Songs, St. Bernard states that the joining of lips expresses the embrace of souls. And to get to the crux of the matter, this is the message that I believe is alluded to by the kissing and embracing couples in paradise in our visual texts.

The metaphor was sustained by the humanists in their writings, such as Marsilio Ficino's passages about the ecstatic and reciprocal nature of love, where an exchange of the lovers' souls takes place. Pico della Mirandola unequivocally posited the kiss as the joining of souls and allowed it legitimacy in the representation of divine love.

To complete the circuit back to religious texts and practices, it can be recalled that the kiss of peace was from early Christian times a part of the mass, bestowed after the priest intoned the "Pax vobiscum."[23] St. Augustine associates the kiss of peace exchanged among the faithful during the mass's celebration with the communion of divine love obtained through the Eucharist. And it was a real kiss shared on earth that was understood to allude to the embrace of divine love: "As your lips approach the lips of your brother let not your heart withdraw from his."

St. John Chrysostom presents a similar view of the import of the kiss when its meaning is extended into the symbolic realm of spiritual love: "[T]he Lord wants our souls to kiss and our hearts to embrace." For these reasons, it was considered particularly heinous that Judas betrayed Jesus with a kiss, because it was a sacred and sacramental sign of love. In his frescoed version of the *Betrayal* from the Life of Christ in the Arena Chapel, Giotto shows the perfidy of the traitor's abuse of this sacred sign, as Judas puckers his lips and moves toward his victim, as a signal to the soldiers to apprehend Christ.

In contrast, Parmigianino imagines the young St. John in the act of kissing the child Jesus in the Uffizi's *Madonna and Child with Saints* from around 1530. The Christ Child responds to the enveloping embrace of John and turns to receive the kiss even as he affectionately grasps his cousin's chin, a motif often used to express carnal desire, but here sanctified. The artist does not shy away from the display of a sensuous tenderness in the exchange, but rather makes it a fundamental theme of the image, since John indulges a proper expression of love for Christ in a gesture to be followed imaginatively by devout believers and in a real gesture during the mass.

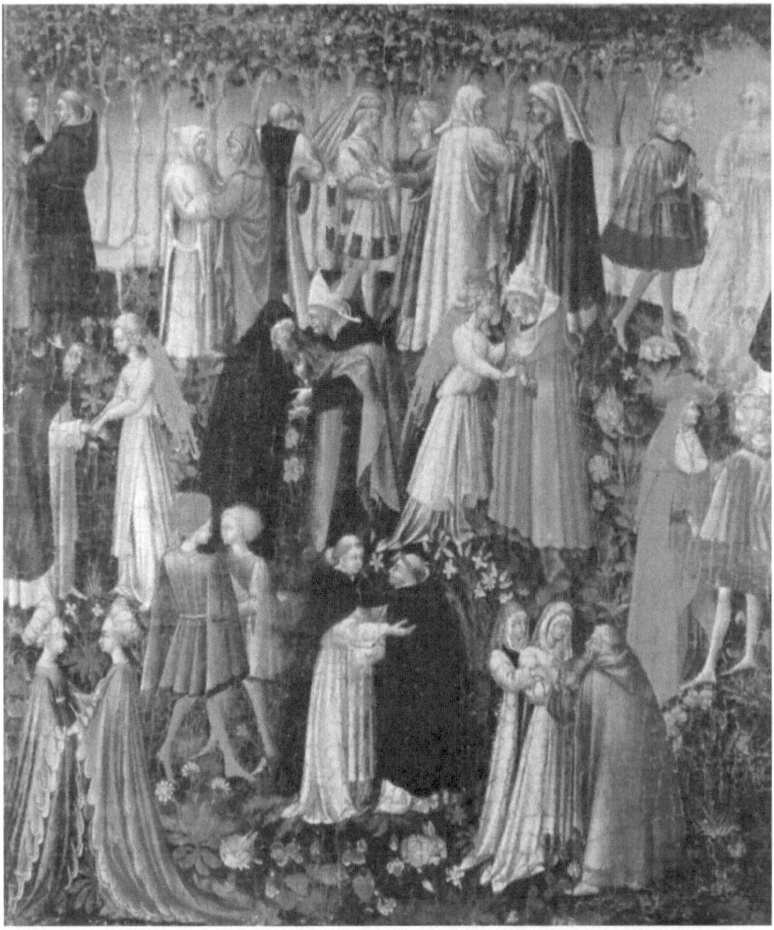

11. Giovanni di Paolo, *Paradise* (fragment), c. 1445. New York, Metropolitan Museum of Art. Photo courtesy of the Yorck Project (license: PD-Art-Yorck Project. GFDL).

In the Holy Family grouping that Agnolo Bronzino painted for the Panciatichi family around the midpoint of the sixteenth century, a kiss that the young John the Baptist is about to bestow on the infant Christ is accompanied by an even more daring gesture of physical tenderness. John's right hand moves across the chest of the contentedly sleeping baby so that thumb and forefinger are in position to caress the nipple exposed by the thin fabric that drapes the infant's torso. This action forms a strong point of focus in the grouping of the two children, yet the strangeness of the gesture within a sacred scene has kept modern comments on the motif to a minimum. The overall tone of the scene is deeply contemplative, with Mary and Joseph regarding the exchange with expressions of introspective meditation. They are viewing a mute, symbolic declaration of spiritual love, expressed through the medium of corporeality, as flesh touches and stimulates the Beloved's flesh, to communicate the intensity of feelings inhabiting the soul. The solemn moment is given further weight by analogy of the extended, sleeping body of the infant Christ to the future image of his full-grown figure limply displayed in death, partially draped in a winding sheet. But in the painting's present moment of innocent sleep and its contemplation, the love that the Savior will eventually demonstrate through his death is now transmitted from John to his Redeemer.

This type of imagery was possible in a symbolic system that made a crucial distinction between love that begins in the noble attraction of incarnate beauty, evolving into a path toward the highest spiritual realms and the fleshly seduction that starts and ends in lust. Because the difference was so clear and differentiated within Renaissance cultural discourse, the distinction could on occasion be willfully blurred for dramatic or comic effect. Anton Francesco Grazzini achieved a virtuoso treatment of this distortion in his raucous hymn of praise for Donatello's *St. George*, by apostrophizing it as though the statue were a live youth, the poet's object of desire.[24] Grazzini begins by thanking God for finding this little fellow who grants him a life of serenity. He has no fear that the young man will haunt taverns or bordellos; and this Ganymede is out of harm's way in the matter of doctors of Greek and Latin, even though he is formed as perfectly as can be. Best of all, this San Giorgio will never grow old or get hairy:

> May Donatello always be blessed in the heavens, land, sky, water and fire for making a youth so fair. Who from day to day, growing ever so slightly, will not suddenly change in face or outfit, nor will a beard make him ungainly and worthless. I will not be forced every three or four years to find a new demigod.

In addition to the teasing animation and profanation of the figure, in the midst of jocularity Grazzini makes a reference to a philosophical idea that we have explored in a more serious way, the function of looking as a conduit to loving:

> Now, certain fools could say to me that they are of another opinion from mine; that I am speaking childishly, because the sweet pleasure of love consists solely in touching; and they don't take seeing seriously.
>
> Such people can be called beasts, as philosophy states so well; but I don't want to go down that path. It is enough for me that my desire is contented in seeing; nor do I yearn for more. And then everyone follows his own fantasy.

Renaissance culture, in both its solemn and playful manifestations, put prime significance on the sense of sight. Human vision was ennobled by the ability to apprehend beauty, both as visceral pleasure and as a bridge to exalted levels of spiritual contemplation, which were the paths that humanity could take in pursuing the quest for divine perfection. The easy movement from physical beauty to sexual seduction was accepted as part of earthly experience and not only as a means of imagining the splendor of the realm beyond the earthbound, but as a path of movement toward transcendence of it. Given the popularity of art that took this tactic and for all of the theological legitimization that sustained it, there were always some who were uncomfortable with the strategy.

As cultural values changed along with the religious reform movements, isolated dissent swelled into systematic denunciation; what had been mainstream consensus became a contested current. The battle around the censorship of art focused on the representation of the eroticized body, and for a compelling reason. Art that uses sexual imagery to construct and convey matters of consequence has undeniable immediacy. It is this very impact that will be maligned as destructive from a different point of view. The debate, which recurs throughout history, was engaged with particular intensity in the second half of the sixteenth century, one of the many cultural, religious, and social conflicts that so deeply marked the period.

Notes

Early formulations of this material were presented in talks given at the Center for Advanced Study in the Visual Arts and at Villa I Tatti, and I thank the directors of these institutions, Elizabeth Cropper and Joseph Connors. In the autumn of 2002 I was fortunate to have the enthusiastic reaction of Salvatore Camporeale to my thesis regarding carnality and spirituality. This essay is dedicated to his memory.

1 Giulio Romano to the officials of the Steccata in Parma in 1542, in Ferrari (1992), 977–78; my translation.
2 Stortoni (1997), 227.
3 L. Steinberg (1997).
4 Gilio (1961).
5 Symonds (1914).
6 Affò (1784), 71–73.
7 Ekserdjian (2006), 78.
8 Vasari (1996), 409, life of Fra Giovanni da Fiesole.
9 Ristori (1986).
10 Caglioti (2000).
11 Andersson (2008), 128.
12 Nagel (2000), 17.
13 Alberti (1991), bk. II, ch. 40, 75.
14 Vasari is quoted in Wohl (1999), 75. I am indebted to his chapter 2 for furthering my own ideas about *ornato*.
15 Wohl (1999), 67.
16 Camille (1992).
17 Camille (1992), 43.
18 Knowles (1831), 2: 235.
19 Condivi (1976), 48.
20 Dempsey (2000).
21 However, see Hub (2005), 103–30, for an interpretation of the theme in a Neoplatonic key.
22 Bloch and Bloch (1998), 137.
23 The following discussion of the kiss in Roman Catholic liturgy is based on Perella (1969).
24 Grazzini (1882), 526–29; my translation.

HOW WORDS CONTROL IMAGES

THE RHETORIC OF DECORUM IN COUNTER-REFORMATION ITALY

Robert W. Gaston

WRITING A HISTORY of decorum's role in the visual arts of sixteenth-century Europe should first require reflection on our own attitudes to this significant critical category. Decorum is not a suprahistorical concept that persists unchanged in the Western tradition. Contemporary notions of decorum form a dense semantic field that varies considerably in its inflections of meaning in diverse cultures. In considering decorum's role in contemporary art history, we may begin from the fact that the freedom of artists to represent whatever they saw fit had become dogma enshrined in late-twentieth-century art theory. Modernism had been concerned with the decorum of the representable, challenging the sacrosanctity of the art object and its depicted subject, as those phenomena had been defined by the humanistic art tradition. The art history industry of the twentieth century that historicized modernism did, however, control the limits of that movement's transgressions in sexual representation, through censorious selection of what was judged suitable for exhibition, lest certain works detract from the art-loving public's almost religious reverence towards the artists.

Postmodernism's response to the decorum of both the old master tradition and modernism has occurred in performance and body art. These art practices seek to fascinate, disgust, sexually excite, or confuse the onlooker in order to force an "interrogation" of what art is, or should be, all this taking place within the gaze of an audience whose presence makes the work or event "real."[1] Performance art shatters the limits of humanistic artistic decorum, in which the decorously arranged nude (e.g., not showing detailed genitals or excessive body hair) is iconic. Yet performance or body art's antidecorum remains a normative system of appropriateness, in which savvy audiences usually play by the rules in touching by invitation and observing artists' bodies, despite the occasional life-threatening audience intervention.[2] In current mainstream art theory, no one believes that government or arts-committee censorship, or even self-censorship by the visual artist, could be justified.[3] Nor does this theory give credence to what a society in general might regard as "suitable" for viewing. Such a criterion (what is considered decorous by "men and common opinion") featured in Lorenzo Valla's definition of decorum in his humanist lexicon, *Elegantiae* (1444).[4] But in our world, where an artist like Joel Peter Witkin can employ parts of corpses to reconstitute and satirize Christian iconography, a concept like decorum seems an outmoded category, a historical relic, despite its subtle omnipresence in the norms and precepts of the actual practice of art.[5] Yet without decorum's lingering presence as the polarized anchor for parody, postmodern art would make little sense.

Approaches to decorum in modern art historical literature have tended to be conservative and repressive.[6] By understating the transgressive potential of censored and uncensored imagery through an agreed-upon system of euphemisms and by masking the tacit moral consensus until recently exercised within the discipline, the literature on artistic decorum has served to perpetuate repression. In linking Renaissance decorum theory directly to the classical tradition of rhetoric, which was apotheosized by humanism and subsequently incorporated into Western notions of civilized behaviour, modern art history has until lately projected the narrow conviction that judicious choice of genre and consistency within its limits is what decorum is really about.

The most influential early-twentieth-century text was Julius von Schlosser's *Die Kunstliteratur* (1924). Schlosser shrewdly regarded Renaissance decorum as a curious "mixture" of ideas, arising initially from ancient rhetoric but recontextualized in the utterly different cultural ethos of the Italian Renaissance.[7] Schlosser was patently hostile to the concept of artistic decorum itself, to "the tyrant of Renaissance aesthetics" as he called it. He valued Leonardo's *cognizioni pratiche* on the indecorousness of some Quattrocento religious images, contrasting these comments with the "grey theory" of Alberti, which his own famous department had published in a critical edition. Schlosser saw Horace's *Ars poetica* as the "bible" of the decorum theorists, drawing (lesser, mannerist) artists and theorists inexorably towards Gian Paolo Lomazzo's *Trattato dell'arte* of 1584, whose decorous recommended figures, he said, "recall the rigid masks of the *commedia dell'arte*" – despite the fact that Lomazzo's descriptions of movements (*i moti*) of the body in erotic excitation and pain constitute a unique corpus of a practitioner's observations. Behind Schlosser's negative appreciation of decorum lay his friend Benedetto Croce's conviction, voiced in his *Aesthetic* of 1908, that the "doctrine of the sympathetic" engendered pseudo-aesthetic appraisive concepts such as the "dignified" and the "decorous," ideas that in his view belonged to a traditional "pedagogic or moralistic-utilitarian" approach to art, to a "capricious metaphysical and mystical aesthetic." For Croce, the "true artist's" selection of theme could not be blamed, only "the manner in which the artist treated it."[8]

Anthony Blunt's *Artistic Theory in Italy, 1450–1600* (1940) ransacked Schlosser's book and adopted his hostility to Alberti's theorizing, as well as his affection for Leonardo's practical gleanings on decorum. Blunt's strongest contempt, doubtless engendered in the disdain of the Cambridge "Apostles" for Western humanism in the 1930s, was reserved for Giovanni Paolo Lomazzo's *Trattato* (1584) and Giovanni Battista Armenini's *De' veri precetti della pittura* (1586), which, he said, "devote their attention to the minutiae" of the artist's training: the artist must now learn "by absolute rules."[9] Rensselaer W. Lee's more important study, *Ut Pictura Poesis*, published as an article in the same year as Blunt's book, also tied Renaissance artistic decorum to the doctrine of Horace's *Ars poetica*, and in a critically pejorative manner:

> [F]rom Horace ... came those ideas of decorum that fill *many a dreary page* of sixteenth and seventeenth century criticism and were, at least in part, responsible for the artificial and formulated expression of a Lebrun.[10]

Lee's restriction of decorum terminology to *convenevolezza* and *decoro* – using Lodovico Dolce's *Aretino* (1557), Bernardino Daniello's *La Poetica* (1536), and Leonardo's notebooks – was calculated to establish the primacy of his Horatian reading.[11] Lee expressed surprise at "the empirical" Leonardo's summation of a decorum theory like Alberti's, given his "eager interest in the infinite variety of nature, but really because "the concept of decorum ... was not one to encourage artistic originality."[12] Lee viewed the Cinquecento critics as having a pernicious influence on the development of the visual arts:

> [T]hey were enjoining ... [artists] to follow the typical formalized, reduced to static and convenient patterns that a person of good taste and good sense (*he need possess no great imagination*) would accept as appropriate symbols for the actions and emotions of people of such and such an age, sex, profession, situation in life, or whatever it might be.[13]

Lee was aware that the notion of "specific conformity to what is decent and proper in taste, and even more in morality and religion" was "not so specifically defined by Horace." But for Lee, the critics Dolce and Gilio da Fabriano exhibited a "severity of judgement," "in keeping with the spirit of the age," in condemning "in the name of Horatian decorum" works of the "heroic artist" Michelangelo. Lee considered justified the distaste of these critics for the mannerist figure style and praised Gilio, despite his "theological pedantry" and "painful misunderstanding of the grandeur of Michelangelo's profoundly personal interpretation" of the *Last Judgment*, for identifying the mannerists' "unseemly" representation of the body.[14] Like Heinrich Wölfflin and several other scholars of mannerism after him, Lee preferred the High Renaissance with its "blameless" Michelangelo (to use Wölfflin's term), or even the baroque, as providing "more adequate forms of expression" than those offered by the mannerists.[15]

Lee's distaste for Lomazzo and similar gatherers of decorous examples "piled up from books"[16] was actually a disparagement of less "worthy" categories of knowledge. This critical disdain for the treatises that followed the Council of Trent's decree on images of 1563 arose from the conviction that "the clerical culture of late-Cinquecento Italy was perversely intrusive and intellectually inferior."[17] Lee referred to a "temporary impoverishment of humanistic values that accompanied the breakdown of the Classical Renaissance in the sixteenth century, and the policy of the Church to press the arts into the service of morality and Christian dogma."[18] Yet not everyone shared Lee's negative view of decorum as a critical category. Rosemond Tuve warned in 1947 that "post-Romantic and modern criticism has tended ... to consider decorum as a matter of barren rule." She understood, correctly, I believe, that "propriety or decorum was the basic [critical] criterion in terms of which all the others were understood." A scholar of English Renaissance literature, she knew that "the grounds for Elizabethan insistence upon decorum" were not "a certain reverence for poetic etiquette, trivially defined, and for 'literary' diction, in and of itself.[19]

E. H. Gombrich's account of decorum in his *Symbolic Images* (1972) propagated the "decorous" view of the concept.[20] Gombrich argued that the genre of Renaissance representational programs "was based on certain conventions ... closely rooted in the respect of the Renaissance for the canonic texts of religion and of antiquity." The art historian must have a "feeling for the kind of programme" that a patron "was likely to impose on an artist," for "what is or is not possible within a given period or milieu." The notion of decorum afforded "the principles by which these subjects were to be used in given contexts." Gombrich noted that Lomazzo "has a list of suggestions for various types of places" and "an even longer list of Biblical and ancient subjects for court buildings ... palaces ... fountains and gardens." While Gombrich hinted that we were "lucky" that such principles had been articulated, in fact he had an aversion to textbooks on how to do art history, and one senses his discomfort, as a student of Schlosser, with Lomazzo's prescriptions for artists.[21] For an artist and patron, Gombrich advised, decorum was a straightforward matter: "a simple principle of selection which is easy to discern." This was "the principle of intersection" between a subject and a context. This might be given "even richer interaction" by choosing a subject that contained " a moral lesson," but this would remain essentially simple. To this structure Gombrich added "the predilections and aptitudes of the artists concerned." Gombrich's account exhibits the rational historicity that he prized in researching Renaissance culture. It also deliberately understates how close to the borderlines of the transgressive some Italian artists from the mid-Quattrocento onwards operated in their religious images, where vividly depicted bodies interacted provocatively with viewers in their gazing and among themselves in touching and self-display. Artists themselves pushed the limits, and their patrons, both secular and ecclesiastical, seem not to have discouraged them, at least until Savonarola and later the critics of Michelangelo made their presence felt.

Phillip Fehl's learned collection, *Decorum and Wit* (1992), was symptomatic – in its avoidance of defining decorum in an art historian's book about decorum – of an assumed, discipline-specific understanding of the phenomenon and its functions within works of artistic genius.[22] Fehl's key decorum term was "dignity," one that Croce had identified as belonging to decorum's semantic field. However, given dignity's linguistic severance in English from its original Latin connection (as *dignitas*) with *decus*, *decor*, and *decens*, it could easily be reclassified as an aesthetic term floating free of its implications of fitness. The dignity of the "great" artist and the dignity of his "treatment" of pictorial subjects are topics with powerful, almost mystical resonances for readers in the old master tradition of art historical scholarship.[23]

The research into "manners," "courtesy," "politeness," "deportment," and "ceremony" that followed the English translation (1978–82) of Norbert Elias's *Über den Prozess der Zivilisation* (1939) has, with its Foucaultian glossing, deepened suspicion against "polite" discourse of any kind. Elias's *The Court Society* (1983) intensified English-language use of the term "etiquette" – for Elias the means by which court society represents itself to itself, but in common English parlance, trivial social rules – to cover the entire range of discourses and practices associated with decorum and politeness.[24] And scholars stimulated by an abundance of decorum terms in Elizabethan rhetorical treatises have lately investigated how texts of classical and medieval rhetoric were adapted to the needs of English readers. George Puttenham's words, "decency," "discretion," "seemliness," "comeliness," "agreeableness," and so on, are recontextualized synonyms for Cicero's two kinds of decorum: the social and (what we would call) the aesthetic.[25]

These profitable inquiries have led to a reassessment of decorum's role. As Richard Lanham shrewdly commented in 1991:

> From the perspective of postmodern thought, one can ... see more clearly that decorum is a *creative* as well as a *pious* concept, that it *creates* the social reality which it reflects. Decorum ... amounts to a pious fraud, the "social trick" par excellence. We create, with maximum self-consciousness and according to precise rules, an intricate structure of stylistic forces balanced carefully as to perceiver and perceived, and then agree to forget that we have created it and to pretend that it is nature itself we are engaging with. Rhetorical theory has spent endless time discussing how to adjust utterance to this pre-existent social reality without reflecting on how that reality has been *constituted* by the idea of decorum.[26]

In keeping with Lanham's idea but tacitly drawing on Foucault's analysis of "representing," Robert Williams's *Art, Theory, and Culture in*

Sixteenth-Century Italy (1997) takes decorum in the visual arts into questions of political power, aesthetic representation, and the cultural ideology of humanism. Perhaps Williams's most important observation on decorum is that it was "both restricting and empowering":

> We tend to think of decorum as the means by which the imagination of artists and viewers was controlled, "disciplined," accommodated to contingency – especially the arbitrary order of the political and social world – yet it was also the means by which that contingency was given the appearance of ideal order: It represents the projection of an artistic principle into the world beyond art.... Though decorum is a means of bringing the order of the illusion into line with the order of the world, and thus makes art reaffirm that order, it also reconfigures the world by grounding that order in representation: It thus offers, however tenuously, the possibility of reconstituting the order of things according to the demands of the imagination.[27]

This reading of decorum's ordered empowering of representation is, however, grounded on the assumption that the concept had been fully developed "in ancient rhetorical theory," meaning chiefly that of Aristotle and Cicero.[28] In fact, ancient decorum theory was both a body of technical definitions of numerous cognate terms in rhetoric manuals and a source for practical applications in Greek and Latin texts from the sixth century B.C. into late antiquity. Even the most familiar of the ancient concepts, *to prepon* and *decorum*, have a "supple and dynamic character" and are antithetical to "a doctrine of uniformity and repetition."[29] That decorum terms could adopt different cultural significations in rhetorical topics is also made clear in fifteenth- and sixteenth-century texts that adapt for new uses the authoritative texts from Graeco-Roman antiquity, from early Christianity, and from medieval philosophy, theology, and canon law.

In Lorenzo Valla's *Elegantiae* we encounter a smooth interchangeability of words, a semantic consistency. For Valla, using solely Roman rhetorical sources to define *decor* is to identify "a kind of *pulchritudo* [beauty] derived from the *decentia* of things and persons to both place and time, whether in action or speech."[30] Bartolomeo Fazio, however, chose to limit the meaning of *decens* to "the gait and posture of the body,"[31] suggesting that he was drawing meaning from the medieval ecclesiastical textual tradition on deportment. Valla's "linguistic empiricism"[32] marks his analytical approach, but it is one still rooted in classical examples. Michael Baxandall noted that the Italian humanists had to deal with classical and medieval Latin, and with Trecento and Quattrocento Italian, but their "classicism committed them to a thorough purge" of "the debased vocabulary of medieval Latin."[33] When, however, Valla turns to another word within decorum's lexical range, the impersonal verb *convenit*[34] (it befits, it is fitting), while he cites examples from classical Latin,[35] he suppresses something he must have known: that *convenit, conveniens est,* and *non conveniens est* had been terms of judgment applied for centuries in Scholastic logic and that the Italian verb *convenire* had, since the thirteenth century, played a significant role in the poetic and prose discourses of the *volgare.* The cultural cogency of phrases like *mi conviene, ti conviene,* and *quello che conviene* has remained largely unnoticed – as a consequence of their being treated as rhetorical flourishes, as nonsubstantive elements of the discourse.[36]

Just as St. Ambrose adapted the decorum stream in Cicero's *De officiis* from its original context in the Roman aristocracy's *mos maiorum* into a guide suitable for the Christian clergy in his own *De officiis ministrorum,*[37] so early-sixteenth-century scholars repositioned the language of decorum for their own polemical and educational purposes. An instructive example occurs in John Colet's *Commentary on First Corinthians,* chapter 11, in which the English exegete (1467–1519) brilliantly deconstructs St. Paul's rhetorical craft for his Oxford audience by using arguments from fitness drawn from both Ciceronian and medieval rhetorical traditions. Colet opens with an axiomatic preamble lifted from the medieval papal chancery's tradition of using decorum concepts to empower arguments ("In Christ's Church it is most especially fitting [*maxime convenit*], and ought, surely, to be kept as an established and fixed custom, that disciples should obey their teachers ... without dispute. For otherwise order will be upset, and ugly deformity will show itself"). Colet then uses Cicero's (and most likely also Ambrose's) decorum terms (*quod decuit, quod decet, decere,* and the *honestas–decorum* coupling) to show how Paul "circuitously" and "in cryptic manner" persuades Corinthian women to cover their hair by treating the matter "from the standpoint of propriety [*honestas*] and fittingness [*decorum*] in dress." For Colet the veil is thus the sign (*signum*) of woman's fitting subjection. Colet's disclosure of Paul's epistolary rhetoric in the deliberative rhetoric of his own lecture is indicative, in its subtle melding of Scholastic and classical argumentative techniques focusing on decorum, a pragmatic new rhetoric that Reformers would use in treating the issue of religious images.

When the German theologian Hieronymus Emser wrote supporting images in churches in 1522 in answer to Andreas Karlstadt's treatise of 1520 calling for the removal of such *Bylder,* he appealed to St. Paul's urging Christians to adhere to the "regulations and laws you have been taught" (in 2 Thess. 2:15, 3:6), saying:

> Therefore, no man should scorn Christian law, for all the succeeding popes, bishops, prelates and, above all, the Christian councils have for all time the self same power and authority to decree and establish *what is appropriate, useful, and pious* for Christendom that Peter and Paul and the others enjoyed.[38]

Emser's grouping of "appropriate, useful, and pious" was a variant of a triadic conceptual linkage that surfaces amidst Paul's injunctions against knowingly eating idol meat in 1 Corinthians 10:23: "All things are lawful [*exestin*] for me, but all things are not expedient [*sumpherei*]: all things are lawful, but all things edify [*oikodemei*] not." The Vulgate transposed Paul's sense as follows: "omnia mihi licent, sed non omnia expediunt; omnia mihi licent, sed non omnia aedificant."[39] For Cicero *licere* meant both what was allowed by law (*lex*) and what was in accord with Roman moral codes, but he leaned towards the good citizen having regard for what is becoming (*quid deceat vos*), rather than for how much is legally permitted (*non quantum liceat vobis*).[40] The contrasted pairing of *licere–decere*, which Quintilian also acknowledges in his handbook on rhetoric, is paralleled by the pairing of *licere–expedire*: what is not expedient (*expedit*) in the courts is not permitted (*liceat*) in the schools of rhetoric; and the orator must keep in mind what is becoming (*quid deceat*) and what is useful or profitable (*quid expediat*).[41] In Emser we perhaps see his reading of Paul through the lens of Quintlian's rhetoric and, as his learned editors note, his application of the belief "that the tradition and the authority of the Church have a relevance equal to that of Scripture, a principle defended vigorously by the sixteenth-century Church in answer to the *sola scriptura* of the Reformers."[42]

The Paduan-trained German Protestant theologian Thomas Gechauff (Venatorius) published his *De Virtute Christiana* at Nuremberg in 1529, including a chapter titled "De Honesto & Decoro Christianorum." Gechauff was mesmerized by the logical sequence linking the terms *rectum*, *honestum*, and *decorum* that derives from Graeco-Roman Stoic thought and is transmitted to the European Renaissance through Paul, Ambrose, and Scholastic theologians.[43] If what is "right" is also "honourable" and therefore also "fitting" in the eyes of the world, then the theologian must turn to Christ's and Paul's teachings (as developed by Ambrose and the Scholastics) positing an interior and an exterior decorum. Gechauff argues that both are necessary for the virtuous Christian, who as in Paul's world should live a quiet, charitable, and inconspicuous life, but the interior decorum exemplified in Christ's own life ought to be rated above that of the "lovers of mere external decorum [*solum externum illud decorum amantes*]."

These exegetic, theological, and rhetorical considerations, and not just the texts of Aristotle, Cicero, and Horace, underpin much of what is written about the decorum of images in the sixteenth-century debates. A scholar with phenomenal linguistic range like Erasmus offers an impressive variety of decorum terms applied in many branches of learning. For Erasmus, decorum concepts used in rhetoric must have a linguistic appropriateness to topic and context. But he notices that what is judged appropriate in cultures consists of elements both "natural" and "conventional."[44] His critique of religious images in his *Enchiridion* (1503), and of all "exterior" religious practices that he subordinates to his interiorized model, is tempered by the pragmatic conviction that "it is not fitting even for adults in the faith to disdain them [likenesses of Christ and certain ceremonies], lest they injure the weak by their example."[45] In his *Ecclesiastes* (1535), his manual of Christian rhetoric,[46] *comparanda* from the visual arts, emphasizing their power to move and to instruct – texts in rhetorical handbooks from Cicero onwards – are glossed with excerpts from the patristic sermon corpus, so as to magnify the persuasive power of the visual over the aural.[47] But the authority of Scripture is never really under threat in these moments of comparative rhetorical generosity. Erasmus counsels that decorum must be exercised in moving the spirit with images, and while allowing that the *rhetor* has affinities with the painter, he chastises unskilled painters for breaching decorum in matters of historical fact and behaviour of persons (*rebus ac personis*).[48] And he implies that there is a level of superior pictorial skill in making sacred art that can remain beyond censure: the greatest artists are self-regulating.

While the Catholic supporters of religious images in Germany in the 1520s attacked images they regarded as sexually stimulating, as scholars have noted, "this was never an important issue for the Reformers," who were preoccupied with scriptural, theological, and philosophical grounds for opposing images.[49] When in 1553, while the Council of Trent was in suspension, Luigi Lippomano, the Reformist bishop of Verona, published a vernacular handbook seeking to "stabilize" Catholic teachings for the laity, he blamed the *libertà dei pittori* for introducing into churches images that "incite vanity and sexual desire, rather than forms of piety or religion."[50] Lippomano, with his Oratorian background, linked *pitture lascive* and *sculture dishoneste* with other abuses in churches, such as polyphonic singing, organ music, secular and love songs, inappropriately dressed women, and sloppy liturgical performance, indicating that he held the clergy partly responsible for what artists depicted in sacred places.[51] Giuseppe Scavizzi has shown that Catholic theologians had gathered to discuss the veneration of images in Rome as early as 1522 and that their treatises were riddled with contradictions. It was by no means clear in the 1550s that Trent could produce a coherent position, and was still uncertain in 1563. Scavizzi observes that the patristic, Byzantine, and Scholastic arguments adopted in various combinations by the Catholics made resolution difficult, while they sought to maintain the "sacred quality" of images against iconoclasm.[52]

For the Italian clergy whose churches had been filled with altarpieces and frescoes by mannerist artists working with the largely nude body types propagated by Michelangelo and Raphael's workshop, the image question threw into relief particular aspects of visual decorum. Some clerical critics were familiar with humanist artistic theory, stemming from Alberti's treatises on painting and architecture. Alberti's emphasis on narrative images that are *digna* (worthy, appropriate, decorous) may seem to arise directly from classical rhetorical handbooks. However, this language has as much to do with a "new" decorum theory that emerges in the late medieval Italian communes, in the papal and episcopal chanceries, and in the linguistic practices of the authors who create their literature in the *volgare*, to which Dante, significantly, grants its own *dignitas*.[53] Important in our present discussion is that Alberti's *De Pictura* sought to suppress the bodily, earthy, sexual dimensions of the painter's craft in a way that predetermined a repressive discourse about the nature of painting for the entire humanistic art tradition.[54]

Let us return momentarily to an issue raised by Lee's analysis of Renaissance decorum. What Lee craved from the Cinquecento critics was "[the] consistent attempt of aesthetic criticism to discover relationships of form between the sister arts."[55] Today, however, we should be sceptical about the perceived benefits of the sister-arts trope and conscious of the manipulative rhetoric of ekphrasis, as well as the hierarchical power relations between artists and writers during the Renaissance. Unreflective use of the trope fails to unmask the strategies of humanist scholars in making their rhetorical topic the visual skills of artists. We should substitute an "agonistic" model that acknowledges the intense competitiveness between verbal and visual representation, and the almost universal belief in the theoretical superiority of the literary arts in early modern Europe.[56] We remain vulnerable to the sister-arts trope because modern art historical ekphrasis, with its exacting stylistic description and minutely descriptive iconographic analysis in the present tense, transposes the visually represented narrative into the reader's present experience. This epideictic rhetoric crafted from aestheticized description defines with *auctoritas* the limits of the expressive (or inexpressive) behaviour of the image's protagonists. Its ekphrastic decorum seeks to reconstitute the work of art textually within the discipline's decorous descriptive limits.

Vasari's enticing ekphrasis in his *Lives* still exercises decorous authority, having the additional persuasiveness of being set within seductive biographical tropes. While there are passing hints in Vasari that artists experienced real bodily desires, the sexual activities of artists, now becoming known from criminal records, were strictly minimized.[57] Vasari's defence of artists in his 1550 edition against the viewer ignorantly interpreting the beauty of saints in images as lascivious projections upon appropriately represented subjects has an escape clause in the post-Trent 1568 edition: "However I would not have any believe that I approve of those figures that are painted in churches in a state of almost complete nudity, for in these cases it is seen that the painter has not shown the consideration that was due to the place."[58] But Vasari did not revise his judgment of religious pictures he had earlier praised. And in his system of decorum Michelangelo, the "divine" genius, could operate outside of the rules of art established by lesser artists.[59] Lodovico Dolce, writing in Venice in 1557 on Michelangelo's *Last Judgment* figures, which in his speaker Pietro Aretino's view "display their backs and fronts in an immodest way," still ("with all due respect") regards them as "unworthy" [*indegna*] of this *santissimo luogo*.[60]

Dolce balances Michelangelo's licence to possess "a freedom which one would not concede to anyone else at all" against the writer's "freedom to speak the truth." Dolce would allow artists to produce classicizing erotica, or even pornography such as Giulio Romano invented for *I Modi*, so long as such images were kept out of public squares and churches.[61] But I cannot believe that Dolce would be unaware of the moral categories of a local Catholic Reformer like Lippomano or of the critiques by members of the Roman Curia in the 1540s of the *Last Judgment*.[62] While Dolce's decorum terminology remains predominantly that of Italian vernacular humanism (*degno–indegno, convenevolezza–licenza, honestà–dishonestà*), his judgment that Michelangelo's nudes in the pope's chapel were to be considered *indegna* to the holiness of the place is very close in this awareness to the Dominican prelate Ambrogio Politi's ecclesiastical language of decorum on this issue, published at Venice in 1551 in his commentaries on St. Paul's Epistles.[63]

Let us now turn briefly to the Trent decree on images. As John O'Malley has noted, the late date in Council proceedings suggests that the matter was deemed of lesser importance than "doctrine" and even "discipline." He rightly states that "the decree turned out to be a balanced and concise summary of traditional thinking.... [It] defended images and their veneration" and urged bishops to "encourage placing images of Christ and the saints in churches as well as in other places." While the text "says nothing about images being aesthetically pleasing," it does warn against their representing false doctrine and being an occasion for superstitious practices and "anything lascivious." And O'Malley justly observes that while the decree "opened the door for bishops, inquisitors, and theologians after the council to move in to ensure that paintings were historically, doctrinally, and morally correct," it also left room for artists and their patrons to continue to adorn religious places with images.[64]

The Trent decree yields instructive information when approached through the diverse traditions of decorum terms.[65] Scavizzi states, in assessing the work of his predecessors, that the decree on images in fact first concerns itself with the invocation and veneration of saints and their relics.[66] But to be strictly precise, Session 25 begins with the decree on purgatory, allowing for *suffragia* for the dead, masses, prayers, almsgiving, and other works of piety to be practiced under the rules of canon law pertaining to testators of foundations. That is, Trent's ecclesiastical logic first perpetuates the legal basis for the liturgical practices associated with images connected with high altars and private chapels in churches and private dwellings. The chief purpose of those images was to facilitate communication with Christ and his saints through private prayer and liturgical observances, beliefs grounded in the doctrine of purgatory. It seems curious, though, that the decree's terminology gives decorum words such a minimal role. Moreover, Schroeder's now classic English translation interpolates decorum inflections to make its presence stronger, in a way that has suited art historians.

When Schroeder translates "such zeal and care should be exhibited by the bishops with regard to these things that nothing may appear that is disorderly [*inordinatum*] or unbecoming [*praepostere*]," he gives the latter term (which means in classical Latin "in a reversed order, distortedly, irregularly") an inference of fittingness that is not warranted.[67] Schroeder again interpolates decorum in translating "quasi festi dies honorem sanctorum per luxum ac *lasciviam* agantur" as "as if the festivals in honor of the saints are celebrated with revelry and *with no sense of decency*."[68]

Decorum's antithetical companion term in Cicero and Quintilian's rhetorical works, *inhonestum*, is used in the decree and, in being coupled with *profanum*, implies that the decorum of classical antiquity's represented body is presupposed. The decree's use of "Holiness becometh (*deceat*) the house of God," from Psalm 92, explicitly refers to what is fitting in a church, in the tradition of conciliar edicts on liturgical behaviour and of medieval rites for consecration of a church. But the sheer linguistic awkwardness evident in describing works of art that are "confusingly arranged" (*tumultuariae accommodatum*) shows the decree's authors struggling to meld a classical Latin decorum term, *accommodatum*, with one of Livy's favourite words for military confusion.[69] The *inordinatum–accommodatum* antithesis in the decree has overtones of classical rhetoric, but it is more likely received through Scholastic theology's adaptations to theories of ecclesiastical polity than flowing without mediation from classical rhetoric. In the 1563 decree we see the Catholic Church's new language of decorum, constructed by the bishops from bits and pieces of diverse traditions, just as Calvin's was using the medieval *Libri Carolini* for his novel purposes.[70]

We have known since Paolo Prodi's masterly survey of 1962 that the 1563 images decree was enforced only in certain Italian dioceses in the following fifty years, notably in Milan and Bologna.[71] But less attention has been paid to Jedin's review of Prodi, in which he traced adumbrations of the Trent decree in Catholic conciliar legislation of the previous century or so, thereby giving a more graduated perspective to the decree's emergence and, correctly, in my view, basing its rhetoric, at least in part, in ecclesiastical legal traditions.[72]

The first Italian publication after 1563 to address *sacre imagini* was Giovanni Andrea Gilio's 1564 dialogue on the "errors of painters regarding history." Paola Barocchi's republishing, in 1986, of this dialogue, together with the companion dialogue on the "letterato cortigiano" and Gilio's legal-antiquarian *discorso* on the terminology of inhabited places, effectively recontextualized the dialogue on images, challenging the proponents of a post-Tridentine decline in intellectual quality.[73] The dialogue genre appears to lock the discourse into humanist rhetoric, as does the emphasis on the classical and papal precedents cited for Cardinal Farnese's *magnificenza* in his architectural patronage.[74] But the dialogue is riven with discomfiture of the sort that Paul Grendler noticed among the midcentury *poligrafi*, who saw everywhere, like Gilio, "mendacious histories, ignorant poets, untrustworthy rhetoricians, and inept painters."[75] Yet Gilio is curiously comfortable with new discoveries. Those of Columbus and Magellan in cosmography are fascinatingly juxtaposed with the achievement of Michelangelo, who is said to have established the *forza* and *vaghezza* of art because he was not content with the *maniera del pingere* of the painters of his day.[76] In Gilio's work we see a cleric still deeply attracted to both humanist and Scholastic thought being forced to deal with a heritage of art and ecclesiastical patronage that suddenly appears less secure. It is therefore not surprising that the destabilizing case of Michelangelo comes to dominate Gilio's subsequent dialogue on sacred images.

Modern reactions to Gilio's critical intervention tells us as much about anticlericalism, allegiance to humanist art critical rhetoric, and the unbridled worship of Michelangelo as about Gilio's intellectual world. Gilio employs the adaptable dialogue genre but frames it with a pastoral poetic invention that presupposes a critique of pictorial verism as represented in poetic description. Roland Kanz interprets Gilio's critical linguistics as belonging to "die inquisitorische Sprachpraxis."[77] But this is not wholly convincing, given that Gilio is patently wrestling with classical, patristic, medieval, and humanistic discourses pertaining to sacred images. An art lover, who supported the Trent decree and witnessed his patrons grandly exploiting visual representation, Gilio was in a tricky position vis-à-vis decorum. Those patrons commissioned works that were inventive, but "regolato" in terms of Horace's decorum.[78] He rightly saw, however, that Michelangelo's works were both transgressive in essence and paradigmatic for lesser artists.[79] The patristic polarity between a sophisticated clergy, who understood why the unlettered faithful needed images but held deep reservations themselves, would just not work for Gilio, although Gabriele Paleotti did adopt that view two decades later.[80] Gilio instead struggled with the difficult argument that while Raphael and the "ingenious" Michelangelo had restored painting to its *vera imagine*, subsequently lost by ignorant painters, Michelangelo had nevertheless erred in certain respects in his late paintings. Preceding these two artists lay centuries of work by "noble and learned" artists who understood "proper and fitting decorum" (*il proprio e convenevole decoro*).[81] For Gilio, contemporary (mannerist) artists lack the requisite *avertenza*, a decorous prudence or accuracy in subject matter.[82]

Gilio's opinion that a ruthlessly historical depiction of the bodily damage inflicted in Christ's Passion and in martyrdoms would produce a "cosa nova e bella" seems absurd to those of us who, armed with hindsight, know that most Italian artists resisted trading selection of moment and beauty for ghastly historical verisimilitude.[83] Artists told Gilio that such images would be "against the decorum of art."[84] Gilio yearned for art's power to be harnessed to a newly conceived sacred history based on authentic sources.[85] For the modern secular critic this constitutes an unwarranted subjection of artistic freedom to Catholic ideology, despite the fact that Gilio was, with professional authority, commenting on perceived "abuses" in art designed for sacred places. His listing of "errors" in iconography, which for him detract from the *reverenza* believers should have for sacred images, is only with difficulty seen by the modern art historian as a component of a program of religious reform. And the term *reverenza* is scarcely recognizable today as one of the most evocative words from the semantic field of decorum in the Cinquecento.

The rhetorical comparison of image and book was fundamental to the Reformation and Counter-Reformation debates about the role of images. For modern art historians these issues can appear to be less challenging, given that the "power" of images (representation) has lately surfaced, along with an awareness of the affective responses of observers.[86] The equivalence in power (*potestas*) of poetic language and visual images was claimed disingenuously by Horace. But when the Belgian theologian Johannes Vermeulen (Molanus) opened chapter 2 of his "worthy" (*dignum*) *De Picturis et Imaginibus Sacris* of 1570 with Horace's *ut pictura poesis* idea, he grounded it in the Council of Trent's decree on images, using rhetorical comparison.[87] Just as obscene or heretical images should be prohibited by law, so should books of that sort.[88] What the Church tolerates in books, so should it tolerate in images.[89] And just as religious images and sculpture produced purely for profit should be removed by secular magistrates, so should the authors of lascivious and obscene books be punished by bishops.[90] Molanus used procedural argument from fitness to justify the chronological order of his discourse (*certo convenienter ordine preocedatur*), beginning with the *antiquitas* of image veneration.[91] He adopted the rhetorician's technique of applying what was "probable and fitting" (*probabiliter & convenienter*) in allowing artists to import appropriate narrative details into a sacred image that were absent in scriptural accounts.[92] But it is the embedding of the decorum terms in the persuasive rhetoric of *comparatio* that makes the play on polarizing *pictura* and *narratio* convincing for the reader.

The patterns of reception and redeployment of decorum terms in the image debate I have identified here could be fruitfully explored throughout many other treatises. Neither ecclesiastical history nor art history has yet deeply investigated how the decorum concepts encapsulated within the rhetorics of the debate have been made persuasive in their rhetorical applications in texts. My argument is that the decorum concepts – which are drawn from ancient, patristic, medieval, and early modern rhetorical traditions – disclose their cultural meanings to us only if they are taken as they appear on the page, in their rhetorical embeddedness. The sheer complexity of the language of decorum in the image debate is indeed daunting. But to acknowledge this difficulty is surely the first step towards a more profound comprehension of what the debate was really about.

Notes

1 See R. Schneider (1997); A. Jones (1998).
2 See Goldberg (1988), 165, on Marina Abramovic's *Rhythm O*, 1974: "[S]he permitted a room-full of spectators to abuse her at their will for six hours.... [A] loaded gun held to her head finally caused a fight between her tormentors, bringing the proceeding to an unnerving halt." Also see R. Schneider (1997); A. Jones (1998).
3 Cf. Coetzee (1996).
4 Baxandall (1971), 10. Baxandall omits Valla's "hominibus" ("to men") from the text he translates; cf. Valla (1540), 125–26.
5 See Celant (1995).
6 I include my own "Decorum," in *The Dictionary of Art*; see Gaston (1996). Some innovations appeared in Ames-Lewis and Bednarek (1992). Cf. also Horn-Oncken (1967); Mildner-Flesch (1983); Mildner (1994).
7 Schlosser (1956), 447–48.
8 Croce (1969), 51, 85–87; see also Lönne (2003). O'Malley (2000), 34–35, notes Croce's use of *Controriforma*, in his *Storia dell'età barocca in Italia* (1929), "to signify the decadence of Counter-Reformation culture and society."
9 Blunt (1978), 149.
10 I cite Lee (1967), 34; my emphasis in all quotations.
11 See Lee (1967), 35, n. 145. Cf. Haussherr (1984), 40, who assumes the concept came directly from "antike Literatur und Architekturtheorie."
12 Lee (1967), 37.
13 Lee (1967), 36.
14 Lee (1967), 40.
15 Wölfflin (1953), 202.
16 Lee (1967), 73.
17 Quoting Gaston (2003).
18 Lee (1967), 40.
19 Tuve (1947), 192, 193, 196.
20 Gombrich (1972), 7–11.
21 See Gaston (1998a).
22 Fehl (1992).
23 On *dignitas* see Hellegouarc'h (1963), 388–421.
24 Elias (1983), 100ff. The bibliography includes Javitch (1978); Greenblatt (1980); Knox (1991); Prodi and Penuti (1994); Arditi (1998).
25 Puttenham (1970), ch. 23, 261ff. There is a new critical edition: Puttenham (2007). See Attridge (1986); Rebhorn (2000).
26 Lanham (1991), 46.
27 Williams (1997), 17–18.
28 See Williams (1997), 85. On medieval *ordo* see Michaud-Quantin (1970), 85–103.
29 Mouchel (1990), 28.
30 Baxandall (1971), 10.
31 Baxandall (1971), 10, gives Fazio's text.
32 Fubini (1990), 66; see Mack (1993), 170, 174, 208, for decorum terms.
33 Baxandall (1971), 9, 13, 48.
34 Valla (1540), 125 r–v.
35 Cf. Lewis and Short (1969), 462–63.
36 Battaglia (1964), s.v. "conviene," 715–19, esp. sec. 17 at 718.
37 On Cicero see Pina Polo (2004).

38 Mangrum and Scavizzi (1998), 55, my emphasis.
39 For the early Latin Bible variants see Tischendorf (1872), 2: 518.
40 Cicero, *Philippic*, XIII, vi, 14.
41 Quintilian, *Inst. orat.*, II, xiii, 8; V, x, 40.
42 Mangrum and Scavizzi (1998), 55, n. 20.
43 Venatorius (1529), bk. I, ch. 17, 60v–63r.
44 On decorum terms see Chomarat (1981), 916, 1011.
45 *Enchiridion*, XIV, 5th Rule: Erasmus (1963), 114. See also Rummel (1995). On Erasmus's attitude to images see Eire (1986), 50.
46 Erasmus (1991); the best critical study remains O'Malley (1985).
47 Erasmus (1994), bk. III, 88.
48 Erasmus (1994), bk. III, 98.
49 See Mangrum and Scavizzi (1998), 93.
50 Lippomano (1553), 173v.
51 Lippomano (1553), 183r.
52 Scavizzi (1992), 63–70.
53 Dante (1968), 170–72.
54 Gaston (1995).
55 Lee (1967), 62.
56 For a critique of the "sister-arts" trope see Gaston (1998b); on ekphrasis, Gaston (1996–97); see also Cooper (1998).
57 See Rocke (1996); on Vasari's sexuality see Gaston (1995).
58 Blunt (1978), 125–26; cf. Nagel (2000), 192.
59 See also Kanz (2000).
60 Dolce (1969), 162–63.
61 Dolce (1969), 163–65.
62 De Maio (1978), 17–63. Cf. Pozzi (1967), 257, on Dolce's humanism.
63 De Maio (1978), 48, n. 15: "Nam haec membrorum nuditas indecentissime in aris et praecipuis Dei sacellis ubique conspicitur." The terms *decens* and *indecens* had clear liturgical applications in the traditions of conciliar edicts.
64 Quotations from O'Malley (2004a), 220–22.
65 I cite *Sacrosancti et Oecumenici Concilii Tridentini* (1824), 304–308.
66 Scavizzi (1992), 75.
67 *Canons and Decrees* (1978), 214–17; Lewis and Short (1969), 1426.
68 Schroeder's translation was disseminated in Klein and Zerner (1966), 119–22.
69 Lewis and Short (1969), 1913.
70 See Ugolnik (1989).
71 Prodi (1962).
72 Jedin (1963).
73 Gilio (1986); Barocchi's introductory essay is crucial.
74 See Cox (1992), 68.
75 *Dialogo ... De li parti morali appertenenti a' Letterati Cortigiani, & ad ogni altro gentil'huomo*, in Gilio (1986), 7v. Cf. Grendler (1969).
76 Gilio (1986), 31r.
77 Kanz (2000), 505.
78 Gilio (1986), 79v.
79 Gilio (1986), 116r.
80 See P. Jones (1995), 134.
81 Gilio (1986), pref., 69r.
82 Gilio (1986), 69v.

83 Gilio (1986), 87v.
84 Nagel (2000), 158.
85 Gilio (1986), 88v.
86 See D. Freedberg (1989), a pathbreaking study.
87 I cite Molanus (1570); see Hecht (1997), but also Herklotz (2000), 48–49.
88 Molanus (1570), pref., 15r.
89 Molanus (1570), ch. 21, 50r.
90 Molanus (1570), pref., 15r.
91 Molanus (1570), ch. 3, 19r.
92 Molanus (1570), ch. 13, 35v.

"LA CUSTODIA DEGLI OCCHI"

DISCIPLINING DESIRE IN POST-TRIDENTINE ITALIAN ART

Maria H. Loh

THIS ESSAY IS about blind spots, about looking beyond the usual frames of viewing, about the things we do not see, whether it is because our view of them has been blocked or because we simply fail to notice them at first. I begin, therefore, with two partial images. The first, a fractured part of a lost whole, is a small early-sixteenth-century oil painting in Vienna that depicts a cupid sitting by himself on the ledge of a low wall set in front of a stereotypically Venetian landscape (Illustration 12). The second, a reproduction of a lost whole, is a black and white photograph of a destroyed painting, an oil on copper attributed to Correggio, *Reclining Magdalene* (Illustration 13), formerly in Dresden.

The *Cupid* belonged to a larger painting with a reclining Venus. In the lower left corner of the reduced canvas, the remains of the missing figure's thigh can still be seen. The putative original would have resembled something like Titian's *Sleeping Venus*, whose cupid was overpainted by a nineteenth-century restorer.[1] The fragment would have easily slid into the corner of such a painting (Illustration 14). The *Reclining Magdalene*, in contrast, represents a different kind of loss. The scrutiny of the connoisseur's eye has simultaneously placed this image in the hand of Correggio and removed this specific body from his authorship. Attribution was already an issue in the seventeenth century, for as Filippo Baldinucci pointed out, collectors erroneously attributed the invention to Cristofano Allori because both he and his students painted the image "many, many times," suggesting an active interest in the theme on the part of early modern artists and collectors.[2] Other painters, like Domenico Fetti, were known to have copied it, too, while Sisto Badalocchio and Giovanni Lanfranco drew much inspiration from the *concetto*, and Annibale Carracci painted a similar picture also in oil on copper.[3] In the eighteenth century, Charles de Brosses saw the Correggio when it was still in Modena and described it as "the little Magdalene, as big as your hand, which is fixed onto the wall and hidden in a little cupboard, because it is eminently portable and

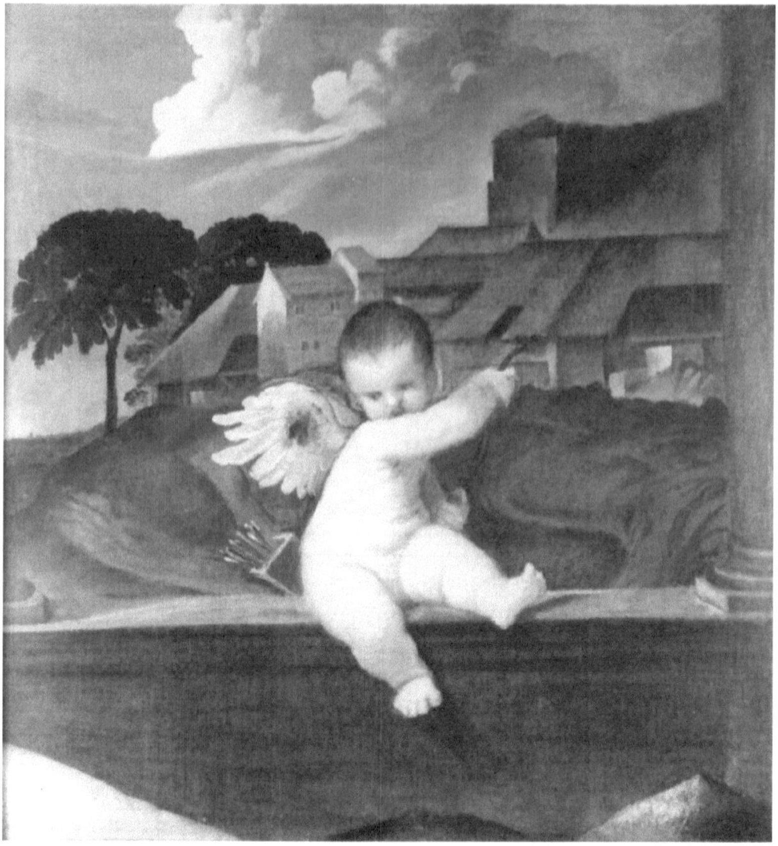

12. Workshop of Titian, *Cupid*. Oil on canvas, 76 × 74 cm. Vienna, Gemäldegalerie der Akademie der bildenden Künste (Inv. 466).

deliciously stealable."[4] Sometime in the middle of the twentieth century, the "deliciously stealable" painting disappeared from the Dresden Gemäldegalerie and is now known only through its reproductions.

Neither attribution nor iconography, however, is my focus. The lost images tell us a far more engaging story about the changing conditions of reception, about how works are transformed both physically and iconographically by altering perspectives, and about how artists shape and are shaped by these changes along the way. For instance, while the copy after Correggio in the Galleria Palatina in Florence is generally identified as one of Allori's "many, many copies" (Illustration 15), it differs from the supposed original inasmuch as Mary Magdalene's saintly attributes (skull, crucifix, and urn) are staged more prominently in the lower left corner. In Allori's post-Tridentine copy, clear and identifiable signs precluded the possibility of iconographical ambiguity, reflecting a shift in both artistic strategies and spectatorial expectations.[5] With the wave of moralizing treatises written after the closing of the Council of Trent in 1563, representations of the body increasingly came to be read as sites of contestation. The classical female nude, which had been acceptable before, suddenly posed new threats. The image that was previously read with pleasure became a source of anxiety. Paintings of female bodies, in particular, fell victim to censure within the new classificatory system that was shifting into the foreground, and it was stipulated in no uncertain terms that looking at indecent pictures of this kind could lead to the soul's ruin.

The Council of Trent was frustratingly terse on the question of images, relegating its comments to a subsection of the twenty-fifth and final session. In rather hackneyed terms glossed from a well-established early Christian discourse against iconoclasm, the Tridentine authorities defended the necessity of images as devotional aids for illiterate worshippers. Visual representation served as "salutary examples" that cultivated piety and that "excite [the viewer] to adore and love God."[6] The underlying concern of the Catholic Reformers, therefore, was to control the passions of the viewer so that their excitement would be directed towards spiritual rather than base desire.

In spite of the brevity of the Tridentine decree, it provided two conclusions that would be taken up by post-Tridentine authors. The first was a warning against idolatry and a stipulation that "superstition," "filthy lucre," and "all lasciviousness" were "to be avoided, in such ways that figures shall

13. Correggio, *Reclining Magdalene*. Oil on copper, 29 × 39.5 cm. Formerly Dresden, Staatliche Kunstsammlungen, Gemäldegalerie Alte Meister.

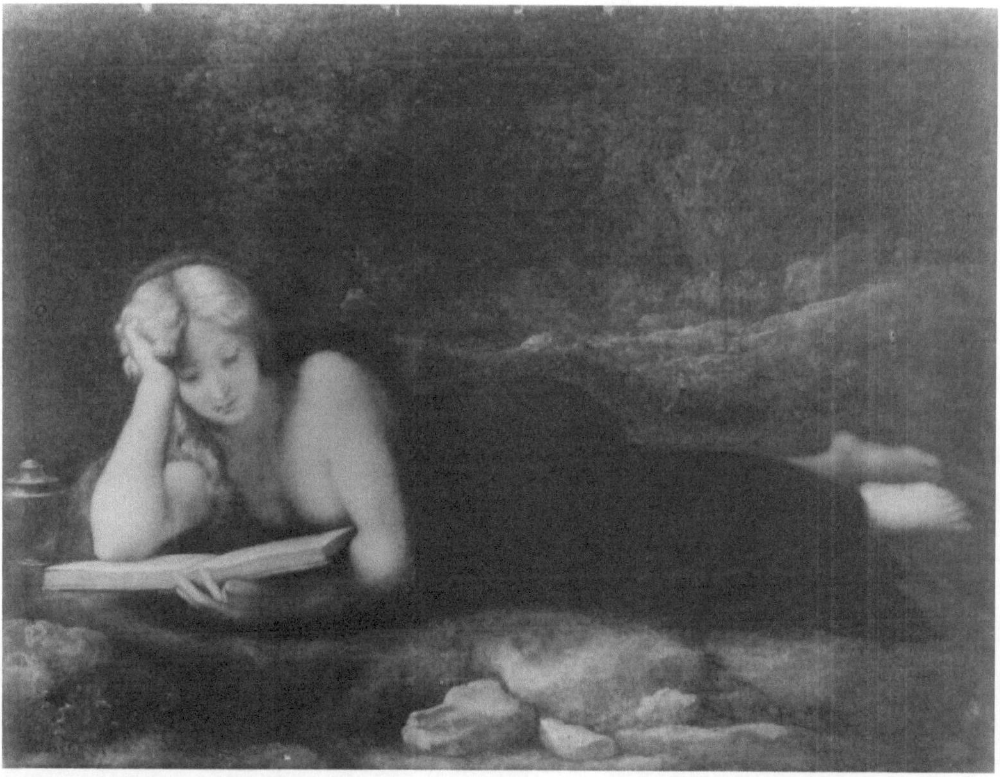

not be painted or adorned with a beauty exciting to lust."[7] The Council was cautious to underline that images in and of themselves were not considered dangerous; instead, the danger lay in the excitable eye of the weak beholder. A second a priori upheld the belief that the large majority of viewers were weak and imprudent: the "uneducated" and "unlettered," it was argued, were prone to error, seeing with the "eyes of the body" rather than those of the soul.[8]

In 1582 Gabriele Paleotti, for one, would identify four categories of spectators: painters (*pittori*), the educated (*letterati*), the uneducated (*idioti*), and Christians (*spirituali*).[9] The well-intentioned *spirituali* who applied "exterior things to interior things" always with the soul in mind were further contrasted with impious *sensuali*, who "embraced things in order to satisfy the senses."[10] However, the majority, Paleotti concluded, were *idioti*, and it was to the needs of this naive, fallible majority that devout artists were expected to address themselves.[11] Good discipline in the ranks of the empowered minority would ultimately facilitate the moral education of the disenfranchised mob.

The *Cupid* and the *Reclining Magdalene* embody two strategies in the reformation of the disobedient gaze of the *idioti*: the first through blockage and physical alteration – blinding the eye from what it should not see; the second (and more interesting approach) through allegory and

14. Author's reconstruction of Illustration 12.

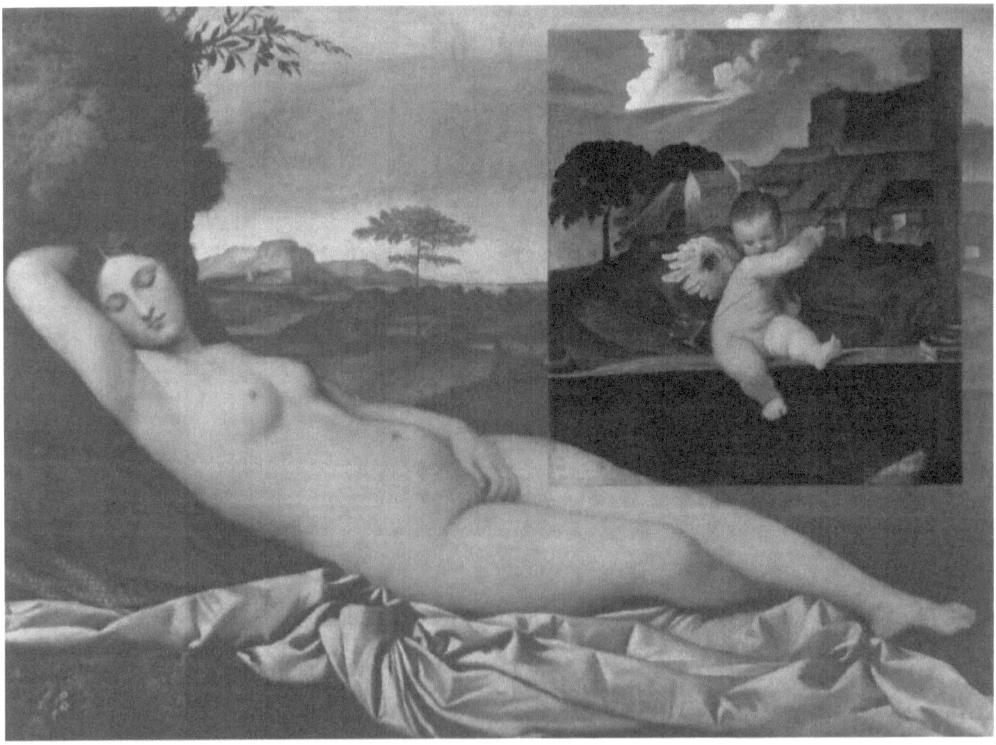

conceptual alteration – educating the viewer to see beyond the physical evidence before his or her eyes. The physical alteration of paintings was a common, though often irreversible, solution in the campaign to reform the spectator's behavioural patterns. In one episode recorded in Giovan Domenico Ottonelli and Pietro Berrettini da Cortona's art treatise, we read of Cardinal Berlingerio Gessi's "painting of a lascivious Venus with a Cupid in the guise of a graceful child, a most excellent work by the famous Titian," which nevertheless "excited immodest thoughts amongst those that saw it."[12] As a result, the cardinal had the figure of Venus removed and kept the cupid. Without necessarily attributing the *Cupid* in Vienna with Gessi's Titian, this anecdote gives us a very good idea of how the larger picture slipped out of sight for subsequent viewers.

In retrospect, despite the physical obliteration of the Venus, the vestiges of the Titianesque *Cupid* can be interpreted as both a successful and an unsuccessful act of iconoclastic censorship: successful because it resulted in the permanent destruction of the work of art as it was originally designed and because the offending body was removed; unsuccessful because the missing Venus had not been completely eradicated and because the presence of the cupid inescapably implied the Venus. Different versions, replicas, and copies of such images were so ubiquitous in the sixteenth century that it would have been virtually impossible not to envision the Venus that was so violently amputated from the

15. Cristofano Allori, *Penitent Magdalene*. Oil on copper, 29.6 × 43 cm. Florence, Galleria Palatina.

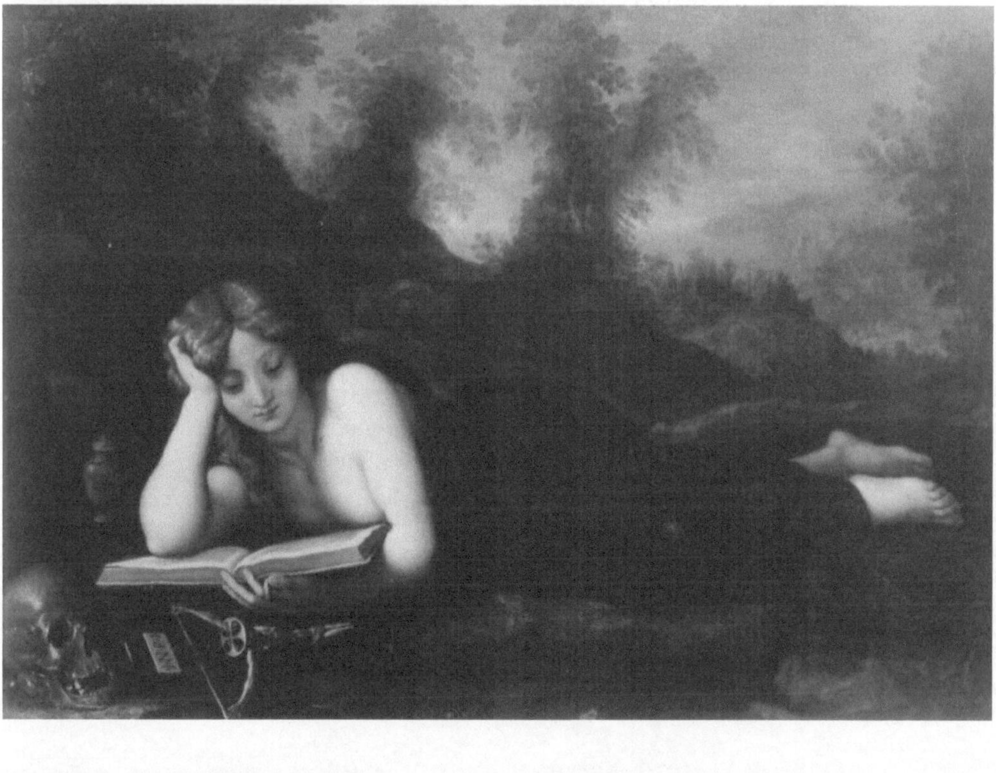

canvas. The *Cupid* operated, in this sense, like a relic: it was physically part of a lost original artefact; moreover, it stood in a metonymic relationship to the larger conceptual entity from which it was extracted. Absence was in the end another form of presence, and it would have been hard for the viewer to resist filling in the obvious blank.

Wandering intentions posed a problem in the push towards iconographic clarity and fixity in early modern Italy. The Counter-Reformation, as many historians have pointed out, was the age of the confessional and a period of intensified social disciplining.[13] Rather than fetishizing the forbidden object, the subject was instructed to look upon the abject object as an external agent that could only cause harm to the undisciplined spectator; it was not things, but the self, that required reform. In other words, rather than simply destroying false idols through iconoclasm, one aspect of the Catholic response was to define and demonize certain types of artworks as intolerable to the virtuous Christian viewer – to co-opt desire and convert representation and eroticism to virtuous ends. It was precisely the disciplining of the peripatetic and overcompensatory imagination to which Counter-Reformatory authors would devote so much energy. Instead of stimulating lascivious thoughts, painting, it was dictated, should provide a blueprint for a "well-disciplined life."[14] The diverse strategies of hermeneutic containment that move from the *blinding* of eros to the *conversion* of eros encouraged the spectator to become his or her own primary censor as well as the censor of others, establishing a society of self-surveillance that governed itself from within. Yet artists and collectors were not completely constituted by the social structures that sought to control them, and it remains to be determined to what extent this enterprise was a success or failure.

THE BLINDING OF EROS: "LA CUSTODIA DEGLI OCCHI"

The *Cupid* fragment and the lost *Magdalene* bear testament to the fraught relationship between the iconoclastic and allegorical impulses inherent in the internalized, self-initiated, and preemptive attitude. The complexities of these strategies of censorship can be further unpacked through a close analysis of Gian Domenico Ottonelli and Pietro da Cortona's *Trattato della pittura, e scultura, uso et abuso loro* (1652). Although it is a rich source of historical anecdotes and miscellanea, the *Trattato* is usually seen as a belated effort to participate in a debate the outcome of which had long since been determined. Julius von Schlosser maligned the *Trattato* as one of the first manifestos aligning art with politics, adding that "the odor of the sacristy" was all over it, a view confirmed by modern scholars who perpetuate the view that "there is really nothing in this work that has not been said seventy years earlier."[15]

Contrary to the impatience revealed in such criticisms, the *Trattato* is an extraordinary document, advertised as a collaboration between theory and practice. Cortona's participation in the actual writing of the treatise was probably somewhat limited, although many of the opinions can be securely attributed to him.[16] In all likelihood, Ottonelli consulted the artist, who offered advice, provided anecdotes, gossip, and rumours, and allowed his name to be used as a sort of celebrity endorsement of Ottonelli's book (the book is also introduced by a letter of praise from Il Guercino). The promotion of the *Trattato* as a co-production of "a theologian and an artist" was, nevertheless, an ingenious strategy in the campaign to educate and win over the hearts and minds of a heterogeneous readership.

The prominence of Paleotti's *Discorso* is one of the primary reasons the *Trattato* has been overlooked. The *Discorso* was first published in Italian in 1582 and translated into Latin two years later in order to reach a larger audience. According to the ambitious plan mapped out in the introduction, the treatise was to include five parts: book 1 provided a definition, history, and typology of the "image"; book 2 listed the most common types of abuses or misuses of images; book 3 would have concentrated on the question of "lascivious" and "dishonest" images; book 4 promised to discuss "in minute detail" specific works of art in Bologna and other Christian cities; book 5 intended to provide practical advice to priests, family men, and painters. Scholars tend to cite Paleotti's *Discorso* as the most innovative and influential of these early post-Tridentine texts because he was an eminent member of Trent (his *Diarium* remains an authoritative account of the sessions of the Council) and because the *Discorso* was one of the first attempts to expand on the official position taken by the Council. It is, however, an incomplete project. The last three books were never written.

This is where the significance of Ottonelli's treatise becomes evident. The discussion of the *Trattato* will be framed here at one end by Paleotti's *Discorso intorno alle immagini sacre e profane* (1582) and at the other end by *La Pittura in Giudicio overo il bene delle oneste pitture e'l male delle oscene*, written in 1696 by another Jesuit, named Carlo Gregorio Rosignoli. If Ottonelli's treatise inspired little critical ink, Rosignoli's *Pittura* has suffered a worse fate, generating virtually no interest amongst scholars. Written 133 years after the closing of Trent, it is largely a reiteration of the *Trattato*, itself consciously modelled after the *Discorso*. Repetition, however, is instrumental in the construction of consensus and the naturalization of ideological positions; the three texts, then, should be read like folds in the same swathe of cloth rather than repetitive summaries of the same argument.

As with the *Cupid* fragment, the importance of these texts is diminished if they are read on their own. Consequently, Ottonelli's text can be interpreted as the larger picture into which Paleotti's unfinished project fits, for the *Trattato* very nearly repeats the structure proposed in the *Discorso*, expanded to six books covering definitions and discussions about painting and "images," as well as providing advice for painters, patrons, spectators, and ecclesiastical authorities. Moreover, all three projects were themselves part of a larger pedagogic program, specific to each author, which focused on reforming social behaviour in relation to early modern "pop culture." Rosignoli's *Pittura in Giudicio* belonged to a group of short treatises, including one on curbing obscenity in speech and another on the nefarious effects of gambling – *La Lingua purgata overo discorsi in emenda del parlare osceno* (1694) and *Il Giuoco di fortuna overo il bene e'l male de' giuochi* (1700). Ottonelli's *Trattato* followed his critiques of the moral responsibilities and dangers of theatre and opera – the *Risposta al quesito che male sia l'andare à Conversatione in casa di una persona poco modesta* (1645) and *Della Christiana moderatione del theatro* (1652). Paleotti's *Discorso* complemented another text for post-Tridentine preachers – the *Istruzzione* (1578).[17]

Nevertheless, there are significant differences between the treatises. In contrast to Paleotti's somewhat theoretical dissertation, Ottonelli directed his handbook to a wider readership. Ottonelli's position on obscene images is largely in agreement with that of earlier authorities; his tone of address, however, is much more conversational, often relying on anecdotes and allegories to make the point. When Paleotti's *Discorso* was translated in 1584 into Latin, it reached a larger readership of a certain social category. Ottonelli's strategy was less elitist. The approach was not to assume that the audience was dominated by *idioti*, but instead to be accessible and flexible so that all readers from the lowest common denominator to the educated elite could share a common ground. Unlike Paleotti's more rarefied and didactic text, the *Trattato* could engage different individuals at different levels of instruction. Rather than condensing the practical advice into one final chapter (as Paleotti had projected), Ottonelli's *Trattato* expanded this discussion into four chapters that are the heart of the book. These describe numerous and various types of everyday circumstances. There are sections, for instance, on whether it is a sin for artists to paint on feast days and for patrons to keep obscene paintings in their homes, how to be a good judge and critic, how to encourage artists with "sweet words" rather than brutality, and so on.[18] Much of the *Trattato* is composed of citations taken from previous authors, re-presented and explained in an accessible way to reach the broadest audience possible. Hence, what Paleotti accomplished through translation Ottonelli achieved through style and Rosignoli accomplished through scale, condensing the key points of the debate into a palm-size edition.

Ottonelli's more egalitarian disposition was perhaps a positive outcome of his Jesuit training (the same can be said of Rosignoli). In the first chapter of the *Trattato*, Ottonelli provided a working definition of "immodest images" as

> those images that move us with great efficiency to dishonesty. For the most part, they cause impure thoughts in the soul of the spectator.... Such images must not be painted, nor tolerated because incredible harm can happen to the souls of spectators who look upon them. They are things

that make you see incorrectly, that corrupt the mind, and that incite repulsive pleasures.[19]

This passage is a fascinating example of the virtuosity and dexterity of Jesuit rhetoric. Ottonelli expands his definition through a dialectical presentation of two extant definitions. The first passage is drawn from the writings of a certain Benito della Serna, who proposed that the labelling of *l'immagine poco modesta* should be limited to those pictures that represent "dishonest acts" rather than to any image that might "become lascivious on account of the spectator's dirty thoughts."[20] Della Serna's position is immediately contrasted with a second passage, taken from Bernardino Rodriguez Agostino, who underlines that a lascivious image can be "a Venus or an Adonis in which the impure parts are shown, regardless of whether they are covered by a beautiful veil."[21] It was enough that these *parti impure* were suggested, for wayward spectators could fill in the missing parts. For Della Serna, dishonesty was inherent in the end results of representation rather than in the process of reception. For Agostino, dishonesty was often produced unexpectedly in the act of reception regardless of what was represented. Vigilance, therefore, was to be directed at the individual subject and at internal behaviour (rather than at objects and external realities).

Preventing spectators from seeing "incorrectly" was the ideological work that these authors were trying to accomplish. And early modern viewers did respond in this manner; it was not merely the hypercautious ravings of ecclesiastics. Looking at one of the many versions of Titian's *Venus and Adonis*, Lodovico Dolce wrote to the Venetian nobleman Alessandro Contarini that "no one [is] so chilled by age or so hard in his makeup that he does not feel himself growing warm and tender, and the whole of his blood stirring in his veins."[22] The artistry demonstrated in Titian's brushstrokes, he added, mirrored the beholder's desire to brush his hand across the skin of the painted body.[23] The perennially controversial Pietro Aretino wrote to Federico Gonzaga about the imminent arrival of Jacopo Sansovino's Venus statuette, which was "so true to life and so living that it will fill with lustful thoughts the mind of anyone who looks at it."[24]

Remarks like these may have been acceptable in the rarefied pre-Tridentine context of the northern Italian courts where these artworks were first seen. The same comments recontextualized in a different social milieu or historical moment, however, would only confirm Ottonelli's fear that while the weak were naturally inclined to err, even a virtuous, learned spectator might unexpectedly slip from "delight" to "curiosity" to "carnal thoughts," thereby endangering the purity of the soul.[25] It was crucial, therefore, to take extreme measures, for the "guardianship of the eyes" would prevent the graver sin of the "fornication of the eyes."[26] Rosignoli would return to this theme in a chapter entitled "La custodia degli occhi è custodia del cuore" (XIV.1). "What the eyes do not see," he explained, "the heart does not desire." To further illustrate this point, Rosignoli described how the virtuous eyes of St. Lodovico remained "brilliant and resplendent like two diamonds without [any signs of] corruption" years after his death and how St. Filippo Neri was able to maintain his "virginal innocence" on account of the "custodianship of his eyes, which never gazed upon the faces of women or upon immodest paintings, even though Rome presented him with so many."[27]

But what was it about the nude body that the Church found so threatening that it had to be literally covered up? From a theological point of view, the awareness of nudity pointed to an awareness of sin. Christian attitudes towards the body were established, on the one hand, upon the simple body–soul dichotomy that vilified the corruptible body as a burden to the soul and, on the other hand, upon an emphasis on how the coupled knowledge of sexuality and death resulted directly from humanity's fall from grace.[28] However, while the abject body was the terrestrial prison where sexuality, desire, and death converged, it was also the only vessel through which the sensate soul could attain spiritual knowledge.

The tension between prelapsarian unity and postlapsarian loss brings us to a second reason for corporeal abjection and has to do with the confusion between psychological and physical desire. Quoting Canon 100 of the Trullan Synod (convened by Justinian II in 692), Johannes Molanus reminded in his attack on nude imagery:

> Wisdom bids you take care that your heart is kept safe and your eyes do not stray, for the sensuality of the body easily spreads to the soul. We therefore forbid hereafter the making in any way of pictures which offend the eyes, corrupt the mind and kindle base pleasures. And if anyone should try to do it, he must be excommunicated.[29]

And this is where the true danger of lascivious images makes itself clear. Rosignoli explained that images of nude Venuses can "pervert the imprudent and those with poor dispositions." The effect on the spectator, he concluded, is as destructive and permanent as the effect on the victim who confronts the Medusa's gaze.[30]

Like a guide, the user's *Trattato* proposed a range of adjustable answers for different scenarios. We have already heard from Ottonelli how Cardinal Gessi's *Venus and Cupid* was cut down. Philip II, king of Spain and patron of Titian, is said to have kept his mythological *poesie* behind curtains in the Escorial, while his successor, Philip III, reportedly ordered the removal of a nude *Susanna* proclaiming to those in the room, "I am not a friend of nude paintings."[31] More drastic measures were also common. The Austrian emperor Ferdinand II is said to have ordered some obscene paintings to be burned.[32] Another owner of an "obscene Venus" had his statuette melted down so that the gold could be distributed among the poor.[33] In another passage we are told about a bishop who removed the three nude goddesses in a painting of the judgment of Paris that was in his villa so that Paris's beauty could be contemplated "without scandal to its viewers."[34]

Representations of the nude body moved the beholder to respond to the simulacrum as if it were a real body, mistaking the representation for a living and breathing body. These types of individual remarks and cautionary tales conform to a classical topos derived from Pliny's tale about the Cnidian Venus, a statue so beautiful that an obsessed man immorally "stained" her in the dead of night. This kind of unacceptable behaviour was not gender specific. In Girolamo Morlini's *Novellae* (1520), a woman is overcome with lust at the sight of a statue with an erection and is discovered copulating with it in the public square the next morning.[35]

These stories address two problems: first, the transgressive infiltration of private sexual activities into the public domain; second, the unexpected corruption of unpremeditated offenders through sensory contact with artworks. Instead of moving the viewer to piety and elevating the soul, the sight of the nude body turned the viewer towards lust; rather than being inspired to do good deeds, the viewer was unexpectedly imprisoned by unfulfilled physical desires. This state was akin to a certain form of madness or, to quote Ottonelli's succinct formula, "[L]ust and idolatry are closely connected for one follows the other."[36] Honest works such as portraits could take on their own uncanny power when misused by their owners. Ottonelli related several stories about men who went mad and literally died of desire for an unattainable woman whose portraits they secretly kept in their rooms.[37] Their inability to distinguish the image (the portraits) from the original (the beloved woman) was another case of pictures inadvertently leading to idolatrous behaviour.

The efficacy of images to quicken action points to a third reason that visual representations of nudity were perceived as a danger. The power of erotic titillation endangered the very structure of the disciplinary society. The ideological implications of subversive images of any kind ultimately concern the maintenance of social order and rigid hierarchies. At bottom, censorship was about power, about controlling who got to see what and under what circumstances. Lascivious images posed a controllable threat to the rarefied male members within the aristocratic court, but the real danger lay in the unavoidable entry of nonmembers into these exclusive circles. Ottonelli specified that although "virtuous spirits who were experts in the things of art" might understand and even enjoy pictures of all kinds, "an indecent Venus" nevertheless posed a serious danger to "spectators of unstable virtue" because "with great efficiency, [these pictures] could move spectators to commit grave sins that would compromise their chastity."[38] As a result, it was better to err on the side of caution than on that of negligence.

Not surprisingly, Ottonelli's *Spettatori poco stabili nella virtù* comprised those groups on the periphery of social power: women, children, servants, the uneducated, and the poor (a mix of Paleotti's *idioti* and *sensuali*).[39] The infantilization of the disenfranchised is made clear by Rosignoli in the section where he uses the massacre of the innocents to allegorize how representations of "immodest figures" function as "homicidal arrows" that "massacre" the soul. In another passage, he uses the metaphor of the foolish butterfly that is drawn to the light but inadvertently throws itself into the flames to explain how reckless young men looking at paintings of ideal beauties in states of undress might similarly set themselves on fire.[40]

Another strategy for circumscribing the *poco stabili* was to feminize them. In Vasari's life of Fra Bartolomeo we are told that a painting of St. Sebastian had to be removed from public view after it was discovered "through the confessional" that, rather than aiding devotion, the naturalism of the male body had caused female viewers to sin.[41] The process of removal occurred in stages: first it was taken out of the church; next it was placed in the chapter house; and finally it was bought by Giovan Battista della Palla, who sent it to the king of France. In the *Trattato*, Ottonelli alludes to another case recounted in Raffaello Borghini's *Risposo* in which Baccio della Porta's Florentine St. Sebastian was removed from the Chiesa de' Padri Predicatori for similar reasons; Rosignoli, drawing from Ottonelli, who was drawing from Borghini, repeats the same tale in the *Pittura*.[42] *Letterati*, too, were prone to such behaviour; however, this type of psychological response was essentialized as typically feminine. Again, in an elaborately constructed passage, Rosignoli quotes Possevino's discussion of Plato's *Republic* as an amplification of the directive outlined in the decree of the Council of Trent to suggest that looking at images of female nudes would cause the soul to "become effeminate" and "inclined to wickedness."[43]

Images were efficient carriers of information and powerful instruments of persuasion. In the end, the reason images were so beneficial was precisely the reason they could potentially be so dangerous. And here the two domains of censorship and propaganda blur into each other. Ottonelli warned that "images were more noxious than books," for an image could annihilate the beholder's chastity in the "blink of an eye."[44] Rosignoli repeated that obscene images were far more efficient corruptors of innocence than dishonest words because the former "lasted longer, were more alluring, and more frequently exposed to the eyes, which of all the senses was the most intense and also the most vulnerable to bad impressions."[45] "The eye," Ottonelli wrote, "is the path to divine love."[46] But the same pathway was also open to vice: "The Devil," he warned, "sends the plague and his venom to the soul by way of the eyes; and when Temptation fails, the Devil uses painting."[47]

EROS UNBOUND: TALES OF CONVERSION

Destruction was an easy solution in the censorship of obscene images. However, as with the fate of the mutilated *Venus and Cupid* fragment, it also had a dangerous whiff of iconoclasm. In addressing the *poco stabili*, Ottonelli, therefore, presented *una spirituale transformatione* as an alternative:

> [Giovanni Paolo Sanfelice] had a beautiful painting in Naples of a nude Venus, with a Cupid at her side who held a pointed arrow in his hand, which he used to strike the goddess with sweet blows of love. It was a work by a famous painter and was cherished by the Signore for its high perfection and noble artistry. However, fearing scandal from the weak in virtue, he kept the painting in a back room, and it was always carefully covered by a drape so that it was not seen by everyone in public. This gentleman died and the painting, along with his title, went to Giovanni Francesco, the nephew of the deceased. Reflecting upon the danger the painting might have on certain persons in the house and to others who might accidentally see such a frivolous and obscene painting, Giovanni was not satisfied with the back room solution nor by the method of covering it with a sheet. Instead, he resorted to more rigorous means, performing a spiritual transformation. He ordered a worthy painter to dress the nude body with a hairshirt, to add a skull near Venus' head, and to place a rod instead of the arrow in Cupid's hand. In this manner, rather than a lascivious Venus, those who saw the work were persuaded that they were looking at a penitent Magdalene, who was receiving saintly instruction from an angel so that she could repent for her grave and dishonest sins.[48]

The Sanfelice story is valuable, for it introduces an ingenious solution concerning the inevitable circulation of paintings of female nudes, which simultaneously endorses the iconophilic position of post-Tridentine Catholicism: conversion through the very materials of art.

This is where the artist comes back into the picture. These texts were as much directed to clerics and patrons as they were to practitioners of painting. The aim of the post-Tridentine authors was to effect reform from within – to discipline the artists rather than directly censure their art, to instil the fear of God into them rather than incessantly check up on them. Painters who did not conform were accordingly demonized:

> Immodest painters are hunters working for the Devil. With dishonest paintings and many other channels, they ensnare the eyes of the careless spectator. It is incredible how much evil is caused by these lascivious images, these Altars of Hell where one sacrifices ones eyes, thoughts, and hearts to the Devil.[49]

The melodrama of this passage is reiterated in another section where Ottonelli comes out and directly categorizes painters of "dishonest things" as heretics.[50] In other words, not only did obscene images corrupt the hearts of collectors and prey on the innocent viewers in their household, they also put the soul of the artist at risk. Indecent paintings, Ottonelli warned, were invented by Satan so that he could "stimulate the soul of some painters to employ their minds, their hands, and their brushes in order to lead the human senses astray with filthy pleasures and to incite these painters to a licentious life, from which would follow eternal damnation."[51]

It was not always easy to be a virtuous painter. We learn from Cardinal Cesare Baronius about a painter who tried to paint a sacred story over an image of a Venus. "The Devil," however, "who was residing in that dishonest painting jumped into the painter's hand causing him torturous agony and it was decided that he would have to cut off his hand"; the painter, clearly unhappy with such a decision, sought the help of a priest, who anointed his hand with holy oil, which freed him from the devil's hold.[52]

The moral of the story is twofold. First, it underlines the duty of the Christian artist to serve God by painting virtuous images that inspire piety, devotion, and good works rather than to be the instrument of the devil's harm in painting lascivious images that might lead him and others to ruin. Instead of following the drastic advice of the biblical phrase "If the eye offends you, pluck it out and if the hand offends you, cut it off," the artist, the patron, and the spectator were instructed on how to discipline the hand from creating offensive images and the eye so that it would learn to blind itself from obscene subjects. Second, this passage instructs the reader that, in the face of trouble and doubt, one should always seek the guidance of a religious authority.[53] The Council of Trent, while laconic about the larger issue of defining what was acceptable and unacceptable, was nevertheless very clear about underlining the importance of institutional guidance and control: no one, it decreed, shall "be allowed to place or cause to be placed any unusual image in any place or church ... unless it has been approved by the Bishop."[54] Although this passage is concerned primarily with the maintenance of decorum in public works such as altarpieces commissioned by private families and corporations, the underlying conclusion that it reinforces is the authority of church officials in matters of judging the moral value of artworks.

But how much of the official rhetoric was internalized and how much of it was simply negotiated in practice? Did artists cower before the declarations of the Tridentine authorities? Vasari, for one, didn't seem to be fazed much by the hype, responding in the life of Fra Angelico that the hypersensitivity of censors only served

> to reveal their infected and corrupted souls, which draw evil and dishonest desires out of these works. If they were lovers of honesty, as they seek by their foolish zeal to show themselves to be, they would achieve the desire for Heaven from these works.[55]

This may have just been typical Vasarian lip-service for he did himself make noticeable changes elsewhere in the 1568 edition of the *Lives of the Artists*, published five years after the closing of Trent.[56] At the same time,

Vasari's passage was sure to reflect the opinion of at least some artists as well as patrons at the time. In either case, it was clearly not the type of response that the Church had hoped for. Vasari's remark articulates a knowing perception of the Church's paranoia in its attitude towards the danger posed by images; yet in doing so, it simultaneously reinforces the belief that sin is in the eyes of the *beholder* (reception) rather than in the content of the *work* (representation).

One of the artists that Ottonelli and Rosignoli return to on more than one occasion is Bartolommeo Ammannati. In 1582, towards the end of his life, the Florentine artist addressed an impassioned letter to the Accademia del Disegno in which he sorrowfully expressed his regret for the lascivious images he had made in his youth and the spiritual harm his works may have caused the virtuous men and women of Florence.[57] It was an unforgivable sin, he lamented, to adorn public monuments with sculptures of suggestive nymphs and lustful satyrs because "with a single glance of the eye" such images were able "to move a soul that is otherwise gentle and healthy to excited and filthy thoughts."[58] What is particularly striking about Ammannati's letter, however, is the public and civic nature of his autocriticism. In decorating public monuments with female nudes and satyrs, the Florentine sculptor claims to have set a horrible example for his viewers and to have committed a terrible crime both against the body politic and against God.[59]

Ammannati's figures on the Triton Fountain in the Piazza della Signoria in Florence were accessible to any passing viewers regardless of their class, sex, and age. In his mind, he felt that he had grievously compromised the innocence and greatness of the Florentines. Perhaps this sense of guilt explains why Ammannati felt compelled not only to apologize for his indiscretion, but also to insist on a full public confession. He writes, "I want to write and confess and correct my talents publicly."[60] Then he stipulates that he wishes to "confess" not so that he may be excused but in order to right the offence that he has committed. Finally, he emphatically acknowledges responsibility for his own actions. It is as if Ammannati has internalized the rhetoric and the discourse of the post-Tridentine Reformers.

The Florentine painter Francesco Furini provides another interesting case study, for he urged his friends to burn his paintings after he became a priest around the age of forty.[61] Prior to his conversion, Furini was celebrated for his highly eroticized female nudes, which were so alluring that "any prudent and chaste soul," as his biographer pointed out, would be scandalized.[62] Like Mary Magdalene, Ammannati and Furini are exemplary Christians, for they are *converted* sinners who have judged their own acts and thoughts to be dissolute and who have subsequently turned to a renewed life of greater moral integrity. More significantly, they enact this conversion as a demonstratively public act of self-criticism and autocensorship. Ultimately, the Church did not need to do anything but wave its blessing over the penitent artists and uphold them as exemplars of virtue.

In both the *Trattato* and the *Pittura*, individual scenes from the lives of the artists are often lifted out of context and converted into Christian allegories. Polygnotus, for instance, is praised not for his skill as a canonic Greek artist, but as the first painter of clothed women.[63] Rosignoli (in another awesome demonstration of Jesuit oratorical skills) transformed the story of Parrhasius's curtain into a lesson about the artist's virtuosity in veiling nude figures, and the story of Apelles and Campase from an anecdote in praise of the patron's magnanimity into a cautionary tale about the dangers inherent in looking at beautiful women.[64] As a means to dissuade the artist from painting nudes, Ottonelli explained how Praxiteles might have been praised for his nude Venuses, but his clothed Venuses fetched just as much money.[65] A passage from Plutarch about how ancient artists submitted their works to extensive correction and revision was turned into a lesson on the importance of self-censorship in the devout painter's creative process.[66] Modern artists are also employed to bolster Ottonelli's portrait of the ideal, devout artist: Bronzino, it is suggested, painted modestly clothed women in his old age to make up for the dishonest images he painted in his youth.[67] The deaths of Leonardo da Vinci, Agostino Carracci, and Raphael would be melodramatically restaged by Rosignoli as scenes of repentance.[68]

In spite of the threat of eternal ruin and damnation preached by post-Tridentine spin doctors (and as the larger history of seventeenth-century art will demonstrate), artists continued to create, innovate, and even manipulate form and content. Instead of shutting down the creative impulse, the post-Tridentine impositions of propriety and decorum pushed certain artists to find even more inventive avenues of expression. Ironically, then, a certain form of creative ingenuity was borne from within the prison walls of censorship.

In the Sanfelice story, it was stipulated that a "worthy painter" was asked to repaint the Venus, transforming her into a Magdalene, or, as Ottonelli sanctimoniously concluded, "[A] lascivious image is thus transformed into a saintly one."[69] And even while Rosignoli would praise the "glorious metamorphosis" of Sanfelice's Venus into a penitent Magdalene, from the perspective of the artist this type of iconographical slippage was common currency; it was a standard form of practical shorthand in the workshop (this is evident in the serialized reclining nudes that came out of sixteenth- and seventeenth-century workshops).[70] The collaborative production of Orazio and Artemisia Gentileschi, for instance, indicates how the same form could be emptied of its content and filled with new meanings: in one image a Danaë receives gold coins, while in another that same body becomes Cleopatra clinging to her poisonous serpent. Admittedly, this is still a far cry from transforming a lascivious image into a virtuous one, but artists did perform such conversions. In another example, Orazio Gentileschi transferred the body of Danaë in one painting to the body of the Magdalene in another (Illustration 16).[71]

In the face of post-Tridentine challenges, artists cleverly reinvented new contexts for old forms. As a literary parallel, one might turn to the increased popularity of Magdalene plays in the post-Tridentine period. This theme provided an ideal stage on which Petrarchan clichés could be rewritten as songs and poems of Christian love. Moreover, in an inversion of conventional gender roles, the Magdalene was recast as the lovesick subject and Jesus as the ineffable object of her pains. The very language of the Magdalene plays is built up around rhyming groups common in Italian love poetry. Words like *amore*, *core*, *dolore*, *onore*, and *errore*, however, are now matched with more Christocentric words like *signore* or terms like *peccatore*, which are rife with post-Tridentine significance. Poetic staples like *infiamma*, *ferito*, *lagrime*, and *duolo* were renewed with spiritual connotations.[72] These plays were generally divided into three parts: pre-conversion depravity, the scene of conversion, and post-conversion triumphalism. The first part enabled writers to devote endless lines to describing the Magdalene's face, hair, and

16. Orazio Gentileschi, *Penitent Magdalene*. Oil on canvas, 163 × 208 cm. Vienna, Kunsthistorisches Museum (Inv.-Nr. GG_179).

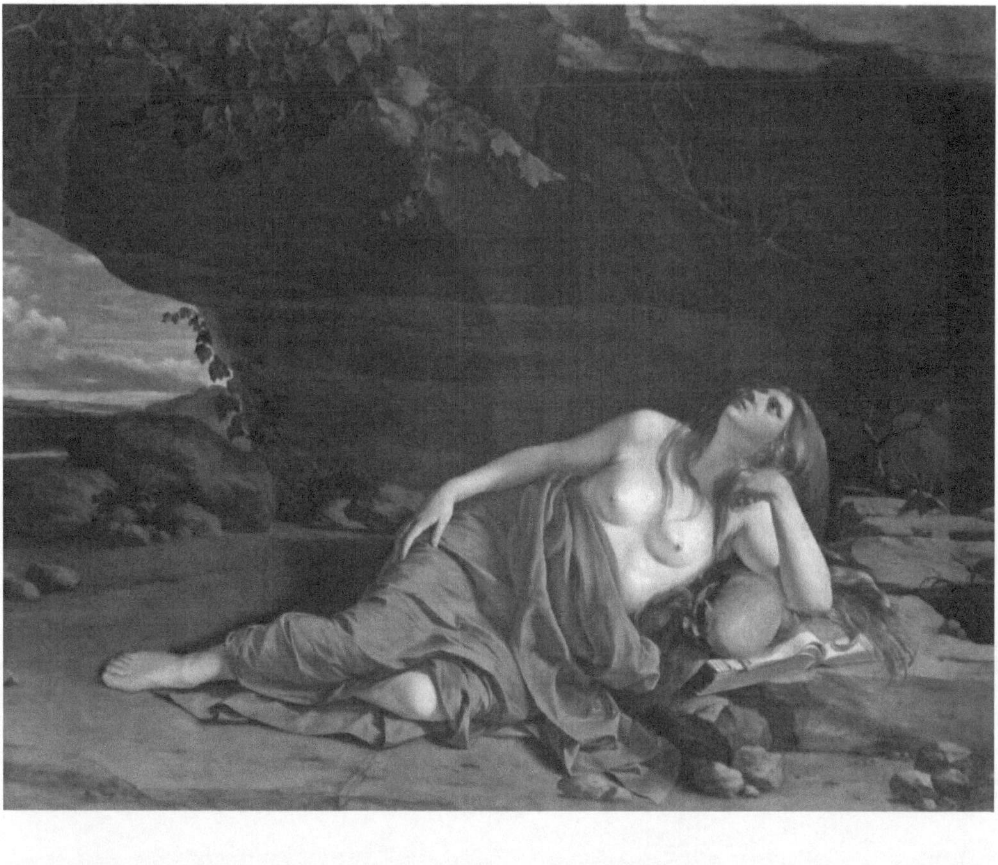

body. Erotic language that would otherwise have been unacceptable was, therefore, given a creative outlet, co-opted for new and highly controlled ends. The second act took certain pleasures in representing the taming of the lascivious screw. And the final act allowed for special theatrical effects. For instance, Giovanni Battista Andreini's play *The Lascivious and Penitent Magdalene* (1617) ends with an angel who appears suspended in the sky and announces, "Yes, Magdalene blossoms from the lascivious Venus!"[73] The self-congratulatory rhetoric of this post-Tridentine morality piece shares a certain resonance in the reclining Magdalene paintings of the seventeenth century and may help to explain the appeal of such images. But victory was not so easily claimed by the censors.

"The obscene body," as Lynda Nead defined, "is the body without borders or containment and obscenity is representation that moves and arouses the viewer rather than bringing about stillness and wholeness."[74] Although Correggio was one of the first Italian Renaissance artists to paint the Magdalene in this pose, Correggio's figure lacked the heightened eroticism of Gentileschi's model. For one, Correggio's saint is represented in the act of reading. She is shown as a modest young woman educating herself: her head is pulled down in front of and enclosed upon her own body; her body is hermetic and self-contained, absorbed in the civilizing actions of self-instruction and spiritual enlightenment.

Orazio's reclining Magdalene, in contrast, fully exploits the sexual tension and iconographical ambiguity implicit in the saintly form. In Orazio's glowing canvas, the sensuous nude is recognizable as a saint only because of the skull and Bible with which she is shown. It is precisely on account of these two small details that we are able to read this figure as a "Magdalene" rather than a "Venus" or just another anonymous indecent nude. Her body language also conveys a completely different message than Correggio's figure (as well as the other Seicento examples by Allori et al.). Orazio's figure is about sensory accessibility and embodied knowledge. In this version her breasts are exposed. Her head is thrown back, lost in ecstatic contemplation, while at the same time opening up the spectacle of her body. No longer engaged in the activity of reading, the figure becomes a passive object to be consumed by the eyes of the viewer.

The advent of the "reclining female saint" in painting at a moment when reclining nudes were looked upon with apprehension provides a clear example of how artists found means to manipulate disciplinary impositions, revitalizing old forms in new ways. It can be suggested here that the artist trumps the censor, although this triumph was also restricted, for writers were quick to co-opt these forms too. Ottonelli could not help but praise such transformative conversions, ending the passage quoted earlier by proclaiming, "The passion of a noble and virtuous soul is so ingenious!" When Rosignoli repeats the Sanfelice story, he similarly adds, "It is an ingenious invention to convert iniquitous and superstitious materials into a subject of piety and religion."[75]

Although it seems that Gentileschi's visual double entendre was especially popular among collectors, it cannot be concluded that all seventeenth-century artists and spectators openly accepted this kind of iconographic instability.[76] For some, the eroticism was clearly too heightened, and the mechanics of self-censorship can be seen moving into play. In one seventeenth-century copy after Orazio's picture executed by Jean Tassel (Illustration 17), the artist has rearranged the saint's hair in order to cover her bare breasts from the viewer's gaze.[77] Ottonelli concluded his anecdote about Sanfelice's *Venus* by noting that "rather than a lascivious Venus, those who saw the work *were persuaded* that they were looking at a penitent Magdalene" (my emphasis).

In the end, both strategies of blinding and conversion failed to erase the potential danger of the female nude from pictorial traditions. If iconoclastic action denied the sight of Venus's indecently exposed body in the Vienna painting and if iconographical conversion encouraged the beholder to identify the reclining body as that of the penitent Magdalene, the early modern spectator could still sense the spectre of the unreconstructed Venus lingering in the shadows and haunting the imagination that could be disciplined but not entirely controlled. The significance of the two partial images with which I began this essay and of the treatises discussed, then, lies not only in the success but more interestingly in the failure of the post-Tridentine disciplinary project. These images and texts can be read as totems of the precarious push and pull that structured the very dynamics of desire.

17. Jean Tassel, *Penitent Magdalene*. Oil on canvas, 105 × 174 cm. Dijon, Musée des Beaux-Arts.

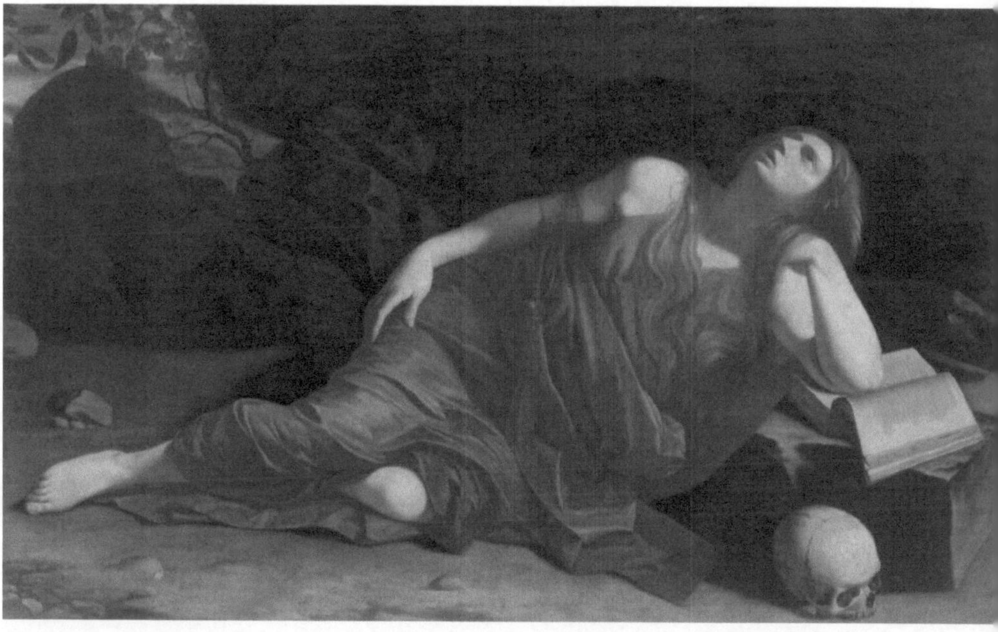

Notes

This project was generously funded by the Joanna Randall-McIver Junior Fellowship, which I held while at St. Hilda's College, Oxford, and by the Leverhulme Trust, which enabled me to complete this during my research leave. Translations are mine unless otherwise indicated.

1 Von Posse (1931).
2 Baldinucci (1974–75), 3: 734.
3 Spagnolo (2005), 22–25. The Carracci painting (now in the Fitzwilliam in Cambridge) shows the Magdalene in a more upright, seated position than in Correggio's model; see Jaffé (1981).
4 De Brosses, quoted in Ekserdjian (1997), 175.
5 See Aikema (1994) for his discussion of Titian's pre- and post-Tridentine Magdalenes.
6 *Canons and Decrees of the Sacred and Oecumenical Council of Trent* (1848), 235; hereafter *Canons* (1848).
7 *Canons* (1848), 235–36.
8 *Canons* (1848), 235.
9 Paleotti (2002), 263–67. *Idioti* is modernized to read *sprovveduti* in this edition; the 1582 original, however, bears the term *idioti* and the 1584 edition reads *idiotae, & vulgares homines.*
10 Paleotti (2002), 267.
11 Paleotti (2002), 266.
12 Ottonelli and Berrettini [da Cortona] (1652), 331–32. The author of the *Trattato* will be referred to henceforth as Ottonelli (1652).
13 See, e.g., Prosperi (1996) and the essays collected in Prodi and Penuti (1994).
14 Ottonelli (1652), 95.
15 Schlosser (1997), 616; Bailey (1999c), 171.
16 For the artist's contributions see Casale (1976). Logistically, however, it seems unlikely that Cortona would have had much time to serve more than as the occasional coauthor. The *Trattato* was published right after the construction of SS. Martina e Luca (1635–50), for which Cortona was the main architect, and in the middle of his most busy Roman period, when extensive fresco work was going on simultaneously at S. Maria in Vallicella (1647–65) and at Pope Innocent X's private palace in the Piazza Navona (1651–54).
17 P. Jones (1995), 138.
18 Ottonelli (1652), 254–60, 292–93, 166–68.
19 Ottonelli (1652), 34.
20 Ottonelli (1652), 34.
21 Ottonelli (1652), 34.
22 Dolce (2000), 217.
23 Dolce (2000), 214.
24 Quoted in Findlen (1993), 63.
25 This chronology is described in Ottonelli (1652), 375.
26 Ottonelli (1652), 369–70.
27 Rosignoli (1696), 227–30.
28 On this see Clifton (1999).
29 Quoted in D. Freedberg (1971), 243.
30 Rosignoli (1696), 85.

31 Ottonelli (1652), 41; cf. Findlen (1993), 54.
32 Ottonelli (1652), 332.
33 Ottonelli (1652), 335.
34 Ottonelli (1652), 332.
35 D. Freedberg (1989), 326–27.
36 Ottonelli (1652), 383.
37 Ottonelli (1652), 381–83; Rosignoli (1696), 224–26 for comparanda.
38 Ottonelli (1652), 324–26.
39 A typical example of this attitude is summed up in Rosignoli (1696), 110: "Trà gli abusi abominevoli, e pestilenti, che regnano nelle case di molti capi di famiglia, uno si è il tener nelle stanze, lotto pretesto d'ornamento, e di splendore della casa, Imagini, e pitture disoneste, non accorgendosi gl'infelici, quanto sieno dannose all'onestà de costumi, massimamente de'loro figliuoli."
40 Rosignoli (1696), 2, 104.
41 Vasari (1966–87), 3: 97.
42 Ottonelli (1652), 180; Rosignoli (1696), 62.
43 Rosignoli (1696), 5.
44 Ottonelli (1652), 36.
45 Rosignoli (1696), 4.
46 Ottonelli (1652), 66.
47 Ottonelli (1652), 40.
48 Ottonelli (1652), 326–27.
49 Ottonelli (1652), 145.
50 Ottonelli (1652), 132.
51 Ottonelli (1652), 8.
52 Ottonelli (1652), 35; cf. Rosignoli (1696), 86–88, for the same story.
53 Cf. Paleotti (2002), 114, for similar remarks about seeking counsel.
54 *Canons* (1848), 236.
55 Vasari (1966–87), 3: 274.
56 Concerning the passage discussed, the 1568 edition includes a long-winded reflection on the question of decorum coded in specifically post-Tridentine terms.
57 Ammannati (1962), 119.
58 Ammannati (1962), 121.
59 Ammannati (1962), 119.
60 Ammannati (1962), 119.
61 Baldinucci (1974–75), 3: 641.
62 Baldinucci (1974–75), 3:631; on Furini see Gregori and Maffeis (2007).
63 Ottonelli (1652), 37.
64 Rosignoli (1696), 165–67, 8.
65 Ottonelli (1652), 46; this point is reiterated in another passage on the importance of Titian's *St. Peter Martyr* altarpiece, in contrast to the popularity of his bacchanals (202).
66 Plutarch, quoted in Ottonelli (1652), 164.
67 Ottonelli (1652), 143, 143.
68 Rosignoli (1696), 11–12.
69 Ottonelli (1652), 323.
70 Rosignoli (1696), 163. On the serialization of the reclining female nude, see Loh (2007), ch. 1.
71 Leonard, Khandekar, and Carr (2001), 6; see also Christiansen (2003).

72 On this theme see Ussia (1988).
73 For details see Zampelli (2002).
74 Nead (1992), 2.
75 Ottonelli (1652), 327; Rosignoli (1696), 164–65.
76 On the different versions from the 1620s see Nicolson (1985).
77 On the French copies see Sterling (1958), 112–21.

RAFFAELLO BORGHINI AND THE CORPUS OF FLORENTINE ART IN AN AGE OF REFORM

Stuart Lingo

A GROUP OF FOUR FRIENDS, escaping the rising heat of May and the cares of city life at a villa outside Florence, discuss the recent paintings that now fill the city's churches and make them its art galleries as well as its religious shrines. One interlocutor, the insouciant Michelozzo, highlights the tensions implicit in this dual function when he admits that he finds an altarpiece in the Ognissanti so bad that "I never go in that church so that I won't lose my taste for painting."[1] The friends' conversation is by turns witty and serious, and occasionally pedantic. Yet at moments it gains an edge, and characters make statements that may still surprise the reader.

Bronzino's *Christ in Limbo* (Illustration 18), a monumental altarpiece completed in 1552 for the important Florentine church of S. Croce, is at once a striking visualization of Christ's incursion into the realm of the dead and a virtuoso artistic performance. Recalling this remarkable scene, Michelozzo exclaims, "[b]efore this panel of Bronzino I feel the greatest pleasure in admiring the delicate members of those beautiful women." Vecchietti, the eldest of the friends, replies heatedly, "[h]ow little Bronzino merits praise in this work, you yourself have shown by admitting that you delight in looking at those lascivious women; considering the[m] ... one cannot help but feel some carnal stimulation, which is completely contrary to what one should experience in the temple of God."[2] Yet Michelozzo will not let the subject drop and later notices that their reflective friend Baccio Valori seems to like the painting as well. Pushed, Valori politely responds, "I delight in regarding those beauties which were given to us by the great giver of all good things." Michelozzo ripostes, "I like your platonic opinion, and if everyone could look with such intention, it would never be necessary to make sacred pictures differently; but I don't know how this continence and holy thinking ... can last in looking at things that so stimulate the senses."[3]

There are a number of such witty yet fraught exchanges in Raffaello Borghini's *Il Riposo* of 1584, the most important art critical text of late Renaissance Florence after Giorgio Vasari's massive *Lives of the Artists*

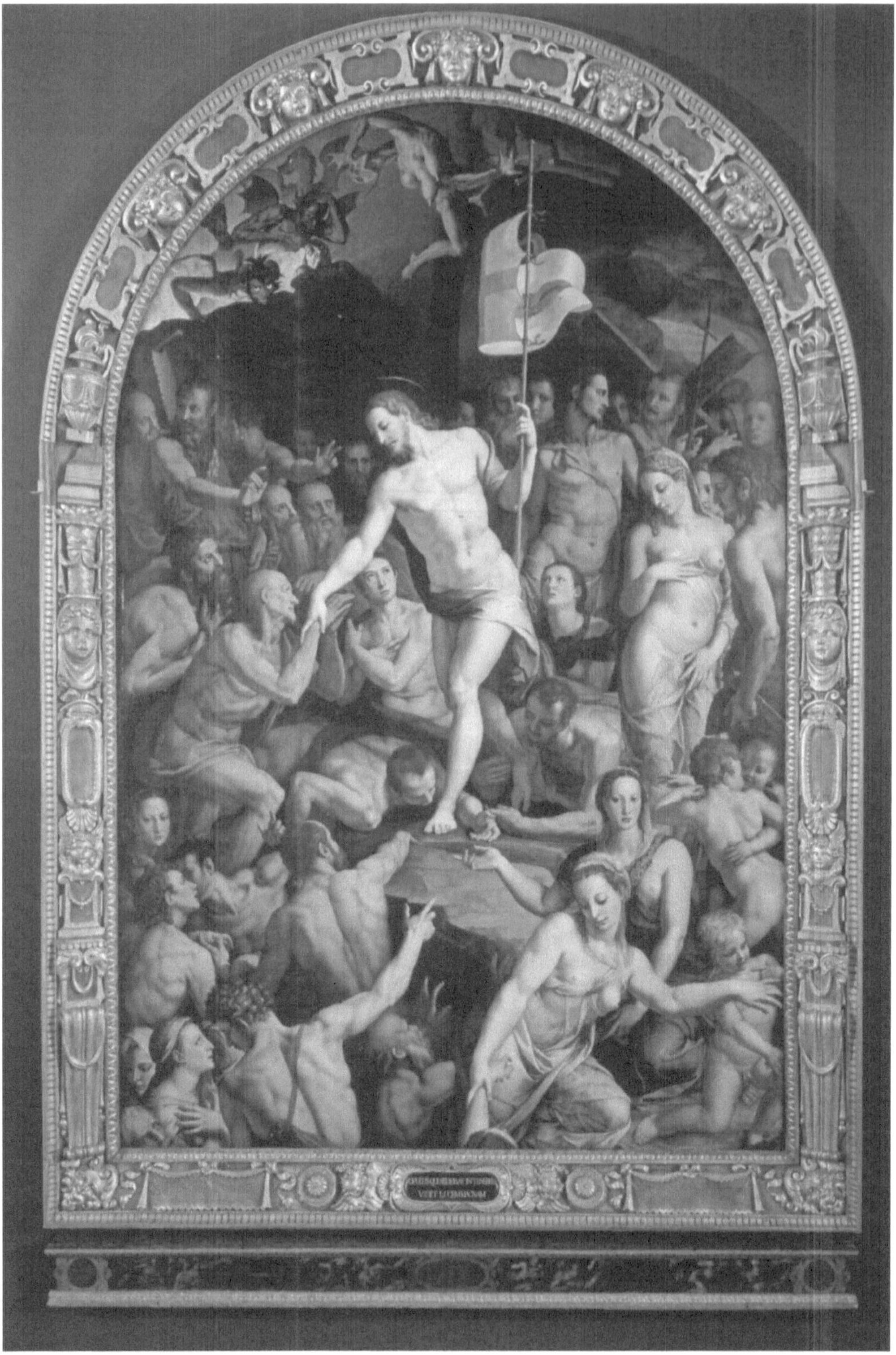

18. Agnolo Bronzino, *Christ in Limbo*, 1552. Oil on panel, 444 × 293 cm. Florence, Museo dell'Opera di Santa Croce. Photo: Nicolo Orsi Battaglini / Art Resource, NY.

of 1550 and 1568. Borghini's work is long and sometimes long-winded, and has often been dismissed as a conservative product of the "Counter-Reformation," principally because of Vecchietti's repeated attacks on modern religious paintings for "lasciviousness" and other failures. Yet the dialogue form allows Borghini to stage a vigorous debate. All the characters express distinctive perspectives, from Vecchietti's moralizing concern to Valori's Neoplatonic appreciation to Michelozzo's frank delight in the sensuality of which later Renaissance painting was capable. Critically, the dialogue refuses to reconcile these views or clearly to privilege any of them. The text does not allow us to determine if Vecchietti represents the views of Borghini (as often assumed), and even the status of Vecchietti's moralizing position becomes ultimately unclear in the unresolved discussions. We are presented in *Il Riposo* with a conundrum, a picture of a culture at odds with itself about the status and purpose of modern art and religious art. This is an impasse that has not been sufficiently interrogated.

It is increasingly recognized that discourses of affect and desire conditioned much creation and reception of art in sixteenth-century Italy. Such discourses were bound up with the ideal of the lovely body as a critical topos for representation – and assumed the rapt presence of the desiring beholder.[4] The ideal of the image as an object and product of desire had become so entrenched by midcentury that it remained potent, and destabilizing, even in those difficult years of religious upheaval and reform during the Council of Trent and the decades that followed. Its elevated temperature can be taken from a text like the *Avvertimenti*, which Ulisse Aldrovandi addressed to his friend Cardinal Gabriele Paleotti in 1581. Paleotti had solicited comment on a draft of his *Discorso intorno alle imagini sacre e profane*, an extended treatise on the appropriate creation and use of images. While the cardinal's text is often assumed to be merely another document of the "Counter-Reformation," it is important to remember admonitions by John Shearman and others that ecclesiastical theorists such as Paleotti were more sophisticated in their culture and thinking than many art historians have tended to imagine.[5] But given that Paleotti was a reforming churchman with definitive aims for painting, some of Aldrovandi's comments seem remarkable. Paleotti's demand that religious images be affecting, for instance, elicited the following response:

> Your Most Illustrious Lordship illustrates very wisely the varied and diverse effects that can be caused by pious and devout images. Concerning this issue, therefore, I will not hesitate to tell you of that statue of the Cnidian Venus, formed of parian marble, which was placed in its temple, as Lucian testifies, and was so beautiful that it drove Charicles virtually insane ... ; running to it he kissed it with his lips, extending his neck upwards as far as he could.... Every hour his love for this beautiful and gracious statue burned more intensely. And if a statue of uncolored marble had this effect, what should works do that are colored and painted in lifelike fashion?[6]

While it seems that the Venus type most closely related to Praxiteles' fabled Cnidia was definitively identified only in the eighteenth century, any nude or nearly nude figure of the goddess would have qualified in general terms, and the *Erotes* (or *Amores*) long attributed to Lucian and cited by Aldrovandi noted specifically the gesture with which Praxiteles' goddess at once shielded and called attention to her sex.[7] Aldrovandi perhaps wisely neglected to mention the "stain" that both the Pseudo-Lucian and Pliny record a young man having left on the statue as the ultimate testimony to an obsessive love. Nonetheless, his decision to employ the Cnidian Venus to illustrate the affective power a religious image should possess seems both unusual and daring – particularly as he quotes not from Pliny's relatively sober account but from the Pseudo-Lucian's more erotically charged narrative that wittily highlights the attraction the statue could exercise on viewers of diverse sexual persuasions.[8] Aldrovandi's tone is open to interpretation; he may be teasing a scholarly friend whose tolerance he trusts, while acknowledging the importance of affect in religious art. But his eagerness to remind the cardinal of the Venus of Cnidos indicates how far ideals of the affecting image had become bound up with concepts of the alluring figure by the later sixteenth century.

The distinctive context of Aldrovandi's text is also a potent reminder of the challenges ambitious artists were increasingly forced to negotiate by the 1570s and 1580s. On the one hand, successful images had to possess the alluring power of the Cnidian Venus; indeed, modern paintings should ravish viewers with even greater force than the most beautiful ancient sculptures. The Venetian art theorist Lodovico Dolce, in a published letter from which Aldrovandi may have borrowed some of his rhetoric, celebrated precisely this achievement in the Venus of Titian's *Venus and Adonis*.[9] On the other hand, Christian paintings had to fuse this stunning affective power with piety and devotion, in forms that carried none of the "lasciviousness" that characterized the sensuous appeal of pagan cult objects – or Titian's mythologies. The gravity of this double bind for modern art had been clear from the unveiling of Michelangelo's *Last Judgment*, which made abundantly clear the extent to which the nude had come to dominate much ambitious contemporary art, even religious art. Period responses reveal that both admirers and critics remarked first on the presence of the body in the work rather than its narrative or religious meaning. Cardinal Cornaro asserted that he would offer Michelangelo "anything he wanted" for a copy of just one of the nudes, for among so many, all were in different attitudes, and all were things "one could not see elsewhere." Giovanni Andrea Gilio, meanwhile, whose *Dialogo ... degli errori ... de' pittori* of 1564 is largely aimed at the *Last Judgment*, agreed that Michelangelo "wanted to show, with so many figures, all the lovely things a body could do by means of twists and other poses" but concluded that "for this feat he cast aside reverence and devotion."[10]

By the time Aldrovandi wrote his *Avvertimenti*, the question of the nude in Christian art had become so pressing that it constitutes one of the leitmotifs of *Il Riposo*. The degree to which this concern haunts Borghini's text has facilitated the historiographic denigration of the dialogue I noted earlier.[11] Yet while Borghini is still too often simply grouped with authors like Paleotti and Gilio, the positions articulated by the interlocutors in his dialogue actually offer a range of perspectives that may alert us to critical aspects of the unquiet relation between the Florentine artistic tradition, its investment in the ideal body, and the exigencies of a changing culture. This is nowhere more apparent than in the extensive discussions of recent Florentine altarpieces in books 1 and 2, the most overtly "dialogic" of the dialogue's four books. Here the works of Bronzino provoke particularly heated discussion as paintings that are often impressive artistically, yet may fail in their religious function because of figural "lasciviousness." Bronzino is usually read as seeking to be a master of the figure – and particularly of the nude – in the great modern Florentine tradition, thereby compromising his ability to articulate a persuasive language for religious art.[12] But the responses to his altarpieces are complex and reveal that more is at stake for Borghini's interlocutors than univocal discourses of religious decorum. Attention to the varied character of the speakers and the distinctive structure of the text allows the richness of these responses, and their implications, to emerge more clearly.

Bernardo Vecchietti, the senior and often the most "conservative" interlocutor, is presented as a Florentine gentleman of sober probity who is also a collector of means and sophisticated taste. He owns the villa in *Il Riposo* and convenes the group of friends. After they have toured his impressive collections and heard about those of Sirigatti, an interlocutor who is a knight of Santo Stefano, collector, and amateur sculptor, Michelozzo asks if the hours of *villegiatura* given over each day to discourse in the shade of the garden might be structured around discussion of the arts. Michelozzo is presented disingenuously as the least knowledgeable among this group of *intenditori* but as having a great desire to learn; he actually emerges as a character with a wicked wit and a sharp eye – and tongue – when it comes to evaluating artistic merit. He thus represents both the "lay" audience of nonartists to whom Borghini explicitly directs his text and that mythic Florentine beholder of "buon occhio e cattiva lingua."[13] Baccio Valori, finally, the fourth member of the group, is a savant with a philosophical cast of mind. Vecchietti, as host and "elder statesman," is commissioned to lead the initial discussion, which is framed as a virtual tour of works in important Florentine churches and concerns "invention," or content: "those parts of painting and sculpture that pertain to philosophy, poetry, and history." This discussion dominates the remainder of book 1. A second discussion, focusing on "those things which pertain to the painter and the sculptor in the practice of their arts," will dominate book 2 and offer new perspectives on the same works; it is led by Sirigatti, the interlocutor with the greatest knowledge of artistic production. This neat division cannot in the end be strictly maintained, but one should bear it in mind when weighing the friends' remarks.

Before Vecchietti initiates the discussion of content, however, the group considers the *paragone* between sculpture and painting – and the Cnidian Venus makes a sudden appearance. The friends remark that sculptors assert that their tactile art can be appreciated even by the blind, and enlist the stories of Pygmalion and of "the Venus of Praxiteles" to demonstrate both the superiority of sculpture's mimetic effect and its overwhelming affective potential. Michelozzo takes this opportunity to reveal the character he will often assume as the dialogue develops. "Truly I do not know ... how the painters will defend themselves against such good arguments. And I, while my judgment in this has little value, would immediately attempt to place myself beside a beautiful sculpture in preference to a beautiful painting, and perhaps, like a blind person, I would find that I had more delight in it." Everyone laughs at Michelozzo's off-color repartee, and when a bantering Sirigatti carries its implications into overtly sexual territory, warning Michelozzo that a heavy marble sculpture could get him into real difficulties in bed, an important undercurrent – or really current – of this far from univocal dialogue is set in motion.[14] Notably, Vecchietti laughs with his friends here rather than assuming the censorious tone he will take in some discussions of images in churches. Further, he has recently praised the exceptional beauty of the sculpture Sirigatti is currently completing: a statue of Venus.[15] While it might be too much to say that Venus presides over the discussions in *Il Riposo*, she certainly weaves through them, a recurring motif of pleasure and beauty.

Vecchietti opens the consideration of invention by relating painting and sculpture: both are created through invention, composition, poses, parts (portions of figures), and color (for painting). He implicitly admits the artificiality of separating invention from the more "formal" aspects of art, as he tacitly acknowledges that artists may play a critical role in invention. But for Vecchietti, this characteristic of modern art and the self-confidence of ambitious modern artists has become a problem, "since it seems to me that the sculptors and the painters, taking too much license, have erred in Invention." Baccio Valori recalls the *Dialogo* of Gilio, and Vecchietti, thanking him, praises Gilio's condemnation of Michelangelo's *Last Judgment*. He initially considers the distinction Gilio drew between genres of painting, and critiques painters who mix genres in ignorant and inappropriate ways. But as the conversation turns to religious art, his remarks descend from the theoretical to focus ever more insistently on the impropriety of the nude figures that had gained new prominence in religious art in the churches of Florence since the works of Michelangelo's maturity.[16]

"Religious art" cannot be stressed enough, however; it would be a serious error to assume that Vecchietti is simply cast as an opponent of the nude

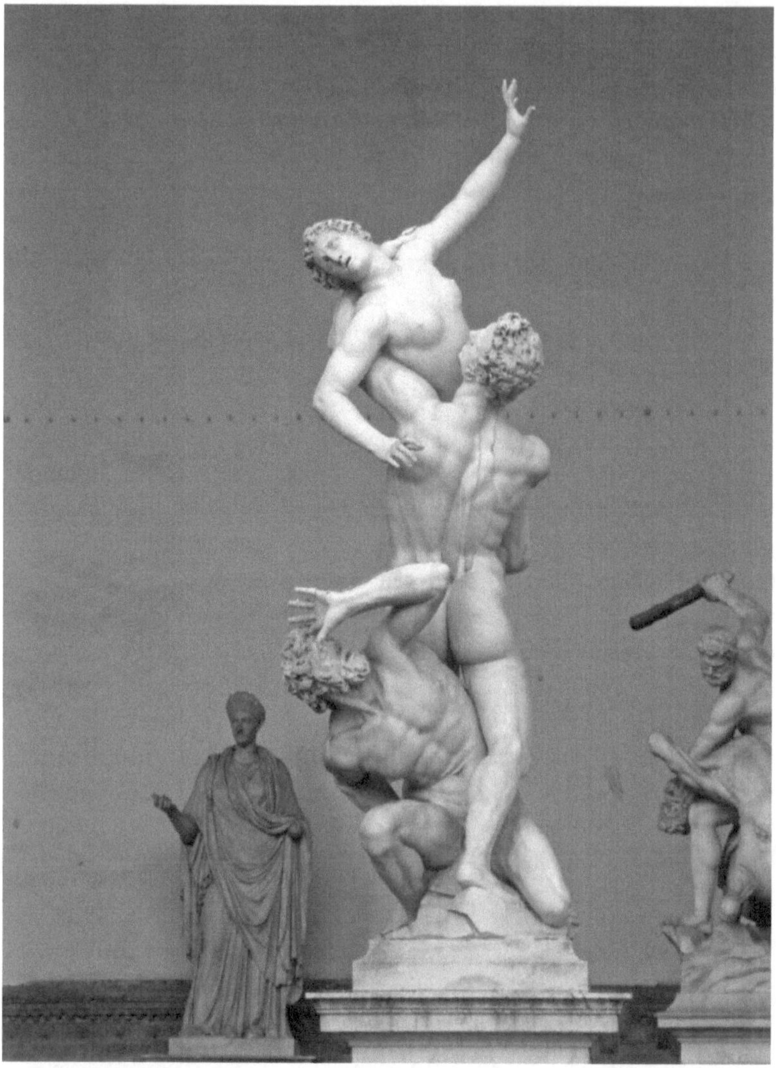

19. Giambologna, *Rape of the Sabine*, 1583. Marble. Florence, Loggia dei Lanzi. Photo: Nicolo Orsi Battaglini / Art Resource, NY.

and the *maniera moderna*. He offers an effusive encomium to Giambologna's *Rape of the Sabine* (Illustration 19), for instance, while acknowledging that this work's origin lay not in the illustration of the ostensible "subject" but in Giambologna's determination to prove himself a leading master of "all the art of nude figures." Indeed, the historical figure on whom Borghini based his character wrote five poems in praise of Giambologna's achievement, published in 1583 – just a year before *Il Riposo* – in a collection celebrating the sculpture. In the dialogue, Vecchietti recites one of his sonnets, and other interlocutors offer examples by Alamani and Pier di Gherardo Capponi. Capponi's sonnet in particular foregrounds the lovely nude as the apex of an art that is inextricably bound up with desire, the lure of the lifelike, and the pathos of the object of desire frozen into marble.[17] Further, the friends have already admired Michelangelo's cartoon for *Leda and the Swan* in Vecchietti's private collection.[18] At the villa, all could chuckle at off-color exchanges about sculptures in bed, and in the piazza they could admire Giambologna's "art." But Vecchietti demands different standards for works in churches. Altarpieces or ecclesiastical frescoes cannot privilege the discourses of art or the prowess of the maker. Scriptural or hagiographical sources must be scrupulously respected in pictorial "invention," artistic embellishments cannot obscure the clarity of the image (which must retain its venerable function as the bible of the unlettered), and figures, far from exemplifying "all the art of the nude," must move viewers to devotion, not to "lascivious thoughts."

The difficulty with Vecchietti's distinction is twofold. All the interlocutors, Vecchietti included, implicitly accept that the art of the figure – and ultimately the nude – is fundamental to the discourses of ambitious modern art. Yet most large-scale public artistic production, particularly for painting, remained religious. It is no accident that the dialogue stages a tour of the major churches of Florence as the way to see the best modern painting. Michelozzo's wry comment that he never even enters the Ognissanti because he finds a painting there so bad dramatizes the attendant problem. Public religious painting is suspended between the demands of devotion and those of the *intenditore*. By probing Vecchietti's attack on Michelozzo's delight before "the delicate members of those beautiful women" in Bronzino's *Christ in Limbo*, we can excavate more thoroughly the conundrum Borghini's characters confront:

> We have already discussed ... how incorrect sacred figures are when made so lasciviously. Now I will say to you in addition that they are out of place not only in the churches, but in any public place, for they give a bad example, and induce vain thoughts.... And how little Bronzino merits praise in this work, you yourself have shown by admitting that you delight in looking at those lascivious women; considering the softness of their members, and the *vaghezza* of the faces of those young women, one cannot help but feel some carnal stimulation, which is completely contrary to what one should experience in the temple of God.[19]

In his vehemence, Vecchietti seems to forget his own recent celebration of the *Rape of the Sabine*, certainly a composition of nudes in a "public place." He sounds unusually close here to ecclesiastical theorists such as Paleotti, who condemned nudity even in domestic secular art (much less public art), and such passages have contributed to the dialogue's indifferent reputation.[20] But Vecchietti responds emotionally to Michelozzo's outré provocation; he patently could not maintain his position, given his published praise of Giambologna. His description of the *effect* of Bronzino's painting is, meanwhile, more sophisticated than it at first appears, and it is telling that he employs *vaghezza* – which denotes a compelling loveliness that could ravish the senses of beholders – as one of his fundamental terms. As I argue in my study of Federico Barocci, the quality of *vaghezza* had become critical to modern artistic production and theoretical discourse, but it was as ambivalent as it was important, for it was freighted with sensual, even sexual, connotations. Agnolo Firenzuola, in his *Dialogo della bellezza delle donne, intitolato Celso* (1548), argues that *vaghezza* bears within it elements of *vagare*, "to wander," and *vagghegiare*, "to desire or long for." While "desire" might remain solely visual, *vagheggiare* had been used since Boccaccio to signal overt physical desire.[21] Gilio specifically attacks "the painter that delights in making the figures of saints nude" as one who values "the *vaghezza* of art ... more than propriety and appropriate decorum."[22] *Vaghezza*'s power is recognized trenchantly by Vecchietti; if one looks at Bronzino's picture, he says, one cannot help but be allured by the *vaghezza* of these figures. This is precisely the difficulty; modern art claims such "Cnidian" powers of compulsion, but in exercising them through the allure of sensuous figures it compromises its status as a vehicle for the representation of Christian mysteries.

Nonetheless, the degree to which figural *vaghezza* retained its power even in the 1580s is emblematized by the fact that Vecchietti's reproof does not prevent Michelozzo from returning to his theme a few pages later. The group, still considering altarpieces in S. Croce, turn to two by Santi di Tito – who figures in *Il Riposo* as an exemplary "devout" artist – and Vecchietti praises them "for the observation of the sacred history [and] for *honestà*," the critical areas in which modern religious images must succeed. Though Vecchietti also admires Santi as a painter, however, Michelozzo repeatedly critiques Santi's pictures precisely for want of *vaghezza*. A discussion of Santi's *Resurrection* reminds Michelozzo of the *Resurrection* by Bronzino in S. Annunziata (Illustration 20), and he derails Vecchietti's moralizing discourse by interjecting, "Having spoken of the Resurrection has made me think of a painting by Bronzino in the Annunziata which depicts this mystery." Vecchietti immediately attempts to forestall this association: "Let us please not speak of that ..., because it contains an angel that is so lascivious that it is an indecorous thing." As we will see, he must indicate the androgynous angel who stands alluringly in a *Venus pudica* pose beside Christ. Michelozzo demurs, but not before making a bold statement: "If I had such a beautiful figure in my house ..., I would admire it very much, and hold it dear."[23]

Michelozzo could be said to appeal to a "decorum of place," admiring Bronzino's figure while tacitly acknowledging that it might be more appropriate in a private domestic setting than in a public and religious one. Yet the difficulty could not be so simply resolved, as Borghini is evidently aware; despite his putative conservatism, he perpetually defers any univocal resolution to the issue of figural *vaghezza*, even in relation to public religious painting. In book 2, some eighty pages after Vecchietti has condemned Michelozzo's delight in the *vaghezza* of the young women in Bronzino's *Christ in Limbo* and his too eager interest in the angel from the

Annunziata *Resurrection*, the group comes around to the *Christ in Limbo* once more. Sirigatti is now fulfilling his commission to discuss the artistic merits and defects of many works considered under the rubric of invention in book 1. Tellingly, Sirigatti takes up the theme Michelozzo had earlier introduced: "I now turn to the panel of Bronzino representing Christ in Limbo, in which I see the most beautiful arrangement, gracious attitudes, the members of figures well understood, colors that are *vaghissimi*, beautiful flesh painting, heads very well done and drawn from life, and everything very well studied, and done with great art." Sirigatti offers somewhat more precise and technical emphases than had Michelozzo, and his stress on the colors as exemplifying *vaghezza* is critical, for it implies the possibility of a "displacement" of the allure of painting from seminude bodies toward more pictorial qualities.[24] But Sirigatti still praises the beautiful painting of flesh and the "members" of the figures that had so excited Michelozzo.

The interlocutors may be imagined to look at Michelozzo, for he immediately and coyly interjects, "I don't have anything to say about this, except that I see Messer Baccio very pleased in looking at it, as I myself am, as beautiful, and *vaga* to behold." This is a remarkable statement; his friends may be imagined to turn to Michelozzo not only because he had been attracted by the *vaghezza* of the young women in Bronzino's panel, but also because in book 2 he has had little but criticism, often harsh criticism, for nearly every work the group has discussed. Indeed, his "I don't have anything to say, except ..." seems playfully intended to make his friends expect another attack. His willingness to then accept Sirigatti's praise of the "art" of the *Christ in Limbo* without even a critique of one figure's form or pose (his most frequent strategies) locates it at the apex of the best modern Florentine painting.

In response to Michelozzo's genial but pointed probing, the reflective Baccio Valori frankly admits that he is entranced, but offers what Michelozzo will identify as a "platonic" assessment: "I take pleasure in regarding those beauties ... which were given to us by the great giver of all good things."[25] Valori here offers a variation of Vasari's defense of contemporary painting against those who interpret "the awkward and inept as devout, and the beautiful and good as lascivious, as some do, who, seeing figures of a young woman or man which are a little more *vaghe* ... than ordinary ... judge them lascivious, not being aware that they very wrongly condemn the good judgment of the painter, who holds the Saints, who are celestial, as much more beautiful than mortal nature."[26] Bronzino's painting can be made to respond to such readings, and may even attempt to stage them. The terribly contorted female demon who twists – or is twisted – in the air directly above Christ's head is certainly cast as an evil-equals-ugly, *sforzato* inversion of the graceful-and-beautiful-equals-good, or at least now redeemed, young women whose forms so arrested Michelozzo's gaze. She is also a demonic parody of

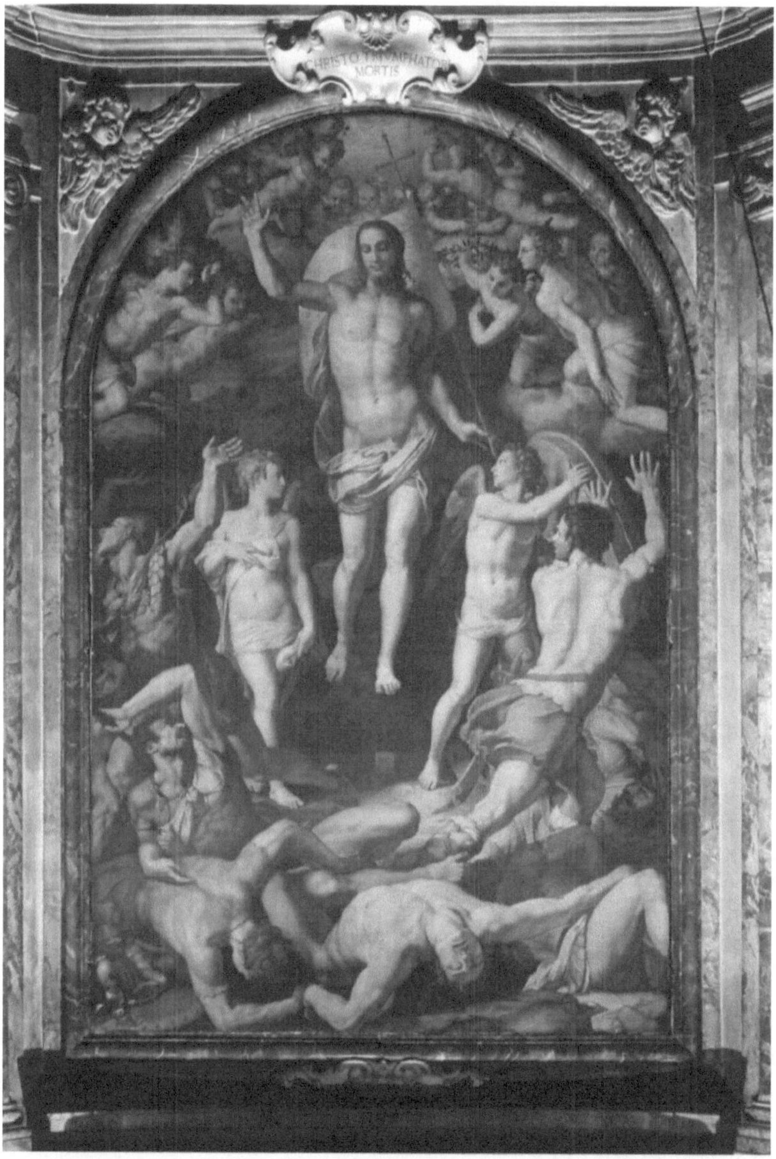

20. Agnolo Bronzino, *Resurrection*, 1552. Oil on panel, 445 × 280 cm. Florence, S. Annunziata. Photo: Scala / Art Resource, NY.

Christ's figure itself, twisted by his triumphant arrival into a pose that is a hopelessly forced exaggeration of his own. But Michelozzo, while insisting on his appreciation of Bronzino's painting, actually undercuts the possibility of maintaining Valori's (and Vasari's) position: "I like your platonic opinion ..., and if everyone could look with such intention, it would never be necessary to make sacred pictures differently; but I don't know how deeply such continence and holy thinking will impact others, or if it does, how long it can last in looking at things that so stimulate the senses." Here Vecchietti again intervenes, dismissing Michelozzo's leading question by returning the group's attention, predictably, to Santi di Tito's *Resurrection*.[27]

Michelozzo has put his finger on the difficulty of holding a "platonic" understanding of Bronzino's painting, but as he has just reminded his friends, this does not lead him to enjoy its beauties the less. Certainly, Borghini casts Michelozzo and Vecchietti as representatives of two poles among possible later-sixteenth-century responses to *terza maniera* religious painting. Yet in foregrounding these extremes, he highlights the tension that viewers could feel between desire and devotion in looking at modern altarpieces, a tension that recourse to ideals of "platonic" looking could not entirely resolve. And while Borghini is often seen as a "Reformer," and wrote after Trent's unequivocal declaration that in religious art "all forms of lasciviousness are to be avoided," he himself may not be entirely convinced by Vecchietti's "Tridentine" positions. Borghini devotes books 3 and 4 to a vast assemblage of lives of artists, both ancient and modern, often recounted with great indebtedness to Pliny and to Vasari. Sirigatti narrates the life of Bronzino. His statements – uncontested by the other interlocutors – effectively stand as the dialogue's last word on the subject. Among the works he highlights are the *Christ in Limbo* and the *Resurrection*. He celebrates without reserve the "many beautiful nudes, both male and female" in the *Christ in Limbo* and concludes that it is "done in a beautiful style, with good *disegno* and *vago colorito*." He then turns to "the panel of the Resurrection of our Lord ..., in which one sees an angel of remarkable beauty."[28] That angel, again.

Indeed, this angel seems to have achieved a sort of "cult status" among cognoscenti in late-sixteenth-century Florence. It is also celebrated without equivocation – and with its pendant figure – in Francesco Bocchi's 1591 *Le Bellezze della Città di Fiorenza*, a guidebook written by a local luminary with numerous contacts with reform circles. The following year would see the publication of Bocchi's *Opera ... sopra l'imagine miracolosa della Santissima Annunziata*, which represents an important moment in the revaluation of the "primitivi." In the *Opera ...*, Bocchi goes so far as to conclude that the late medieval *Annunciation* venerated in S. Annunziata surpasses even the works of Michelangelo and Raphael in what could be termed "the beauty of holiness."[29] Bocchi "rationalizes" this inversion of standard period notions of artistic development by asserting that the *Annunciation*'s most beautiful element, the head of the Virgin, was painted by angels as the human artist slept. Nonetheless, given his encomium of an archaic religious image, it may come as a surprise to read his appreciation of Bronzino's *Resurrection* – an altarpiece from the choir of S. Annunziata itself – in *Le Bellezze*. After describing the figure of Christ ("painted with dignity, and colored in a delightful ... manner") Bocchi proceeds: "Two angels are praised and admired, as they are of the most beautiful appearance; one of them raises the stone of the sepulcher with a gracious movement, and the other, as is fitting, is of a rare beauty, as appropriate to his angelic nature." It seems clear that this second angel, singled out for its "rare beauty" as it stands in a pose akin to that of the Cnidia, was the figure that so scandalized Vecchietti yet had entranced Michelozzo and Sirigatti and here even manages to captivate a *literato* invested in reform.[30]

Bocchi implies that viewers may appreciate the figures from a "platonic" perspective, as he stresses that their loveliness is appropriate to their "angelic nature." Indeed, elsewhere Bocchi elaborates a related mode of argument to assert that the features of Donatello's *Saint George* actually elevate and purify those who gaze upon their perfection.[31] But for a Michelozzo, the sober appreciation of figural *vaghezza* was predicated on the ability to bring *to* the experience of viewing both the appropriate philosophical and theological equipment and unshakeable piety. From Michelozzo's perspective, viewers that could attain this condition were rare, even among the most educated class. Nonetheless, both Sirigatti's final encomium to Bronzino and Bocchi's celebration of the angels in the *Resurrection* demonstrate that in the post-Tridentine years the investment of modern religious art in figural beauty and the ideal nude not only constituted an area of concern, but continued to be desired even by many moderate viewers sympathetic to ecclesiastical reform.

Sirigatti's praise, coming as it does from an amateur artist – and without any justification of the angel's appearance – points toward a further question: How might artists situate such figures in religious painting? I have already noted that Bronzino's *Christ in Limbo* could sustain and even stage a "platonic" reading, and I find much to recommend in the scholarship that perceives the sacred painting of Michelangelo and of Bronzino as enterprises in which the powers of modern art were put to work for religion. Nonetheless, we should consider seriously a remark Vasari makes in his *vita* of Michelangelo. Already in the 1550 edition of the *Lives*, Vasari offers a striking assessment of the nudes in the background of the *Doni Tondo*, who remain an interpretive conundrum for art history (Illustration 21). Following a sensitive reading of the innovative representation of the Holy Family, Vasari concludes, "Because this was not enough for Michelangelo, he made in the background ... many nudes, leaning, standing, and sitting, as a further demonstration that his art was very great." A recent study of the tondo argues once again that the nudes should be read through a Neoplatonic lens and ignores Vasari's assessment. Vasari was writing a half-century after Michelangelo's invention, and his world was very different from that of 1500. I could certainly believe that the young Michelangelo intended his *ignudi* to express something beyond the discourses of art. But it remains telling, particularly for the cultural ambient of Bronzino, that by midcentury Vasari could look back and read the *Doni Tondo* nudes exclusively as figures of art. This does not seem to have troubled Vasari in the slightest. The *Lives* went through a long process of revision and expansion during the following eighteen years, often with intervention by literary friends and advisers. The fact that the passage remains unchanged in the 1568 edition implies that none of the Florentine literati who worked with Vasari found his reading disturbing either.[32] What this may reveal about Bronzino's intentions in the *Resurrection* or the *Christ in Limbo* remains unclear – although Maurice Brock has noted perceptively that the pose of that famous angel not only is derived from the *Venus pudica* but relates as well to the *ignudi* of the *Doni Tondo*, a work much revered in midcentury Florence.[33] In any case, Vasari's comment can reveal something about the contemporary *reception* of these works, a reception that still resonates, though in a different key, some twenty years later in Borghini's dialogue.

It is a commonplace dating back to the sixteenth century that Vasari's *Lives* is at base a celebration of the Tuscan artistic tradition as the most developed and important in Italy, and a defense of it against its rivals and critics. An analogous concern may reveal the invisible thread binding Bocchi's encomium of the archaic S. Annunziata *Annunciation* to that of Bronzino's *Resurrection*; both works, different as they are, help articulate Florentine identity. The *Annunciation* was among the principal miracle-working images of the city, its great healer. Particular works by Bronzino, and particular figures in those works, presented some of the best examples in the city of a very Florentine ideal of pictorial *disegno* based on the cerebral invention of sophisticated compositions and the expert delineation of figures, often largely nude. This vision, embraced and radicalized by Michelangelo to focus exclusively on the art of the body, came to dominate an important strain of modern Florentine art. Yet this tradition had come under attack just at its apogee in Michelangelo's *Last Judgment*, and from two equally dangerous directions.

There was, of course, the damaging critique on the basis of morality and decorum. But there was also a critique that was artistic, and saw Michelangelo's overwhelming focus on *disegno* and the male nude as too limiting in an age in which the achievements of Titian and the Venetians – not to mention Raphael – demonstrated a vast new range of possibility for the modern art of painting. Bronzino himself, in altarpieces like the *Christ in Limbo* and the *Resurrection*, had attempted to (re)expand the field of the Florentine nude to include a non-Michelangelesque range of beauty. But in committing to the nude for public religious paintings, he in essence radicalized Michelangelo's already radical innovation, despite the growing controversy enveloping the *Last Judgment*. Thus, his art effectively became polemical and controversial. Yet while *Il Riposo* stages criticisms of his commitment to the nude, Borghini and other Florentine literati of the late sixteenth century seem to have perceived Bronzino's best paintings and figures as exemplars of a tradition they saw as central and understood increasingly to be under both religious and cultural assault. This is why figures such as the angel in the S. Annunziata *Resurrection* can become "icons" of modern Florentine art. And I would argue that this conviction motivates Borghini's very commitment to the dialogue as a literary form in *Il Riposo*.

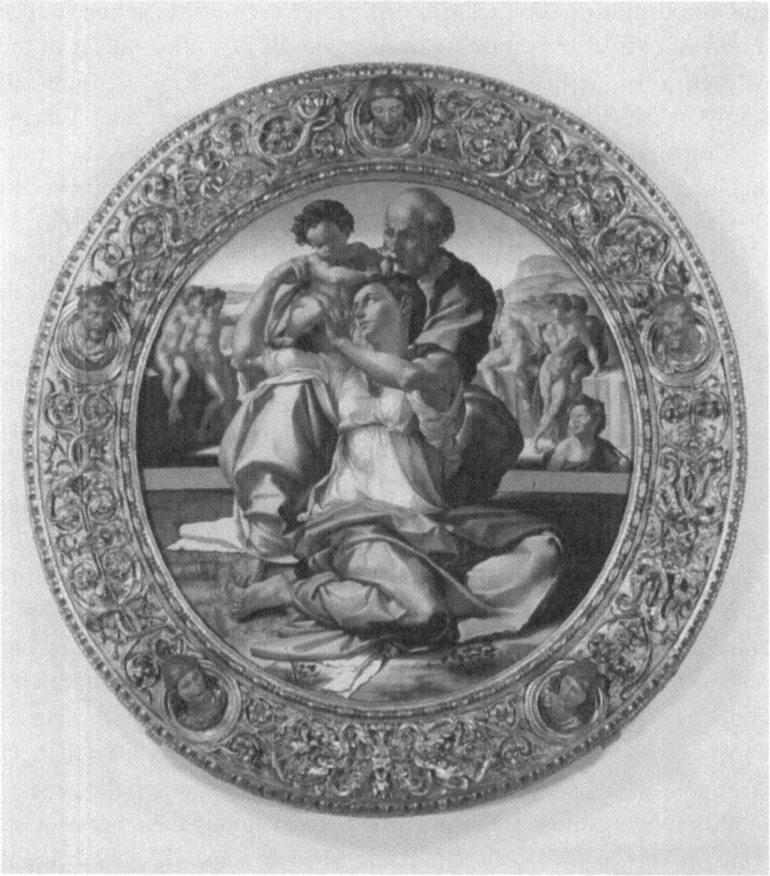

21. Michelangelo Buonarroti, *Doni Tondo*, c. 1507. Oil on panel, 173 cm diameter with original frame. Florence, Galleria degli Uffizi. Photo: Scala / Art Resource, NY.

It is easy to argue that the later sixteenth century witnessed the multiple voices of the dialogue tradition losing their fertile heterogeneity and becoming mere mouthpieces or foils for a dominant authorial persona. In the face of this historiography, Borghini's pointed refusal to articulate a univocal resolution of the religious and social questions raised by Bronzino's altarpieces, or by implication Michelangelo's ideal for religious art, stands as either a corrective or an exception that demands explanation.[34] Perhaps it is something of both.

It is difficult to "close" the dialogic form completely; even Gilio's *Dialogo* is not strictly one-dimensional. Nonetheless, the principal interlocutor, Signor Ruggiero, is a cleric, and when Signor Vincenso defends the nudes in Michelangelo's *Last Judgment* as imitations of the antique and demonstrations of "the excellence of art," Ruggiero mounts a blistering counterattack, decrying the lasciviousness of ancient religion and its imagery, which effectively silences Vincenso. There is no witty Michelozzo riposte in Gilio.[35] In the secular context, meanwhile, Lodovico Dolce's *L'Aretino* of 1557 becomes a polemical celebration of Venetian accomplishments and a refutation of the exclusive cultural primacy of Michelangelo. The Tuscan interlocutor Fabbrini is "reeducated" as the shortcomings of the Michelangelesque manner are exposed, in terms of both decorum and art (Michelangelo's over-insistent focus on the muscular nude). Fabrini, too, attempts to excuse Michelangelo's Sistine nudes as models of art and is subjected to an attack on the master's sense of appropriateness that overwhelms even his harassed "you are being too rigid and moralistic [*scrupuloso*]."[36] Yet in Borghini, the appreciation of Bronzino's figures continues to exist in tension with – and even resists – the discourses of decorum. Reformers and cognoscenti each have their say, but Vecchietti's harshest condemnations, for all the respect and stature accorded him, are not given the last word.

Indeed, Vecchietti's own position on the Florentine nude is ultimately ambiguous, and not solely because of his admiration for Giambologna's *Rape of the Sabine* or of the lovely, even "lascivious" things he treasures at his villa. Predictably, Vecchietti criticizes Bronzino's late and unusual *Martyrdom of Saint Lawrence* (Illustration 22), a monumental fresco for the Medici parish church of S. Lorenzo in which the aged master wrestled one last time with the ideals and implications inherent in Michelangelo's *Last Judgment*: "Bronzino, feeling himself to be particularly excellent in making nudes, painted the Emperor ... surrounded by his courtiers who are all nude, or with very little drapery – a thing that is extremely inappropriate to persons who serve great Princes. Likewise those Virtues, in the guise of most beautiful women, are inappropriate seated among the other people." Thus far, Vecchietti's tone is predictable. Then he adds, "[I]f nonetheless it pleased him to put them in the picture, he should have figured them in the air or in some other place set apart."[37]

These women are not nude, unlike many of the muscular young men around them. For Vecchietti, their inappropriateness inheres in their prominence in the center foreground, where they may confuse the genres of allegory and sacred history (a mixture viewed with suspicion in Gilio's dialogue) and distract from focus on the saint. And it must be admitted that barons who serve great princes do not ordinarily issue commands without their clothes. Vecchietti's critiques could thus be read as conventionally concerned with the integrity, accuracy, and decorum of the sacred narrative. But aspects of his response escape such predictable parameters. For instance, he does not condemn the nearly nude workmen – perhaps "accurate" as portrayals of workers laboring around great heat, but certainly figures that introduce a striking level of exposed flesh into a painting accessible to many viewers of various classes and levels of education. Nor does he seem disturbed by the extravagantly posed river god at the lower right, very much a figure of art in its allusions both to Michelangelo's favorite antiquity, the Belvedere Torso, and to the master's own *Day* in the Medici Chapel in the same church of S. Lorenzo. All these things – nudity, complex poses, self-conscious references to the canons of art instead of

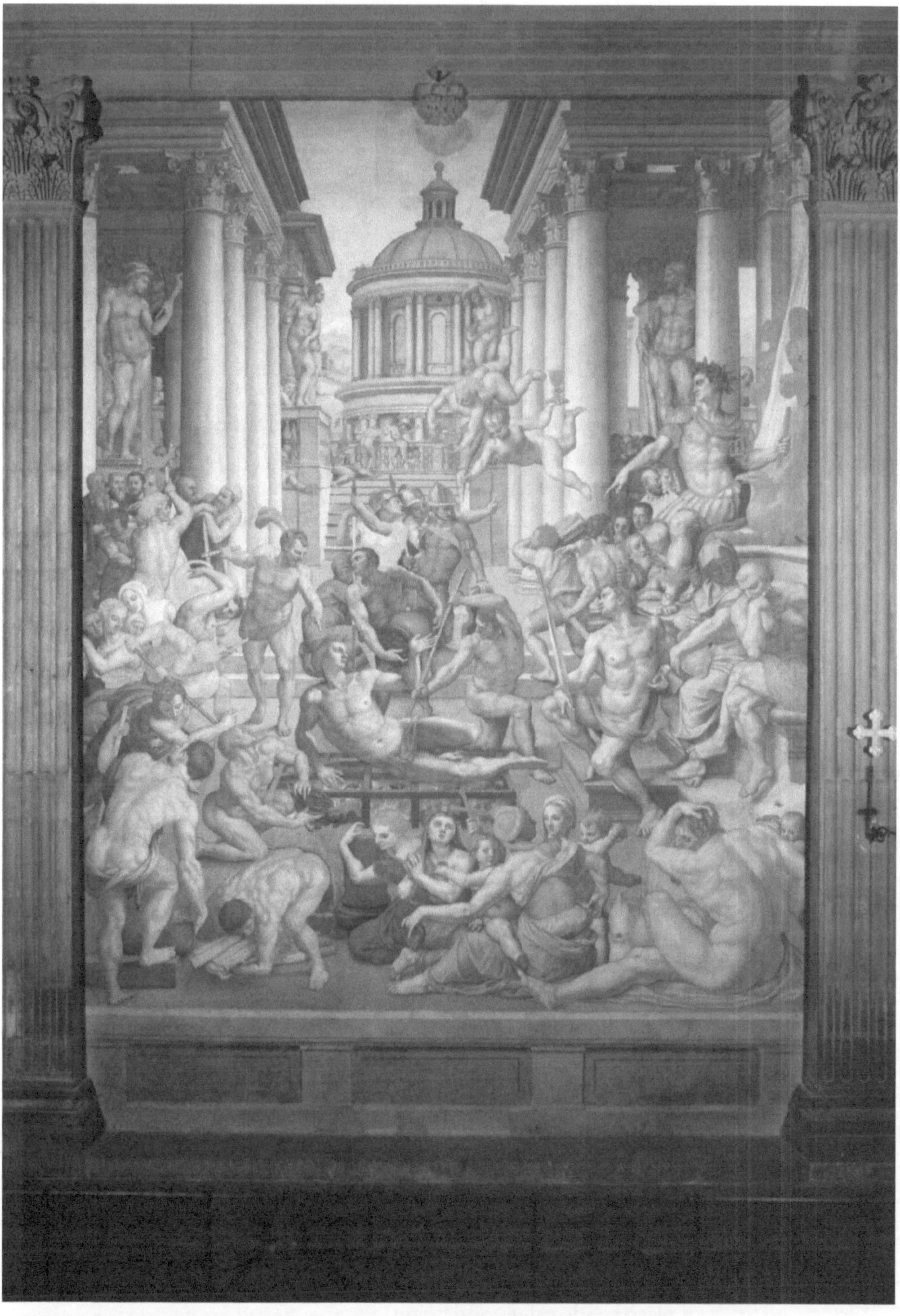

22. Agnolo Bronzino, *Martyrdom of Saint Lawrence*, 1569. Fresco. Florence, S. Lorenzo. Photo: Scala/ Art Resource, NY.

narrative clarity and pictorial decorum – would have scandalized Gilio but pass without comment for Vecchietti (it helps that the god is turned away, his genitalia thus concealed).

In addition, while the young women representing virtues are largely clothed, Vecchietti feels compelled to stress that they are "most beautiful." He virtually cannot help but look at them first as beauties, thus recalling the problem exemplified by Michelozzo's excessive admiration for the "delicate members" of the young women in Bronzino's *Christ in Limbo*. He ultimately accepts their presence, but desires their relegation to the margins of the image. Upon consideration, it becomes apparent that nearly all the figures Vecchietti implicitly accepts among the nudes here are "marginal," literally or figuratively. They may be august, as is the river god; but they are off to the side, separate from the *istoria*. Or they may be participants, as are the laborers, but in this case they are marginalized socially and morally – one remembers that Vecchietti never criticized the seminude figures of fainting and fleeing soldiers in Bronzino's *Resurrection*.[38]

Thus, even Vecchietti ultimately appears compelled to admit that figures of art, quotations from Michelangelo, and bodies by *disegno* are of import even in public religious painting in Florence.[39] It is precisely their importance, critiqued by an ecclesiastical theorist like Gilio but acknowledged by Vecchietti (and Borghini), that occasions such concern in the dialogue about finding the elusive line between artful display and inappropriateness, between lovely beauty and lasciviousness. But the forest of debate and discourse conceals the golden thread. The lack of resolution that haunts the dialogue emblematizes the fate of that Florentine pictorial tradition polemically committed to *disegno* and the body. It was a tradition that had created means that no longer clearly led to the ends still demanded of it, and it struggled to continue to conjoin the increasingly self-conscious theoretical imperatives of "art" with those of devotion. Yet these imperatives of art and taste were so bound up, from Vasari forward, with regional assertions of cultural primacy that discourses of art became as much a part of the "culture wars" transforming sixteenth-century Italy as did the period's notorious religious polemics or – in Florence – the city's political tensions under Medici rule, which Stephen Campbell perceives simmering under Bronzino's theatrical set piece in S. Lorenzo.[40] In this moment when the once dominant Florentine artistic tradition was under increasing religious and artistic pressure, even elite Florentines preoccupied by religious decorum might evince the desire to collect, display, assert, and preserve distinctive glories of Florentine artistic accomplishment: *disegno*, the ideal nude, the power, beauty, and primacy of the figure. Issues of cultural identity were of such import that they could retain and even reassert a place beside values of religion.

Bronzino himself, and certainly Michelangelo before him, may have still believed that there was no necessary contradiction between these impulses: the *forza dell'arte*, the "power of art" and of Florentine *disegno*, might still in their minds provide compelling contours for devotion. The Portuguese artist Francisco de Hollanda, who came to know and admire Michelangelo in Rome, wrote *Dialogues on Painting* during the 1540s that cast Michelangelo as a principal character. De Hollanda's Michelangelo argues explicitly that his style generates the ultimate religious art, as it stimulates a profound intellectual contemplation that can elevate beholders into considerations beyond the simple pieties of tears and pleas that characterized the uneducated and unreflective response to typical devotional images. He goes so far as to link what might be termed an "elite" devotion with the arduous sublimity of his style: "[F]or with wise persons nothing causes devotion to ... arise more than the difficulty of the perfection which unites itself with and joins God."[41] One could imagine a persuasive reading of the *Doni Tondo* that depended equally on de Hollanda's statement and Vasari's, and found no contradiction between them. But by Borghini's time, frustration and hesitation had overtaken Michelangelesque self-assuredness, as cultural and artistic fissures began to fragment the unity Bronzino might still have sought in a painting like the *Christ in Limbo*. Discourses of art and discourses of devotion were both critical. The one was not yet replacing the other; reading *Il Riposo* as revealing the "secularization of art" would be facile and deeply insufficient. But the parameters of an effective synergy between art and devotion were in these years increasingly unclear in Florence, and their relation to one another was confused and easily compromised. For Borghini, only adherence to the open form of the dialogue could both effectively stage and to some extent disguise and contain the uncertain forces in play.

Notes

1 Borghini (1584), 202: "Io non vo mai in cotesta chiesa [replicò il Michelozzo] ch'io non perda il gusto della pittura."
2 Borghini (1584), 109–10; see n. 19 for excerpts of the Italian.
3 Borghini (1584), 187; see nn. 25 and 27 for the Italian.
4 Elizabeth Cropper and Stephen Campbell, in particular, have highlighted these issues; see Cropper (1995); Campbell (2005, 2006).
5 Shearman (1967), 165–70, noted the importance of poetic and rhetorical theory in the thought of some of these writers. See further Dempsey (1982), 55–75, with particular reference to Giovanni Andrea Gilio. More generally, John O'Malley (2000) and others have stressed that the so-called Counter-Reformation was far less monolithic culturally than has been assumed.
6 Aldrovandi (1962), 511–17, 515. Given space constraints, I have reproduced only critical portions of original texts that are easily available. Aldrovandi's climax here is: "E dalla bellezza di questa statua impazzito ..., ogni ora più s'accendeva il suo amore verso tanto bella e graziosa statua. E se una statua di marmo scolorita faceva questo effetto, che dovranno poi fare le colorite e dipinte al vivo?"
7 Haskell and Penny (1981), 330–31. For the text of the Pseudo-Lucian, see *Lucian* (1967).

8 *Lucian* (1967), 168–79. Aldrovandi also adapts his source by eliding the admiring exclamation of Charicles, a speaker in the *Amores*, with the obsessive behavior of the earlier admirer who had stained the statue.

9 Dolce's letter, to Alessandro Contarini, was published in *Lettere di diversi eccellentissimi huomini*, ed. Lodovico Dolce (Venice, 1559); it is reproduced in *Dolce* (2000), 212–17 (quotation 216–17): "Ne è maraviglia, che se una statua di marmo pote in modo con gli stimuli della sua bellezza penetrar nelle midolle d'un giovane, ch'ei vi lasciò la macchia: hor, che dee far questa, che è di carne; ch'è la beltà istessa; che par, che spiri?" An important discussion is offered by Cropper (1995), 187–90.

10 "[P]erché egli più s'è voluto compiacere de l'arte ... che de la verità del soggetto, et ... vedendosi innanzi sì largo campo da mostrare, in tanta moltitudine di figure, tutto quello che vagamente può fare un corpo umano per via di sforzi e d'altri posamenti, non ha voluto perdere l'occasione...; e per questo fare ha messa da banda la devozione, la riverenza, la verità istorica e l'onore che si deve a questo importantissimo e gran mistero." Gilio (1961), 55–56. Cardinal Cornaro's appreciation is recorded in a letter of Nino Sernini, an agent of the Gonzaga, written shortly after the fresco was unveiled: "Ma il rmo Cornaro che è stato lungamente a vederla ha detto bene, dicendo che se Michelagnolo gli vuol dare in un quadro solamente dipinta una di quelle figure gli la vuol pagare quello ch'esso gli dimanderà, et ha ragione per essere al creder mio cose che non si possono vedere altrove" (text in Chastel 1984, 278). Gilio's critique echoes Sernini's conclusion that Michelangelo "put all of his effort into making imaginative figures in diverse attitudes."

11 The incisiveness of *Il Riposo* has been questioned at least since Schlosser (1996), 351. (Schlosser does, however, recognize the work's historical importance.) Some recent scholars have begun to reconsider one-dimensional readings of Borghini; see, e.g., Frangenberg (1990), esp. 77–102; and Hall (1999), 247–48.

12 While Bronzino's commitment to the Florentine tradition is habitually read in terms of the emulation of Michelangelo and Pontormo, the catalogue accompanying the important 2010–11 exhibition in Florence has argued for a Bronzino invested in a very un-Michelangelesque imitative practice focused on the "life-like" and grounded in portraiture; see Falciani and Natali (2010). The catalogue became available after this essay was submitted, and thus I can incorporate its insights only sparingly. I find the reorientation of Bronzino studies invigorating and in many respects convincing. In the context of Florentine literary responses to Bronzino's major public religious works, however, the question of the nude and *disegno* continues to occupy a critical position, and in Borghini both criticism and praise of his religious works frequently focus on the art of the body, which is explicitly associated with artists such as Michelangelo and Pontormo.

13 The phrase is Vincenzo Borghini's; see Shearman (1992), 44, citing Wazbinski (1977), 15. Borghini (2007), 42, reads Michelozzo as a foil for his sophisticated friends (though he argues that Borghini "rather clumsily" attempts to have him develop in the course of books 1 and 2). While this may be the ostensible scenario – and Michelozzo often professes ignorance of specialized points – the dialogue is effectively self-subversive, as Michelozzo's critical barbs leave deep and lasting effects. He is, as well, a conduit for received opinion (almost always critical) of a number of works.

14 Borghini (1584), 28–29.

15 Borghini (1584), 11, 22.

16 See Borghini (1584), 53–81, for a general discussion; critiques of impropriety remain a leitmotif in the discussions of specific paintings that follow from p. 81 through the remainder of book 1, and recur occasionally in book 2. For Gilio and genre, see Dempsey (1982), 55–75.

17 For Vecchietti's praise and reading of the statue's origins, Borghini (1584), 71–73; for the sonnets, 165–69.

18 Borghini (1584), 13.

19 Borghini (1584), 109–10. The critical passages read: "Io mi son fermo, disse il Michelozzo, dinanzi alla tavola del Bronzino ..., e sento grandissimo piacere nel rimirare le dilicate membra di quelle belle donne. Di già habbiam noi ragionato, rispose il Vecchietto, quanto mal fatto sia, le figure sacre fare così lascive.... Perciò quanta poca laude meriti il Bronzino in cotesta opera, voi medesimo dilettandovi nel rimirare quelle donne lascive il confessate; e io son sicuro che ciascuno che si ferma attento à rimirare questa pittura; considerando la morbidezza delle membra, e la vaghezza del viso di quelle giovani donne, non possa fare di non sentire qualche stimolo della carne, cosa tutta al contrario di quello, che nel santo Tempio di Dio far si doverebbe."

20 For Paleotti, see Biancani (1997).

21 For an extended discussion of *vaghezza*, see Lingo (2008), esp. 125–42, with further references (for Firenzuola's importance, 126; for *vagheggiare* in Boccaccio and early modern dictionaries, 127).

22 Gilio (1961), 80: "Tenga per fermo il pittor che far si diletta le figure de' santi nude, che sempre gli leverà gran parte de la riverenza che se li deve. Però compiacciasi più tosto de l'onestà e del convenevol decoro, che de la vaghezza de l'arte." Dempsey (1982) has stressed Gilio's indebtedness to theories of literary decorum.

23 While the angel is androgynous and in a pose that recalls a famous female nude, Bronzino conceived the figure as male; both angels reveal their genitals in the highly finished *modello* in the Uffizi (Gabinetto Disegni e Stampi 13843F; see Brock 2002, 276, for illustration). This was evidently perceived as requiring adjustment in the finished painting. The quotation is Borghini (1584), 116: "Digratia non ne parliamo, replicò il Vecchietto, perche vi è un Agnelo tanto lascivo, che è cosa disconvenevole. S'io havessi cotesta bella figura in casa, disse il Michelozzo, io la estimerei molto, e ne terrei gran conto per una delle piu dilicate, e morbide figure, che veder si possano." Michelozzo occasionally praises Santi; the *Raising of Lazarus* in S. Maria Novella, for instance, is "molto bello" as well as "molto honesto." In book 2, however, Michelozzo cannot resist disparaging its *colorito* as "non ... troppo commendabile"; Borghini (1584), 106, 198.

24 Borghini (1584), 187: "[M]e ne passero alla tavola del Bronzino rappresentante Christo nel Limbo, in cui veggo una bellissima dispositione, attitudini gratiose, membra bene intese, colori vaghissimi, belle carnagioni, teste molto ben fatte, ritratte dal naturale, e tutta molto studiata, e fatta con grand'arte." For an extended discussion of Barocci's experiments with the "displacement" of *vaghezza* from represented bodies into more pictorial qualities such as color, see Lingo (2008), 125–242. Period praise of Bronzino as a colorist is a recurrent theme in Falciani and Natali (2010).

25 Borghini (1584), 187: "Io non ho sopra questa che dir cosa alcuna, rispose il Michelozzo, oltre à che veggo M. Baccio molto compiacersi in rimirarla,

talche ancor io, come bella, e vaga la riguardo. Io mi compiaccio à rimirar quelle bellezze, soggiunse incontanente il Valori, che à noi dal sommo donatore di tutti i beni furono donate, perche con mezi convenevoli le rimirassimo: e considero à così dono quanto al donatore siamo obligati."

26 Vasari (1966–87), *Testo*, 3: 274–75: "Ma io non vorrei già che alcuno s'ingannasse interpretando il goffo et inetto, devoto, et il bello e buono, lascivo, come fanno alcuni, i quali vedendo figure o di femina o di giovane un poco più vaghe e più belle et adorne che l'ordinario, la pigliano sùbito e giudicano per lascive, non si avedendo che a gran torto dannano il buon giudizio del pittore, il quale tiene i Santi e Sante, che sono celesti, tanto più belli della natura mortale."

27 Borghini (1584), 187: "[M]i piace la vostra platonica opinione, replicò il Michelozzo, e se ciascuno con tale intentione le rimirasse, non accaderebbre far le pitture sacre altramente; ma non so come questa continenza, e questo santo pensiero in altri trapassasse, ò trapassato lungamente (mirando cose che tanto allettano il senso) si durasse." Frangenberg (1990), 101, notes this passage but reads Michelozzo (and Borghini) as taking Valori seriously: "Michelozzo nimmt Valoris Auffassung Ernst, in irdischer Schönheit werde ihre göttliche Quelle erkennbar; auch in anderen Schriften operiert Borghini mit neoplatonischer Theorie." I would read the riposte as deeply ironic.

28 Borghini (1584), 536: "In Santa Croce alla Cappella degli Zanchini fece poi la tavola ..., dipignendovi Christo disceso al Limbo per trarne i Santi Padri, dove sono ignudi bellissimi, e maschi, e femine in diverse attitudini, e gratiose." For the *Resurrection*, see 537: "È di sua mano parimente la tavola della Resurretione del nostro Signore posta dietro al coro della Nuntiata alla Cappella de'Guadagni, in cui si vede un'Angelo di tutta bellezza." Frangenberg (1990), 101–102, is virtually alone in noting that the series of discussions of Bronzino's altarpieces concludes not with the criticisms well known in modern historiography, but with this positive assessment. As this issue is not his focus, however, he does not probe Borghini's choices and concludes that, while the dialogue leaves Borghini's beliefs unclear, Vecchietti often appears as the figure of greatest authority. This may be – but I would argue that it is significant that Borghini does not "allow" Vecchietti to object to Sirigatti's encomium. See also Borghini (2007), 738–39, for a brief discussion without interpretation.

29 See Bocchi (1592), esp. 71. For a discussion of the work and of Bocchi's ties to reform thinkers, see Wazbinski (1987).

30 Bocchi (1971), 226–27: "Sono lodati due Angeli, e si come sono di sembiante bellissimo, ammirati; uno de' quali alza la pietra del sepolcro con movenza graziosa: e l'altro, come conviene, è di bellezza rara, e conforme à sua natura di vero angelica." For Bocchi's taste and *campanalismo*, see Shearman's introduction (n.p.). Tellingly, when Bocchi's guide was significantly revised by Giovanni Cinelli in 1677, the passage was retained, despite the fact that Cinelli frequently added editorial critiques of Bronzino and painters of his generation; see Bocchi and Cinelli (2004), 443–44, 145, for a critical editorial addition to Bocchi's description of Bronzino's *Noli me tangere* in Santo Spirito. Williams (1989), 116, has noted that Bocchi himself (as one might expect) often expressed reservations about "mannerist" painting.

31 See Williams (1989), esp. 120; and Barasch (1975).

32 Vasari (1966–87), 6: 13–14, 22: "Né bastando questo a Michele Agnolo, per mostrar maggiormente l'arte sua esser grandissima, fece nel campo di questa

opera molti ignudi, appoggiati, riti et a sedere." A recent study of the tondo is Stefaniak (2008).

33 Brock (2002), 283. In a letter of 17 August 1549, Anton Francesco Doni advises a friend to spare no effort to see the tondo, by the "master of masters." See Bottari (1822), 347.

34 For the understanding that the dialogue became increasingly empty of real debate during the later sixteenth and seventeenth centuries, see, e.g., Cox (1992). A detailed treatment of post-Tridentine censorship and the defense of the dialogue is found in Snyder (1989), 87–133. (It should be noted that historians of dialogue tend to perceive the "Counter-Reformation" as only one among multiple cultural forces putting pressure on what Cox terms the "open dialogue.")

35 Gilio (1961), 37.

36 See Dolce (2000), 161–65 (Fabbri's objection, 162).

37 Borghini (1584), 62: "[I]l Bronzino, che sentendosi molto valere nel fare ignudi, ha fatto l'imperadore ... intorniato da' suoi baroni tutti nudi, o con pochi panni ricoperti: cosa molto disconvenevole a persone, che servano superbi Principi; siccome ancora mal vi si convengono quelle virtù, in forme di bellissime donne, a sedere fra l'altra gente: e se pure gli piaceva il farlevi, doveva in aria o in altro luogo separato figurarle."

38 The one – striking – exception to this observation is the figure of St. Lawrence himself. It is remarkable that Vecchietti voices no criticism of this central, nearly nude and highly artful figure. While Lawrence's relative nudity may be rationalized by the logic of the *istoria*, his marmoreal elegance would have scandalized Gilio even if it could be excused as a visualization of the saint's urbane wit and apparent imperviousness to pain, qualities celebrated in his hagiography.

39 Ironically, in book 2, Michelozzo offers what for him is unusually harsh artistic criticism of Bronzino when he identifies the *Martyrdom* – despite Sirigatti's unequivocal praise – as the product of an elderly, failing artist; see Borghini (1584), 196. Other occasional *artistic* critiques of Bronzino occur, e.g., 194 (the *Resurrection*), 196 (the *Martyrdom of Saint Lawrence*), and 203 (the *Noli me tangere*). Elizabeth Cropper (2010), while stressing the subtlety of the dialogue, reads Borghini as marking the beginning of a decline in Bronzino's fortunes (esp. 24–25). I would agree, but focus here on the repeated attempts in the text to safeguard critical aspects and figures characteristic of Bronzino's art at its best from the growing disaffection with *maniera moderna* religious painting. As I have attempted to demonstrate, Bocchi continues and develops this strategy, leading him at times to make apparently surprising statements.

40 Campbell (2004).

41 See De Hollanda (1903), 240. This and related passages are discussed in Nagel (2000), 192–93. My point is not that De Hollanda directly reflects Michelangelo's views; his text rather provides intriguing period parameters for possible receptions of Michelangelesque art. Agoston (2006), 135–67, has offered a compelling case that De Hollanda cannot be read as a "transcription."

CENSURE AND CENSORSHIP IN ROME, c. 1600

THE VISITATION OF CLEMENT VIII AND THE VISUAL ARTS

Opher Mansour

THE REIGN OF Clement VIII (Ippolito Aldobrandini, 1592–1605) is a notable period of artistic achievement. Caravaggio, Annibale Carracci, and Rubens were all active in Rome during these years, when they produced works that reformulated the sensuous appeal of the religious image. Their syntheses of naturalistic effects and reinvented traditions proved tremendously influential, both in their own right and as precursors of the baroque style.

These achievements, though, bore little relation to direct papal patronage, a fact that is notable in light of the scale and ambition of Clement's artistic projects.[1] These included the rebuilding of the Lateran, the decoration of St. Peter's Basilica, the frescoing of the main audience chamber of the Vatican Palace, support for Cardinal Baronio's restoration of early Christian churches, and other preparations for the Jubilee of 1600.[2] For the largest projects, Clement mostly favoured Giuseppe Cesari, Cavaliere d'Arpino.[3] His most visible patronage, in the mode established by Sixtus V (1585–90), was coherent and purposeful in seeking to project an image of a resurgent Catholicism, with the city of Rome as a living monument to its unbroken historical and apostolic legitimacy.

Clement's artistic patronage did not quite share the ambitions of popes such as Paul III (1534–49) and Urban VIII (1623–44), who accrued cultural prestige by virtually monopolizing the output of the most famous artists. His apparent indifference to the nascent Accademia di San Luca is also notable; the example of contemporary Florence, where the Medici carefully fostered the Accademia del Disegno to enhance their prestige, was not followed in Rome.[4] Accordingly, when collectors like Giulio Mancini and Vincenzo Giustiniani surveyed painting in the city, they saw competing schools and divergent stylistic tendencies.[5] Papal patronage and cultural priorities impinged little on their classification or ranking of these schools.

This essay will argue that the creative diversity of art in Rome around 1600 was due in part to the contradictions of curial cultural politics, which expressed themselves not only through patronage and the embrace of particular artists and artistic tendencies, but also through censorship and through internal and external constraints that precluded the papacy from either wholly rejecting or embracing the sacred art of the Renaissance and its legacy. Its main subject will be the visitation of Roman churches that Clement conducted, which provides the best available guide to his, and his closest collaborators', attitudes to that legacy.

In his influential *Likeness and Presence*, Hans Belting argued for a historical "Crisis of the Image" associated with the Reformation, in which rival conceptions of the image as both a sacred and an artistic object became increasingly difficult to reconcile.[6] In Catholic Italy, the outcome was a synthesis, in which images presented "a double face ... as receptacles of the holy or as expressions of art."[7] Art historians who have examined the intricacies of this synthesis, such as Alexander Nagel in his study of Michelangelo, Stuart Lingo in his monograph on Barocci, and Marcia Hall in *The Sacred Image*, have often approached it from the creative perspective of the artist or, like Gauvin Bailey, by examining the devotional and theological preferences of the patrons.[8] This essay approaches the same problematic from an alternative and often neglected direction: that of the censor, a perspective that draws attention to the limits of consensus and to the difficulty of imposing unity on a society whose conceptions of both the sacred and cultural functions of the image were complex, varied, and evolving.

Clement VIII and his contemporaries were the legatees not only of the art of the Renaissance, but also, as detailed in the introduction to this volume, of a body of theoretical and moralistic writings that sought to define the place of the Renaissance in the reformed, post-Tridentine Church. The *querelle* over Michelangelo's *Last Judgment* ran on into the 1590s.[9] Concurrently, a stream of publications by clerics, including Carlo Borromeo, Gabriele Paleotti, and Johannes Molanus, sought to fill out the grey areas present in the Council of Trent's rulings concerning sacred images.[10] Naturally, the differences of opinion among these writers, and even between them and their antagonists, are much less pronounced than those between Catholic and Protestant polemicists. But even within the Catholic fold there was room for debate. At issue in these writings were questions about the relative claims of devotional efficacy and artistic sophistication; the significance of style; the authority of scriptural texts; the proper scope of painterly *invenzione*; the licitness of classical subjects and forms; the proper relations of painting to their sites and audiences; and the autonomy of artists and patrons vis-à-vis ecclesiastical authority.

The policies of censorship adopted during Clement VIII's reign, and in particular those that accompanied his visitation in the 1590s, provide insight into the degree to which these debates influenced the Curia and the extent to which its members were prepared to impose their views on Catholics who did not share their interpretation of artistic reform. The tension between religious and artistic imperatives emphasized by Belting is only one strand of the muted tensions that emerge from a close reading of the visitation records. As Pamela Jones has shown, responses to sacred art, and particularly altarpieces, in Roman churches were "as varied as members of Catholic society themselves."[11] Some of these variations owed as much if not more to differing cultic practices, to a sense of history and place, a particular personal or communal devotion, or a differing sense of decorum, as to an attachment to a particular aesthetic of religious representations. It is within this matrix of values and responses that Clement's visitation acquires its significance as an art historical study.

The importance of the visitation to the history of the visual arts is sometimes expressed in terms of scale, emphasizing the extent of the destruction and repression it wrought.[12] Such an assessment is only partially true. Clement issued hundreds of instructions mandating the repair and outfitting of chapels, the completion of church decorations, the movement of obstructive altars, and the removal of structures that obscured religious images. This aspect of the visitation says much about Clement's ambition to provide decorous, well-maintained, and clearly organized sacred spaces. However, it has less to say about how his vision of reform stood in relation to the devotional and artistic preferences of others. This emerges only in cases where the pope either encountered resistance or voiced particular objections to the works of art whose removal, modification, or destruction he ordered. These instances, in which some principle of expression or belief is at stake, can justifiably be called censorship. The visitation's records, however, allow us to identify only a relatively small number of them. In this essay, I focus on fourteen instances in which questions of artistic expression were at stake.

Questions of artistic censorship are sometimes approached in a quantitative spirit, on the assumption that it is their scale, thoroughness, and harshness that best reveal the efficacy, or lack thereof, of the post-Tridentine Church. Such an approach aligns the study of artistic censorship with wider debates surrounding the extent and significance of censorship of the printed word.[13] However, the question of coercive censorship's efficacy captures only part of its historical significance. Art history, as a discipline, has traditionally been sensitive to questions of the value, significance, and prestige of particular art objects, artistic styles, and the artists who produced them. The perceived relation to the demands of patrons and of religious and political authorities has played a part in determining how artworks produced within their purview are perceived. The paintings of Scipione Pulzone or Federico Barocci, for example, are often perceived as exemplary attempts to visualize the values of reformed Catholic spirituality; the work of Bernini as answering to the dual spiritual and political claims of the papacy; and the paintings of Caravaggio (not without controversy) as oppositional to ecclesiastical authority. If one accepts that Roman society in the period around 1600 was, within limits, pluralistic and that it comprised different publics who viewed and valued works of art in overlapping but divergent ways, then the ways in which these groups defined, reproduced, disseminated, and valorized their particular visual cultures within what might be referred to as an early modern public sphere become a factor in explaining the historical significance of contemporary artworks.[14]

In this context, an event such as the visitation is significant not only for its concrete effects, but for its discursive ones, as a series of symbolic acts aimed at asserting the dominance of a particular interpretation of artistic and religious norms. Put another way, the visitation shows us not only what Clement VIII did to control religious art, but also what values he sought to foster in this regard within the Curia and how he communicated the (un)acceptability of deviating from those norms to a wider Roman public.

Canonical visitation, a practice of ancient derivation, was greatly reinvigorated by the Council of Trent. The Council called for biennial visitation of dioceses, to promote "sound and orthodox doctrine ... maintain good morals, and ... animate the people."[15] Visitation carried with it the authority to examine and discipline clergy as well as the duty to inspect, maintain, and improve the fabric of churches – to which end the authority of visitors to determine "the ornaments of the church" was placed over the rights of patrons.[16] Trent also vested most powers of visitation in bishops. In the years following the Council, the visitations undertaken by Carlo Borromeo in his Archdiocese of Milan became a model for Reformers. The influence of Borromeo's pastoral example was amplified not only by his fame and prestige, but also by the publication of the *Acta Ecclessia Mediolanensis* in 1582.[17] This incorporated his instructions for visitation, as well as the related text of the *Instructiones Fabricae et Suppellectilis Ecclesiasticae* originally published in 1577.[18] The proliferation and intensification of visitation in the years after the Council made it a key vehicle for the promulgation of its reforms; it has, accordingly, been extensively studied as an instrument of *Sozialdisciplinierung*.[19] The record of Clement's visitation, however, also provides ample evidence for the applicability of "negotiation" (as outlined in the introduction to this volume) as a model for understanding this particular instance of Catholic Reform – at least so far as art is concerned.

Despite the Council's injunctions, visitation in Rome itself had been sporadic since 1564.[20] Thus, Clement VIII was responding to neglect when he promulgated the bull *Speculatores Domus Israel*, establishing the Congregation for the Visitation, on 8 June 1592.[21] In aiming to promote "the veneration of divine things, the maintenance of good morals, correction of errors and the arousal of piety among men," Clement largely reiterated the injunctions of Trent. In practice, by selecting monastic and collegial institutions for inspection, he emphasized the morality and piety of the clergy as his visitation's principal goal.[22] While these criteria largely governed the selection of churches for visitation (see Appendix), Clement would also pay close attention to the fabric and decoration of Rome's houses of worship. *Speculatores* equated the physical upkeep and orderliness of the Church's literal "houses" with the spiritual welfare of the larger "Domus Israel" itself. Though the visitation's activities directly concerned Rome, one of Clement's aims was to make the cleansing of the city an example for the wider Church. Accordingly, the visitation of the four major basilicas was a priority, and the visitation can also be seen as a prelude to the Jubilee of 1600.

While Clement's predecessors and successors were willing to delegate most of the work of visitation to trusted subordinates, this visitation was notable for the extent of the pope's personal involvement. Between 1592 and 1596, he personally led all inspections of buildings and clergy – often requiring repeated visits. His assiduity did not escape the notice of observers, such as the Venetian ambassador, Paolo Paruta, who noted that Clement attended to the visitation of churches as if he actually were a bishop with a single diocese.[23] The chronicler Teodoro Ameyden noted that Clement went so far as to endanger his health in the pursuit of his goals.[24]

One of those goals, as Paruta understood it, was to acquire a reputation for personal goodness.[25] Clement's ecclesiastical career as canon lawyer and diplomat had afforded little scope for demonstrative piety. The visitation allowed him an opportunity to prove himself as a loving and rigorous pastor. Thanks to the example of Carlo Borromeo, this was a role that projected an aura of personal sanctity and of adherence to the cause of reform.[26] Clement's visitation was, accordingly, a very public affair, accompanied by masses, *quarant'ore* devotions, and sermons to assembled clergy; it was closely watched by *avvisi* writers and diplomatic observers.[27] Its decrees, including the censorious ones, must be understood not only as precisely focused attempts to effect change, but also as public, performative acts meant to advertise the reforming character of Clement's papacy.

One corollary of the strongly personal nature of this visitation, of Clement's determination to attend to minutiae, and of the need to balance visitation with his other duties, is that it proceeded slowly. Between 1592 and 1598, the pope inspected 28 churches (see Appendix).[28] By contrast, Cardinal Antonio Barberini would inspect 339 on behalf of Urban VIII between 1624 and 1632.[29]

But while keeping close control of the enterprise, Clement did not act alone. The visitation also comprised (initially) four cardinals, three bishops, and a small staff of theological consultants, a secretary, notary, and legal officers.[30] Of the cardinals, one, Girolamo Rusticucci, the longtime vicar general of Rome, was a member by virtue of his office – the visitation's responsibilities overlapped with that of the vicariate.[31] The identity of the remaining members indicates that the senior echelon of the visitation drew heavily on members of two highly influential and intertwined reforming circles: that of the late Carlo Borromeo, and the friends and followers of Filipo Neri. Thus, in addition to Mariano Pierbenedetti, the cardinals included Alessandro de Medici, a close friend of Neri and Agostino Valier, who was closely tied to both Borromean and Oratorian groups.[32] Of the bishops, Lewis Owen was a former vicar general to Carlo Borromeo and a direct link to the Milanese visitations, while Ludovico de Torres was closely associated with the Oratorian circle and with Cardinal Baronio.[33] As the visitation progressed, this orientation was strengthened by the addition to the visitors' ranks of Carlo Borromeo's nephew and successor, Federico Borromeo, who likewise enjoyed very close links to the Oratory;[34] so did Silvio Antoniano, who became the visitation's secretary.[35]

To guide them, the visitors had a copy of the *Acta Ecclesia Mediolanensis*, which the Oratorian Pompeo Pateri obtained for them at Owen's suggestion.[36] The *Acta*, which incorporated the text of Borromeo's *Instructiones*, contained extensive prescriptions regulating the physical fabric, layout, and equipping of churches. Its attention to the imagery of sacred art was comparatively brief – though not without influence on Clement, several of whose decrees on religious imagery correspond to principles enunciated in the *Instructiones*. Equally if not more revealing of the visitors' thinking is Federico Borromeo's *De Pictura Sacra*, a text that engages far more closely with the visual representation of the sacred and whose composition, as both Barbara Agosti and Pamela Jones have argued, probably began in the 1590s.[37] A number of overlaps between Federico's views in *De Pictura* and the decrees of Clement's visitation strengthen this argument and suggest that *De Pictura* was, in part, a reflection of Borromeo's experiences as a visitor.

While the corrective censorship of existing church art takes up only a small proportion of the visitation's decrees, it is clear from other forms of censorship that Clement issued concurrently that the regulation of religious imagery did play a distinct part in his vision of episcopal reform. Rusticucci, as Clement's vicar general, issued a decree in 1593 requiring the preventive censorship of new church art, which was later reissued by Camillo Borghese in 1603.[38] Another papal official, the master of the Sacred Palace, oversaw the licensing and censorship of prints.[39] While a full examination of these developments is beyond the scope of this essay, the relatively spare use of corrective censorship must be assessed within this broader context of regulation.

The greater part of Clement's censures concerned images that were deemed problematic for their nudity or lasciviousness – a concern that applied to male, female, and angelic bodies alike. Typically, his instructions in such cases were that the images in question be altered and more decently covered up. This was the case, for instance, at S. Maria Maggiore, where Clement ordered that the wooden angels on top of the ciborium that held the venerated icon of the Madonna Salus Populi Romani

(Illustration 23) be "more decently dressed, or removed."[40] At St. Peter's he similarly ordered the reworking of an image of the Magdalene, which decorated a reliquary cupboard in the Chapel of the Holy Sacrament, stipulating that the figure's hair be made denser and longer to cover her nudity.[41] At S. Angelo in Pescheria, Clement ordered the altarpiece at the altar dedicated to St. Lawrence to be replaced or repainted in a "more decent" (*honestiore*) manner.[42]

On occasion, Clement was content to move an image rather than remake it. At S. Maria della Consolazione, he ordered the covering up of a crucifix, with the proviso that it could be moved into the sacristy.[43] On another occasion, while searching the monastic quarters of S. Pietro in Vincoli, the pope came across an image of the Magdalene "of a less than decent type" in the prior's cell. This was, seemingly, a movable devotional image, since Clement ordered that it should be sold.[44] Evidently, where questions of decency were concerned, it was the character of the audience as well as that of the image that was under scrutiny. The prior's Magdalene, while unsuitable for a monk, was acceptable elsewhere. The crucifix in S. Maria della Consolazione, while unacceptable in the nave, was suitable for the more guarded gaze of priests. These decisions demonstrate quite a fine parsing, both of the degree of an image's indecency and between differing groups of potential viewers, distinguishing not only between laity and clergy, but also between different types of clergy.

While some of these instructions concerned relatively small or obscure objects, Clement's objections did sometimes alight on more prominent images. At the Chapel of the Crucifixion at S. Marcello al Corso, he instructed that one of the ceiling frescos, Perino del Vaga's *Creation of Eve*, be more decently covered – which was accomplished by extending her hair to cover her pubic area (Illustration 24).[45] Perino's *Creation of Eve* is a very close variant of Michelangelo's painting of the same subject on the vault of the Sistine Chapel, a painting that Clement would certainly have seen. However, Michelangelo's Eve, viewed more laterally than frontally, is a touch more modest than Perino's.

It was at St. Peter's, at the funerary monument of Paul III, that Clement made his most public censorious intervention. At this time, Guglielmo della Porta's sculpture group stood at the southeastern corner of the crossing (the location, since 1633, of Duquesnoy's *St. Andrew*) and comprised four female allegorical figures – Peace, Plenty, Prudence, and Justice – flanking a statue of Paul III. The monument, in a reduced three-figure configuration, now stands in the tribune.[46]

All the allegorical figures exhibited some degree of nudity, a feature that was emphasized by Vasari in the *Vite*. Prudence was "a matron, young in aspect ... and partly nude"; Plenty was "a young woman ... clothed in such a manner as to show the nude beneath the draperies"; Peace, an older matron, was nude from the waist (Vasari did not consider this detail worth recording), while the youthful Justice (Illustration 25) was "a nude figure

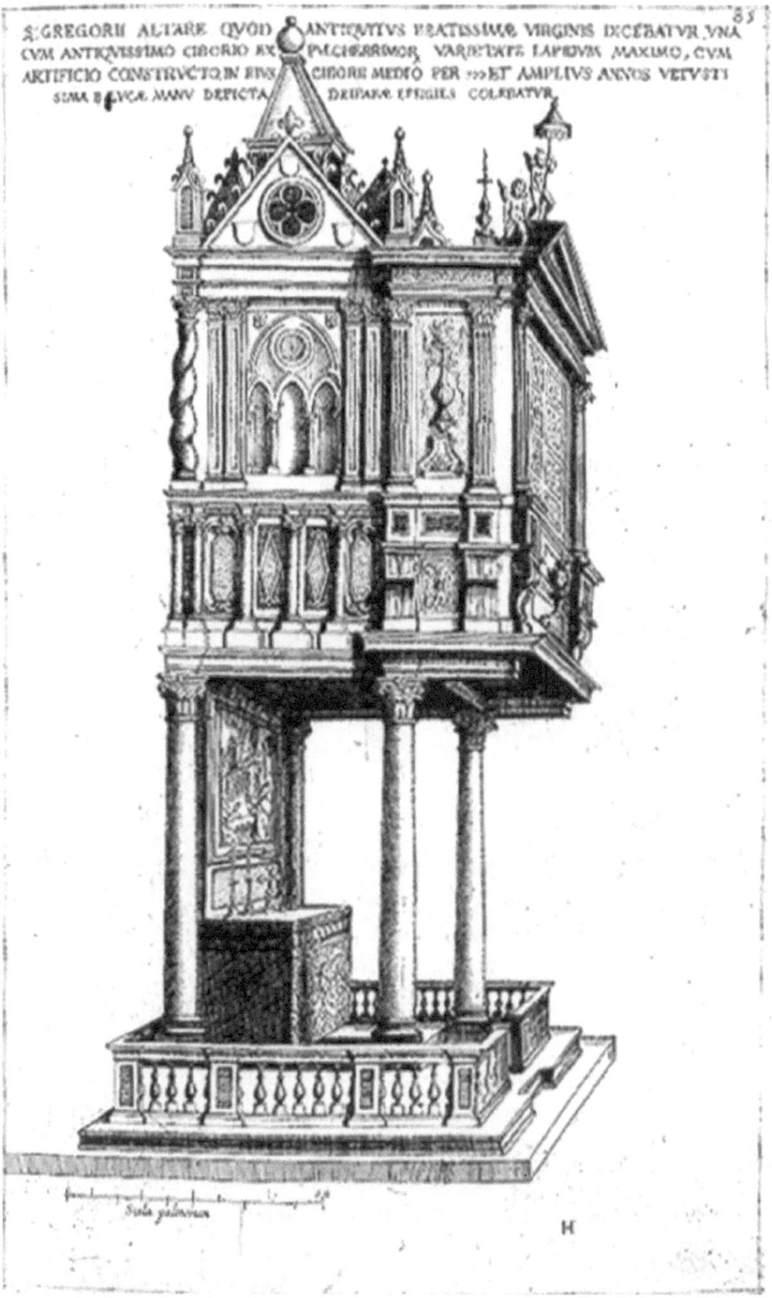

23. Altar of the Blessed Virgin, before renovation in 1603–13. Rome, S. Maria Maggiore. From Paolo de Angelis, *Basilicae S. Mariae Maioris de Urbe*, 1621, p. 85. Photo: British Library.

lying across some draperies ... young in countenance ... and the aspect full of expression."[47] The visitation's records indicate that Clement took an undifferentiated attitude towards these figures, ordering that the statues "be moved, or more decently covered up."[48]

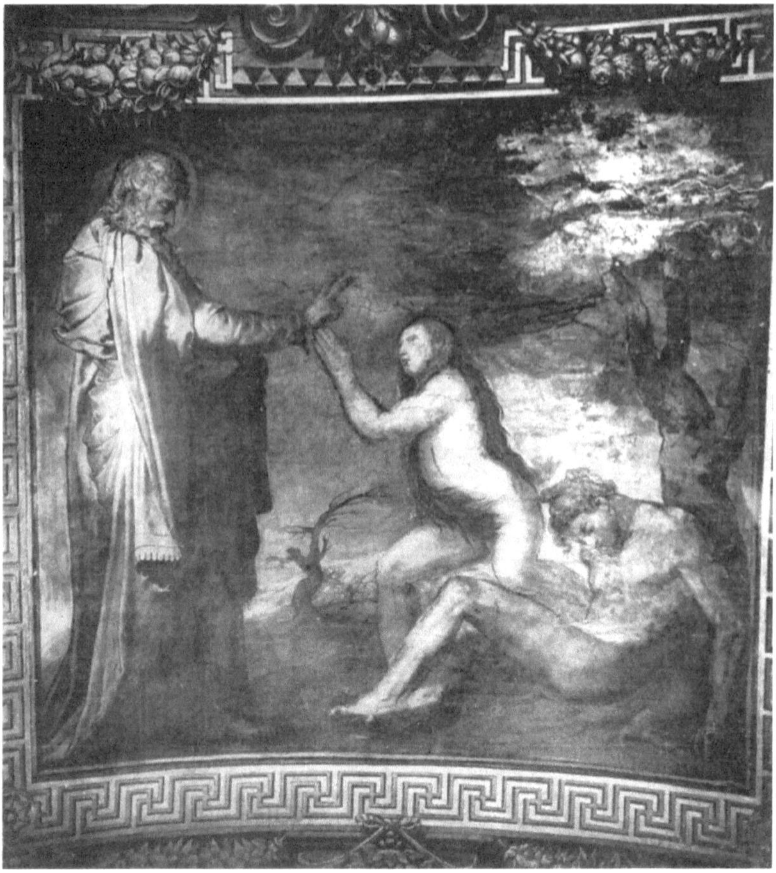

24. Perino del Vaga, *The Creation of Eve*, before restoration. Rome, S. Marcello al Corso, Chapel of the Crucifixion.

This was a measure of considerably more gravity than the redecoration of the door of a reliquary cupboard. Paul III's monument was a prominent Michelangelesque artwork, celebrated and extensively described by Vasari. It was also the monument of a fairly recent and prominent pope, whose family was among the most prominent noble families in Rome, where they were represented by the grandiose Palazzo Farnese and by the person of Cardinal Odoardo Farnese. The cardinal objected, protested that the monument was harmless, and attempted – with some success – to modify Clement's decision. Odoardo paid for a specially cast bronze extension, by Guglielmo's son, Teodoro, which was added to the figure of Justice – evidently the most provocative of the four – entirely covering her nudity (Illustration 25). This work was completed by December 1595.[49] The remaining figures were left untouched and (for the time being) in place. This vitiated some of the worst consequences of the decision for the Farnese, who were able to avoid the diminution of their monument, while satisfying at least some of Clement's requirements.

The mixed outcome of this episode illustrates not only the resistance that corrective censorship could encounter, but the diversity of spectatorial responses that made its effects so uncertain. For Vasari, the nudity of the figures was a mark of their aesthetic value. The eventual solution preserved, as far as possible, the integrity of the sculpture and of the larger group, suggesting that Odoardo, at least, continued to value its artistic qualities alongside (or within) its value as a dynastic monument. The antiquarian Giacomo Grimaldi, who completed his description of St. Peter's in 1620, dissented from Clement's censure, arguing that Justice should, as a matter of clarity and convention, be nude; in so doing, he chose to emphasize the figure's allegorical sense over its corporeal character.[50] On the other hand, the Florentine *avviso* writer who reported on the affair to the Medicean court was sceptical of Odoardo's claims that the marble figure had never incited any onlooker to lust, pointing out that its thigh had been uncovered "fino all'orlo del vaso naturale."[51] In the event, the compromise, considered an act of censorship, backfired. The rumour that *Justice* represented Paul III's mistress, already circulating in the 1580s, survived the covering of the statue.[52]

Another act of censorship with a confused outcome occurred during the visitation of the Gesù, where Clement objected to two recently completed altarpieces by Scipione Pulzone. One of these was the altarpiece of the Chapel of the Seven Archangels, unveiled in 1592, depicting the eponymous archangels in adoration of the Holy Trinity.[53] Clement ordered that

25. Guglielmo della Porta, *Justice*, from the funerary monument of Paul III. Rome, St. Peter's Basilica. Photo: Scala / Art Resource, NY.

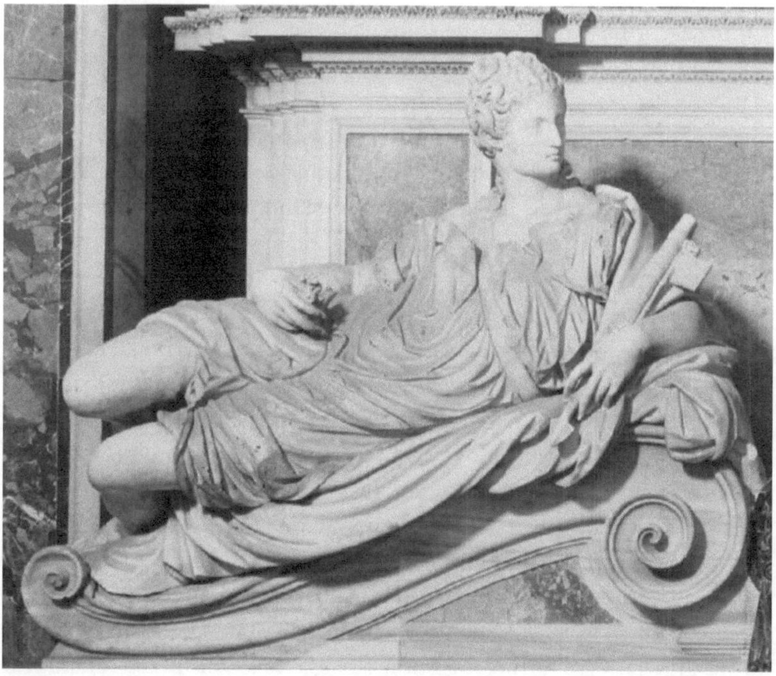

the figures of the angels be more decently covered and honestly depicted.[54] The subsequent course of events is complex and difficult to reconstruct. There is no indication that the Jesuits hastened to comply with Clement's instructions, but the patronage of the chapel did change hands, and with that, its decoration was entrusted to Federico Zuccaro in 1594. He then proceeded to redecorate the chapel in its entirety, repainting the frescoes, as well as providing a new altarpiece. This last was not completed until 1600 and was subsequently repainted by Domenico Passignano in the early 1610s. Pulzone's original is lost.[55]

Pulzone's painting, then, disappeared under circumstances that may have had nothing to do with its condemnation by Clement. Zuccaro had sufficient incentive to efface or replace, without papal encouragement, the work of an artist he regarded as a rival. On the other hand, if the visitation had indeed placed Pulzone's altarpiece under a cloud, this could have encouraged the Jesuits and the chapel's new patrons to replace it and may have informed Zuccaro's decision to clothe his angels almost from head to toe.

That Clement's decision achieved some notoriety is confirmed by the account of the affair given by Giovanni Baglione in his *vita* of Pulzone. Baglione claims that the altarpiece depicted recognizable individuals in the guise of angels and that these were then removed "per cancellare lo scandalo."[56] This does not accord with the visitation records, but it is nonetheless significant, as much for its *inaccuracy* as for the fact of its circulation, even years after the event, in a literary and (presumably) oral form. Like the rumours that continued to circulate after the censoring of the monument of Paul III, Baglione's *vita* of Pulzone (published in 1642) demonstrates that acts of censorship had a persistent, if mutable, afterlife. Baglione's confusion is, as Gauvin Alexander Bailey suggested, not unmotivated.[57] His account of the incident is in keeping with his overall characterization of Pulzone as a painter of portraits whose devotion to naturalism limited his capacity as a history painter.[58] In Baglione's text, the rationale that informed Clement's action is (wilfully or negligently) misunderstood, and the decree itself has become a moralistic element within a larger critical debate.

During the same visitation of the Gesù, Clement issued yet another condemnation of an altarpiece by Pulzone, the *Lamentation* (Illustration 26), then in the Chapel of the Passion.[59] As was the case on a number of occasions, Clement objected to a representation of the Magdalene and ordered that the prominent figure at the bottom left of the canvas "be altered to have a more devout and modest appearance."[60] The figure as it appears today bears no traces of such alteration. Moreover, it is based on the same drawings as the nearly identical figure of the Magdalene in Pulzone's *Crucifixion* in the Chiesa Nuova, a painting for which no form of censorship is recorded.[61] Accordingly, the painting as it appears today almost certainly preserves its appearance as Clement saw it, not as he wished it to be. This raises a further question since, unlike the naked, eremitical

Magdalenes to which Clement objected elsewhere, Pulzone's is fully, and modestly, clothed. The "immodesty" of this figure refers not to nudity, but to decorum and to the close physical contact between the mourning Magdalene and the naked body of Christ, on whose knee she rests her cheek and whose foot she holds and caresses with both hands. Alone of the several mourning women in the painting, the Magdalene also has her hair uncovered and unbound. On Pulzone's part, this seems to be an attempt to assimilate the mourning Magdalene to the Mary who washes Christ's feet with her hair (John 12:3), with whom she was conventionally identified. Clement was surely not insensible to this, but objected to the figure's "immodest" pose and demeanour nonetheless. While Christ's nudity is deemed acceptable and the Magdalene's own dress is unimpeachable, it was the interaction between them that attracted censure.

Evidently, then, it was not nudity alone that determined the visitors' decisions with regard to depictions of saints. While the inadequacy or absence of clothing was a matter for concern because it was "lascivious," it was complemented by a more broadly defined concern for the dignity of sacred persons, under the rubric of decorum. In the words of the *Instructiones Fabricae Ecclesiasticae*, sacred images should express the full dignity and sanctity of their subject, as well as their decorum, physical demeanour, social position, and dress.[62] Federico Borromeo, writing in a more metaphorical vein in *De Pictura Sacra*, argued that decorum was "a kind of luminous splendour, or perhaps a flower growing out of every movement and activity, that refreshes the mind," while its opposite, indecorum, arose in instances where a figure's actions were either inadequate or excessive in relation to this ideal.[63] Both these definitions bring a whole range of pictorial values under scrutiny. In the case of Pulzone's *Lamentation*, it seems the visitors acted out of such an expanded definition of decorum.

Nor was it the only occasion on which they did so. While conducting the visitation of SS. Trinità dei Monti, Clement took exception to the depiction of the Madonna in Daniele da Volterra's *Deposition* (Illustration 27) in the Orsini Chapel (now in Bonfili Chapel), stating that she "lacked patience in suffering."[64] The motif of the Virgin swooning at the cross contradicted the text of John 19:25, in which she is described as standing beside it. Nonetheless, the depiction of a fainting Madonna was popular among Renaissance artists, who took advantage of the opportunity to demonstrate their mastery of the *affetti*. Indeed, Vasari singled out this particular figure for praise, opining that here Daniele "showed the greatest judgement, and [himself] to be the rarest of men."[65]

Clement's condemnation of the figure seems to have been motivated by more than a desire for textual accuracy alone, given the moralistic phrasing of the decree. Federico Borromeo, who was present, expands on this reasoning in a passage from *De Pictura Sacra* seemingly written with Daniele's painting in mind. Modern artists, Borromeo writes, are unable to depict mental disposition properly and, when they attempt to do so, represent "the least appropriate" emotions; in particular they "do not know how to represent the Mother of god in anguish at the sight of the Cross.... Consequently they resort to painting her in a lifeless faint, which ... runs against the authority of the Fathers of the Church."[66]

26. Scipione Pulzone, *The Lamentation of Christ*. New York, Metropolitan Museum of Art. Photo: Metropolitan Museum of Art / Art Resource, NY.

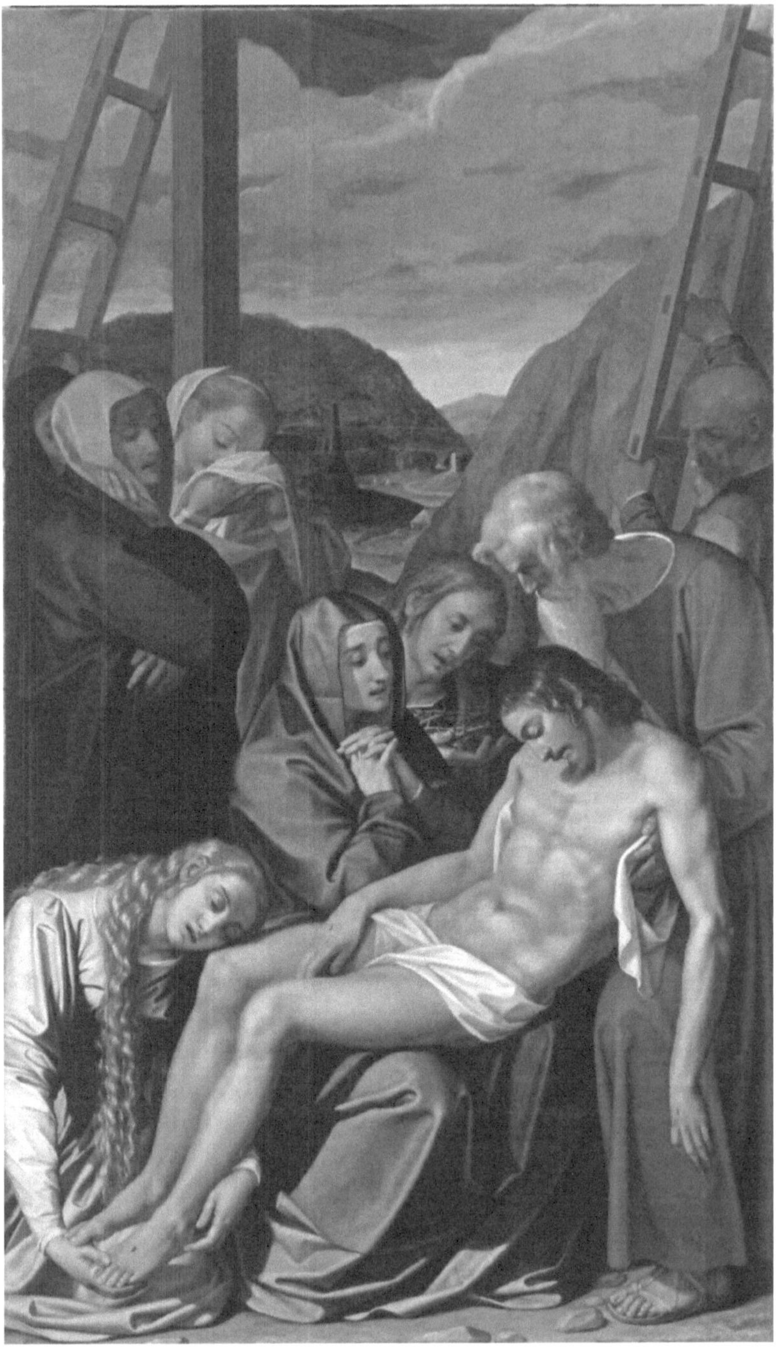

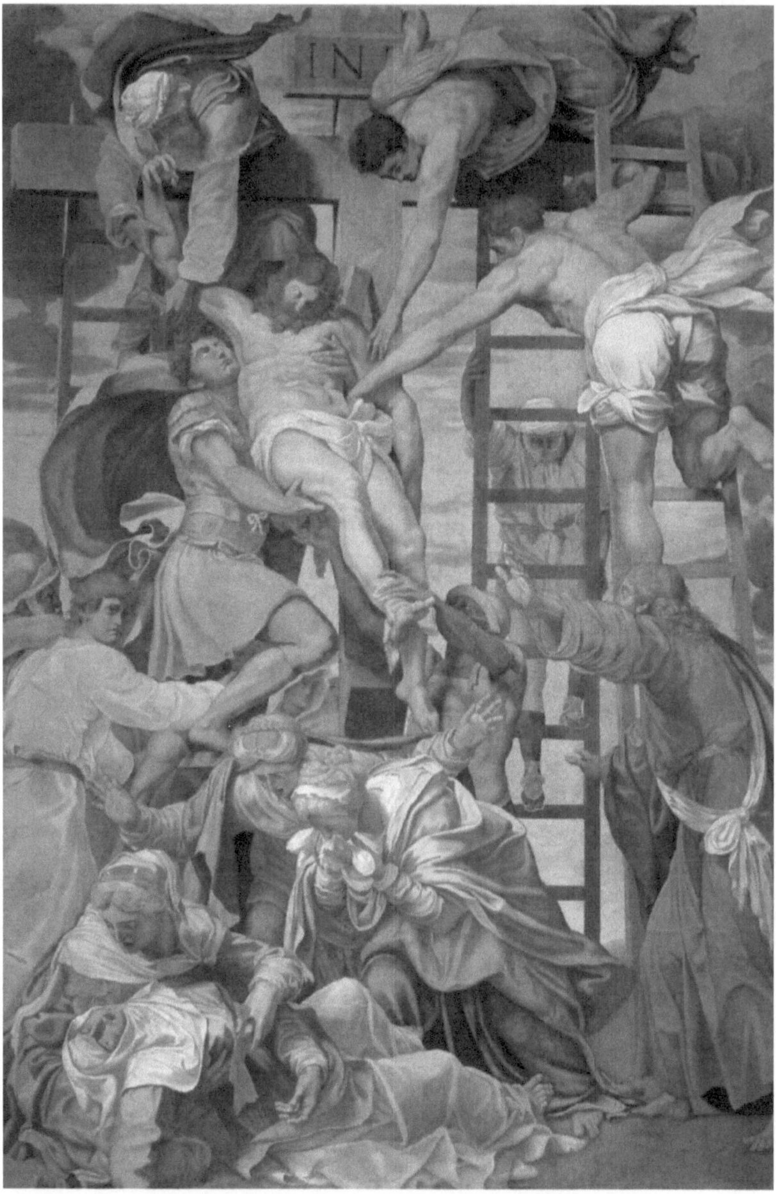

27. Daniele da Volterra, *The Deposition*. Rome, SS. Trinità dei Monti. Photo: Andrea Jemolo / Scala / Art Resource, NY.

Despite Clement's instructions there is, once again, no indication that the extensive repainting that the decree required was ever carried out.

The overlapping of a concern for decorum with a desire for textual and historical accuracy appears once more in a further act of censorship that the visitation ordered in S. Maria Maggiore, this time of a painting that stood at the side of the Chapel of Pope Leo the Great. The painting depicted Leo "extending his hand to a woman"; it was to be erased and replaced by a depiction of him dissuading Attila from sacking Rome.[67]

The incident depicted in the painting was one of the miracles associated with the Basilica's most sacred relic, the *Madonna Salus Populi Romani.* According to the version of the story recounted in the *Golden Legend*, Leo was celebrating mass at the Basilica when, in the course of events, a woman kissed his hand and he found himself involuntarily aroused by her touch. Mortified, Leo amputated the offending member, but later regretted his action after the hand's absence was noticed at subsequent masses. He appealed to the Virgin, by means of the miracle-working icon, and she responded by dispatching an angel who reattached the missing hand.[68] Despite the picturesque nature of the story, it was of considerable importance to the Basilica and its canons, since it was the first and oldest miracle attributed to their principal relic.

Although the painting in question would have depicted no nudity or strictly visual impropriety, it clearly referred to the sexual sinfulness and self-mutilation of a sanctified pope – at a time when Clement was striving to present a devout image of the papacy. This prompted Clement to take harsh measures. It is the only occasion where Clement ordered the outright destruction of a Christian image, in accordance with the Tridentine injunction to remove images that communicated "false doctrine, and ... dangerous error to the uneducated." In Clement's view, the story was false, and its circulation in any form was harmful.

Some authorities, such as Molanus, were inclined to be indulgent of images that inspired popular devotion even if they were historically baseless.[69] However, Clement and his Oratorian fellow visitors were most likely influenced by the views of Cesare Baronio, who regarded such fabricated hagiography as "tares" and diabolic snares, even when related with the best of intentions. Baronio's views on the incident are very clear, since he published them some three years later in the sixth volume of the *Annales Ecclesiastici*, rejecting the story of Leo's hand as "trash, and prattling old fables" of a kind that spread easily among the *vulgus* and the thoughtless, to their spiritual detriment. Baronio did, in fact, lend credence to another version of the miracle, in which Leo's hand had been wounded by an iconoclast, but he nonetheless approved of Clement's decision to have the offending image entirely replaced. Since he states that Clement took the decision after consulting with "learned men," he may very well have been involved in it himself.[70]

The fate of the painting is impossible to determine, but as Baronio makes clear, the target of this particular decree was not so much the particular image as the story that underlay it. In this regard, it was not a success. Paolo de Angelis, a canon of the Basilica, took issue with Baronio's critique in his history of the church, published in 1621. He asserted the antiquity of the miracle, recounted the version that centred on Leo's concupiscence, blandly recounted Baronio's opinion, and proceeded to describe the chapel at which it was commemorated.[71] Clement may or may not have been able to effect some change in the imagery, but the dedication of the altar to the miracle he abhorred remained current.[72]

There was one further occasion on which Clement condemned an image for misrepresentation of sacred history, though on this occasion both the error and the proposed remedy were less severe. At S. Maria Rotonda (the Pantheon), Clement ordered numerous changes to the altars and chapels. At the altar of St. Catherine of Alexandria, he noted that the dedicatory saint was painted in close proximity to the wheel that is her most frequently depicted attribute. In Clement's eyes, this was apt to give the misleading impression that the wheel was the instrument of her execution, whereas it was in fact miraculously shattered, whereupon St. Catherine's martyrdom was accomplished by beheading. Clement ordered that St. Catherine be effaced and repainted at a greater distance from the wheel, to show that she was unaffected by it.[73]

This painting contained no substantive error; it was simply ambiguous. This is the only occasion on which Clement evinced a concern for pictorial clarity in the course of the visitation. Evidently, his decision was taken with uneducated and error-prone spectators in mind, since Clement and his companions were well able to understand the painting's correct meaning.

It remains to consider the relatively small number of occasions on which Clement acted to remove pagan elements from sacred spaces. The paganism of Renaissance art was an area of keen concern for many clerical Reformers. Most proximately, these included Paleotti, who devoted considerable attention to this problem in his *Trattato*, the Jesuit censor Antonio Possevino, and Federico Borromeo.[74] All of these writers concurred that paganism was a form of profanity that should be excluded from sacred space, as something that was not merely different from the sacred, but inimical to it. The quantity of manifestly pagan artefacts in Roman churches was limited – although on one occasion in the visitation, Clement did order the inscription *Diis Manibus* effaced from an altar slab in S. Marcello in Corso.[75] The actual focus of censure was the perceived paganism of Renaissance art and its manifestation in Christian spaces in the form of ornament and allegory.

Grotesques were a particular focus of concern. Not only were they pagan in origin, they also dovetailed with the well-known screed of St. Bernard of Clairvaux against the distracting and irreligious effects of the "deformed beauty and ... beautiful deformity" of Romanesque capitals on their viewers.[76] This argument was revived in the post-Tridentine period. It appears, applied to grotesques, in Carlo Borromeo's *Instructiones*.[77] It was taken up by Molanus and, in particular, Paleotti, who integrated it into his broader argument against paganism.

In keeping with these concerns, Clement on three occasions ordered the removal of grotesques: twice in St. Peter's, where he decreed the removal of "profane images" from the bronze candelabra on the altar of the Holy Sacrament and from the organ Alexander VI had commissioned for the Basilica in 1496.[78] At S. Lorenzo in Damaso, he gave instructions to remove the grotesques around the organ in the Chapel of the Immaculate Conception and to have them replaced with images "more fitting to this sacred place."[79] Clement, however, was hardly fanatical in his opposition to grotesques; in the course of his visitation, he passed over two far more notable examples of ecclesiastical grotesque decoration – Filippino Lippi's Carafa Chapel in S. Maria sopra Minerva and Taddeo Zuccaro's Mattei Chapel in S. Maria della Consolazione – without comment or interference. Whatever particular circumstance, whether of content or location, motivated him to act on the occasions when he did so is impossible to determine.

On one further occasion, at the Della Tolfa Chapel in S. Maria in Aracoeli, Clement took action against an allegorical image. The Della Tolfa Chapel (or Chapel of the Ascension, formerly part of the Della Valle Chapel) was the funerary chapel of Vittoria della Tolfa, Marchesa della Valle, and her husband, Camillo Pardo Orsini, both of whom were represented by busts on facing walls, flanked by allegorical representations of their accompanying virtues: Prudence, Glory, Victory, and Perseverance.[80] Clement objected to the figure of Prudence beside the bust of Camillo (Illustration 28), referring to it as "Minerva," and ordered that it be repainted as "St. Minerva."[81]

"Prudence" did, indeed, display many of the attributes of Minerva, including her aegis, complete with gorgon's head. Minerva's associations with wisdom were self-evident, and the practice of incorporating her image into allegorical schemes was well established. Clement, however, evidently chose to interpret the image literally as a representation of a pagan deity and to propose the equally literal revision of having her repainted as a saint. The decision is difficult to account for inasmuch as it would have been possible to repaint Prudence in less pagan form, paralleling the practice endorsed in Cesare Ripa's *Iconologia* of devising allegorical figures based on Christian rather than classical iconography.[82] Ripa's manual, first published in Rome in 1593, offers a specific Christian substitute for the conventional utilization of Minerva to represent wisdom.[83] Clement's proposal instead addresses the figure not as an allegory, but as an idol, while the proposed remedy, of remaking the "pagan" object, is more closely paralleled by the papal Christianization of pagan monuments such as obelisks and the columns of Trajan and Marcus Aurelius, under Sixtus V. Whereas a revision of Prudence *qua* allegory would have been integral to the existing scheme, a reworking of Minerva as a Christian saint would have left a lasting sign of rupture and of Christianity's triumph over paganism. Rome was full of such signs, and it may be that Clement valued such an image over the unity of the chapel's allegorical scheme. It is by no means clear that others shared this view, however, since there is no indication that this injunction was carried out.

In June and July of 1596, after a period of relative quiescence, Clement redoubled his efforts with a series of monastic visits, though by this later stage he was more concerned with disciplining monks than with inspecting buildings. His other duties were apparently becoming more onerous, as he declared his intention to delegate more of his duties to the prelates.[84] The visitation then continued to the end of July, after which records of its activities are scarce.[85] It certainly became less prominent: with the cessation of direct papal involvement, mentions in *avvisi* tail off.

At this point, when the visitation had been ongoing for four years, Cardinal Paleotti, in the final campaign of his long career (he was to die in 1597) made a determined attempt to change Clement's policy towards the arts. He had been working over the preceding years to revise and complete his *Discorso.* In the preface to this revised edition, he called for the establishment of an index to regulate images, analogous to the one that already existed for books.[86] In September 1596, he circulated a letter to this effect, *De Tollendis Imaginum Abusibus Vovissima Consideratio*, among the Curia.[87] Paleotti argued that the problems with Catholic religious imagery were grave and widespread, that decades of reform had done nothing to improve the situation. He called for the creation of clear and authoritative guidelines and a centralized organization to guide episcopal censorship. In effect, Paleotti proposed a congregation for the censorship of images very similar to the Congregation of the Index.[88]

This was not well received. Clement's secretary of briefs, Silvio Antoniano, circulated a reply that refuted Paleotti point by point.[89] Antoniano was himself a prominent censor and an advisor to the Index.[90] Because of his closeness to the pope, his rejection of Paleotti's arguments should be seen as carrying a papal imprimatur.

28. Niccolò da Pesaro, *Allegories of Prudence and Glory*. Rome, S. Maria in Aracoeli, Della Tolfa Chapel. Photo: author.

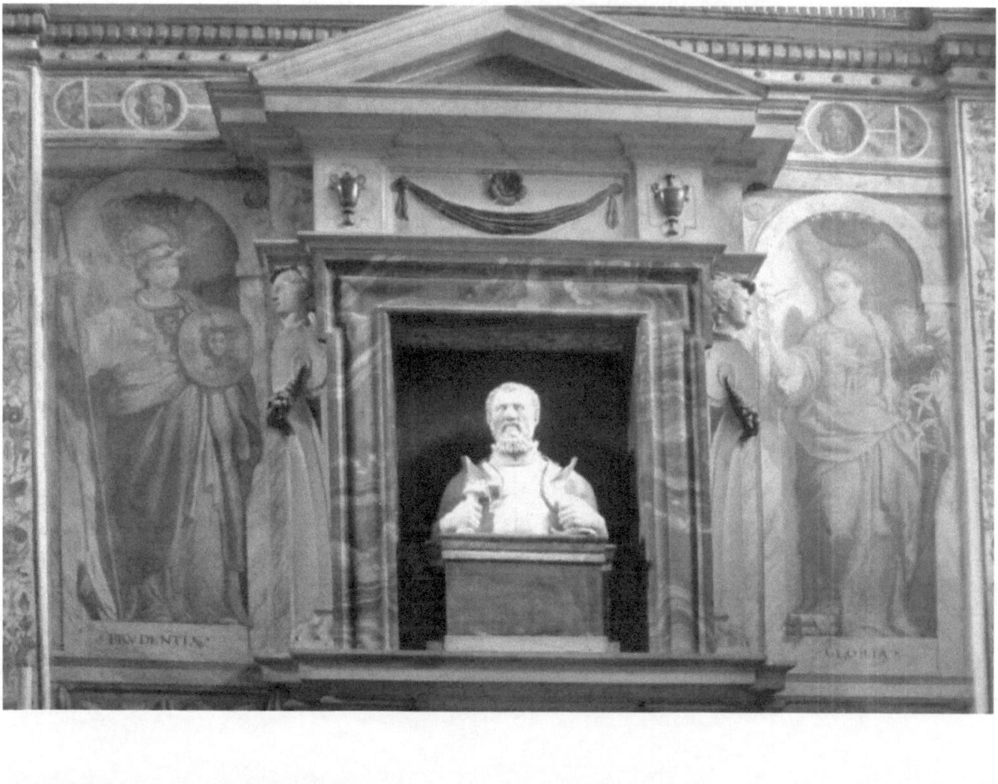

Antoniano denied Paleotti's claims that "abuse" was so endemic and so grave as to require such measures; and he also raised the spectre of iconoclasm, arguing that excessive attention to artistic problems lent ammunition to Protestant critiques of the cult of images, doing harm to the Church.[91] In effect, he argued in defence of Clement's policy of the preceding four years. The pope was committed to a relatively conservative policy of censorship. While he saw problems with existing church art, they did not seem to him to warrant special measures or reforms beyond establishing the visitation and empowering the cardinal vicar to address them. Though Paleotti penned a riposte to Antoniano, his proposal was effectively buried.

The full range of Clement's actions as a censor indicates that while he shared some concerns with earlier moralists and reformers, his concern with "decency" in the depiction of scared figures was predominant. The visitation's actions addressed paganism, grotesques, historical inaccuracies, and a lack of pictorial clarity, but concern with sexual "immodesty" and lack of decorum in the depiction of sacred figures was most prevalent in its decrees.

These last two categories often overlapped, but their rationales could be distinct. "Lascivious" images had the capacity to corrupt their beholders; they were problematic largely because of their effect. Accordingly, Clement sometimes addressed this problem not by destroying or rectifying, but simply by moving works of art, in one case from a lay into a clerical context, in another from a monastic setting into the lay marketplace. The same thinking informed Clement's initial instruction that the statues surrounding Paul III's tomb should be *moved*. There was nothing intrinsically wrong with a nude allegorical Justice – it was her position in St. Peter's that was problematic. That the dispute was eventually resolved by covering the statue does not alter this initial assessment of the nature of the issue.

The desire to make such distinctions indicates some reflection on the character and responses of audiences, as well as a degree of (inadmissible) common ground with Luther's view that the moral virtue (or otherwise) of images lay not in the objects themselves, but in their spectators.

However, the question of the image's effect on the viewer was not always the principal consideration. It was also possible for a visual representation to be problematic because of its indecorous relation not to its audience, but to the subject it depicted.

The concept of decorum, Aristotelian in origin, was introduced into artistic theory by Alberti, who had employed "decorum" (*convenevolezza*) to designate the proper integration of different parts of a represented body.[92] By the later years of the Cinquecento, "decorum" had become moralized and acquired a number of additional meanings. In the sense in which Federico Borromeo employed it, it still designated an appropriate relation between discrete but related things. As this applied to the depiction of saints, however, the salient relation was, as the Council of Trent had reiterated, that between the sacred prototype and the sacred representation; normatively, the latter ought to convey both the truth and the dignity of the former. Where it failed to do so, as was the case with Volterra's fainting Magdalene or the depiction of the miracle of St. Leo in S. Maria Maggiore, the "error" evidently called for alterations to the image itself, not to its mode of display.

A certain antipathy to Michelangelesque art is also evident, inasmuch as Clement condemned works by Perino del Vaga, Guglielmo della Porta, and Daniele da Volterra. Whether Clement actually thought of these as a "school" is unclear, but the artistic vocabulary of Michelangelo's followers clearly did not appeal to him. On the other hand, Clement also condemned two works by Scipione Pulzone, an artist whose naturalism, clarity, and emotive directness have been proposed as the epitome of a reformed style.[93] As a patron, Clement certainly had his preferred artists, and his enthusiasm for Barocci is well attested, but there is little in his record as a censor to suggest that he thought of the regulation of images in terms of the proscription or promotion of a particular manner of painting.[94]

The condemnation of Pulzone's altarpieces in the Gesù, along with the debate provoked by Paleotti in the summer of 1596, is an indication that even among clergy committed to the reform of religious art, consensus was limited. Paleotti clearly found Clement's actions as a censor inadequate. Conversely, for the Jesuits who welcomed Pulzone's recently completed altarpieces into their church, his decrees were evidently unwelcome. Furthermore, other clerics – such as Odoardo Farnese, Giovanni Grimaldi, and Paolo de Angelis – can be found objecting to Clement's actions as excessively harsh. The apparent extent of noncompliance with several of the pope's instructions suggests resistance, or at least indifference, to their execution.

The history of the visitation, then, reveals differences of opinion concerning the need for reform and the best means to remedy "abuses," as well as divergent judgments about the extent to which particular works of art met or contravened the needs of the post-Tridentine Church. While the actual scope of these differences is narrow compared with those that separated Catholics from most Protestant denominations, they were broad enough to generate differing responses both to existing and to new works of religious art even within Rome's clerical establishment. The combination of broad agreement on basic principles, widespread disagreement on their interpretation and implementation, and willingness to make relativistic judgments about the admissibility of images that often revolved around their audience and location rather than their intrinsic properties created an environment in which the doctrinal and moral foundations of the Church's authority to censor were continually reinforced but in which its decrees were sometimes mitigated, disputed, or misunderstood. But for all that any estimations of the papal authorities' willingness to bowdlerize, remove, or destroy existing religious art must be hedged with caveats, the congruence between the judgments recorded in the visitations records, the principles set out in the clerical treatises of the "reform" of sacred art, and even the dissenting proposals discussed between Antoniano and Paleotti, all point to the existence, if not quite of common norms, then at least of a common language of "reform" in which the concerns broached at Trent had come to be codified in a distinctive and well-defined set of concerns. Clement VIII's visitation is as notable for its limits as for its effects, but among those effects is the reproduction and transmission of a developed post-Tridentine discourse on the rights and wrongs of the sacred images into the changing cultural economy of the Seicento.

APPENDIX

Churches Inspected in the Course of the Visitation, 1592–96

Church	Date of First Inspection
S. Giovanni in Laterano	17 June 1592
S. Marco	20 June 1592
St. Peter's Basilica	2 July 1592
S. Maria Maggiore	6 July 1592
SS. Dodici Apostoli	8 August 1592
S. Spirito in Sassia	31 August 1592
S. Marcello in Corso	26 October 1592
S. Maria in Trastevere	21 November 1592
S. Lorenzo in Damaso	n.d.[a]
S. Lorenzo in Lucina	24 March 1593
S. Maria della Consolazione	20 June 1593
SS. Croce e Bonaventura	7 July 1593
S. Maria ad Martyres	26 July 1593
S. Eustachio	1 August 1593
S. Maria in Via Lata	22 September 1593
S. Angelo in Pescheria	6 October 1593
Il Gesù	4 January 1594
S. Maria in Traspontina	5 February 1594
S. Maria del Popolo	5 March 1594
SS. Trinità dei Monti	19 August 1594
S. Maria in Aracoeli	22 February 1595
S. Maria sopra Minerva	19 June 1596
S. Croce in Gerusalemme	22 June[b]
S. Prassede	7 July 1596
S. Pietro in Vincoli	14 July 1596
S. Maria in Trivio	21 July 1596
S. Maria della Pace	28 July 1596
S. Agostino	26 July 1598?[c]

Note: Most information about the visitations' sites, dates, and participants derives from ASV, Misc. Arm. VII, vol. 3, ff. 1–98: *Decreta Sant.mi D.ni Clementis Papae Octavi facta in visitatione Ecclesiarum Urbis.* The document is transcribed, with occasional errors. Accordingly, there is uncertainty over the dates of some visitations.

[a] The date is omitted, but visitations are recorded in chronological order. Clement returned to examine clergy on 15 June 1593 (ASV, Misc. Arm. VII, vol. 3, 55v), which suggests that the original visitation took place in early 1593.

[b] Decrees are omitted but mentioned in *Avvisi di Roma* 1596, BAV, Urb. Lat. 1064, 397r.

[c] This date is an outlier and may be a mistranscription.

Notes

1 Abromson (1981).
2 Freiberg (1995); L. Rice (1997); Chappell and Kirwin (1974); Abromson (1978); Zuccari (1984).
3 Röttgen (2002).
4 Barzman (2000); Lukehart (2009a).
5 Mancini (1956), 1: 310; Giustiniani (1981), 41–45.
6 Belting (1994), 458–90, esp. 458, 484.
7 Belting (1994), 458.
8 Nagel (2000); Lingo (2008); Bailey (2003).
9 As late as 1591, it formed a major component of Gregorio Comanini's *Il Figino*. See Comanini (2001), 84–90, 97. For the course of the debate, see Barnes (1998).
10 Summarized in the introduction to this volume and discussed in detail in Hecht (1997).
11 P. Jones (2008), 325.
12 Zapperi (1994), 53.
13 See, e.g., Fragnito and Rozzo (1997); for an alternative view, see Ditchfield (2004).
14 The classic definition of the public sphere refers, of course, to a particular bourgeois configuration formed in the eighteenth century. For an argument for the applicability of the term to early modern Italy, see Randolph (2002).
15 In chapter 3 of the decree on reform in its twenty-fourth session. Schroeder (1978), 194.
16 Schroeder (1978), 195.
17 Borromeo and Galesio (1582).
18 Borromeo and Galesio (1582), 177–212, as well as earlier decrees concerning the regulation of sacred art (4, 49–51). Note that Borromeo (1977) reproduces only book I of the *Instructiones*, omitting the lengthy lists of liturgical instruments.
19 See, e.g., Nubola (1996) and Turchini (1996), as well as the essays in Nubola and Turchini (1993) and Mazzone and Turchini (1985).
20 Beggiao (1978), 24–32; Monticone (1953); Fiorani (1980); Pagano (1980).
21 Cherubini and Cherubino (1638), 5–6. The Congregation, however, does not seem to have had a continuous existence until its revival by Urban VIII. See Del Re (1998), 364–66.
22 See Beggiao (1978), esp. 79–94.
23 Paruta (1887), 20.
24 BAV Ferraioli 374, 44v–45r.
25 Albèri (1857) ser. 2, vol. 4, 441.
26 Alberigo (1984).
27 Von Pastor (1923–53), 24:148–52; BAV Urb. Lat. 1060–64, passim.
28 The rhythm of the visitation was not constant. Beginning on 17 June 1592, it continued with some regularity until August 1594. Another spate of visitations, now increasingly concerned with monastic discipline, took place in 1596, and a last, isolated visit took place in January 1598 (96v).
29 ASV Misc. Arm. VII, 111.
30 On the identities of the visitors, see Beggiao (1978), 50–53; Macioce (1990), 14.
31 On Rusticucci, see P. Jones (2008), 20–22. On the role of the Vicariate, see Del Re (1976).

32 On Alessandro de Medici, see D'Addario (1972); Tarchi, Nubola, and Turchini (1993). On Valier, see Pullapilly (1992); Tacchella (1972, 1974); BAV, Vat. Lat. 5479.

33 On Owen, see Ughelli (1717), 9: 353, l.43. On de Torres, see Zuccari (1984), 99–100, 108.

34 Borromeo was absent from Rome when the visitation commenced. He first appears in its records on 20 June 1593, initially as a substitute for the absent Rusticucci (ASV Misc. Arm. VII, vol. 3, 58r). He became a regular participant but left Rome again in April 1595, missing the remainder of the visitation. See Gabrieli (1933–34) for Borromeo's whereabouts over the period. For his views on religious art, see especially P. Jones (1993, 1997); on his relations with the Oratory, see Cistellini (1981).

35 BAV Vat. Lat. 5479, 6v.

36 Cistellini (1989), 784.

37 It was eventually published in 1624. F. Borromeo (1994), 1–5; F. Borromeo (2010), x–xiv.

38 ASVR scaff. 64 tom. 38, ff. 68r–168v. Reproduced in Beggiao (1978), 106; see Zuccari 1984, 15–17.

39 See Witcombe (2004), 69–72; Lincoln (2000), 152; Leuschner (1998).

40 "Statuae lignea, quae super ambonem sunt posits, decentius amiciantur, vel inde auferantur" (ASV Misc. Arm. VII, vol. 3, f. 21r).

41 "Armarium Sacrarum Reliquiarum ornatus intus vestiatur et Imago S. Mariae Magdalenae extrinsecus in ea depicta, densioribus, et prolixioribus capillis congetatur" (ASV Misc. Arm. VII, vol. 3, f. 27v).

42 "Imago autem S.ti Laurentii, quae ad Altare est, aut decentiori picturae opere accommodetur, aut hac deleta, alia honestiore specie depingatur" (ASV Misc. Arm. VII, vol. 3., f. 68r).

43 "Imago S.mi Crucifixi velo tegatur, vel in sacristium transferatur" (ASV Misc. Arm. VII, vol. 3, f. 58v).

44 "Et cum in Cella D. fabiani die Ravenna Prioris reperiiset Imaginem B.ae Maria Magadalena minus honesta specie depictam mandavit, ut venderetur, et praetim sacristiae usibus assigneratur" (ASV Misc. Arm. VII, vol. 3, f. 93r).

45 "Quae nuditas in Sacelli fornice depictae decenter contegatur" (ASV Misc. Arm. VII, vol. 3, f. 46r). I am indebted to Michael Bury for correctly identifying this painting.

46 On the history of this monument, see Gramberg (1984).

47 Vasari (1997), 6: 206.

48 "Statuae in monumento felicis recordationis. Pauli Papae III amoveantur; vel quamprimum honestius cooperiantur" (ASV Misc. Arm. VII, vol. 3, f. 29r).

49 Gramberg (1984), 290, 350.

50 Grimaldi (1972), 385.

51 Archivio di Stato di Firenze, *Mediceo del Prinicipato*, busta 4027. Cited in Zapperi (1998), 15.

52 Zapperi (1998), 81–82.

53 For the most comprehensive account of the chapel's history and a summary of the extensive earlier research and arguments, see Bailey (2003), 211–14, 242–47.

54 "Imagines SS.orum Angelorum decentius contegantur, ut modestior consulatur" (ASV Misc. Arm. VII, vol. 3, f. 69v).

55 Although Bailey (2003), 212, has argued that its composition survives in a print by Hieronymus Wierix.
56 Baglione (1995), 1: 54.
57 Bailey (2003), 212–13.
58 Baglione (1995), 54.
59 Bailey (2003), 209–11; Dern (2003), 162–63.
60 "Imago Beatae Mariae Magdalenae hic depictae ad speciem magis devotam, et modestam redigatur" (ASV Misc. Arm. VII, vol. 3, f. 69v).
61 Bailey (2003), 211, n. 166.
62 "De decore sacrarum imaginum: Sacrarum imaginum expression tota prototypi dignitati et sanctitati, apte ac decore, corporis habitu, statu et ornate respondea." C. Borromeo (1962), 3: 43.
63 F. Borromeo (2010), 5, 9.
64 "Reformatur imago B.e Mariae Virginis Juxta Crucem D.ni N.ri Jesu Christi deliquium patientis" (ASV Misc. Arm. VII, vol. 3, f. 84r). For the history of the chapel, see Hirst (1967); Davidson (1967).
65 Vasari (1997), 6: 540–41.
66 F. Borromeo (1994), 39.
67 "Pictura, quae est a latere sacelli, ubi sanctus Leo Papa manum mulieri porrigit deoseulandum deleatur; eiusque loco pingatur imago eiusdem sancti reprimentis eloquentia sua furorem Attilae" (ASV Misc. Arm. VII, vol. 3, f. 22r).
68 Maggioni (1998), 2: 1210–11.
69 Molanus (1996), 112–14.
70 Under the subheading "Exploditur de Leone Favella"; Baronius (1588–1607), 6: 254.
71 Angelis (1621), 245.
72 It remained unchanged in 1621; Angelis (1621), 73.
73 "Pingatur alia Imago S.tae Catharinae, quae longius distet a rota, cui nunc adhaerat, quod constet hoc tormenti genere non fuisse affectam; sed huiusmodi machinam paratam Deo volente fuisse mirabiliter confractam" (ASV Misc. Arm. VII, vol. 3, f. 62r).
74 Paleotti (1582), bk. 2, ch. 10, 289–93; F. Borromeo (1994), 23–24; A. Possevino (1595).
75 ASV Misc. Arm. VII, vol. 3., f. 46r.
76 Rudolph (2000), 11–12.
77 Under the heading "De parerga et additamentis ornatus causa"; C. Borromeo (1962), 44.
78 "Ad Altari S.mi Sacramentis: Ex ceroferareis aeneis auferantur imagines profanae in eis sculptae" (ASV Misc. Arm. VII, vol. 3, f. 27v). The Altar of the Most Holy Sacrament is otherwise known by its dedication to the Virgin and St. Gregory Nazienzus. It stands in the Cappella Gregoriana, the first (and at that date the only) permanent chapel constructed in New St. Peter's, built by Giacomo della Porta for Gregory XIII between 1578 and 1585. It was intended to be the sacrament chapel of the new basilica; see L. Rice (1997), 23–27. The organ was commissioned by Alexander VI in 1496. By 1592, it was located in or near the Cappella Gregoriana; see Antinori (1997), 135. Vasari attributed its grotesque decorations to Amico Aspertini, whose figures, he observed, were habitually "mad" and "capricious." They are now known to have been painted by Aspertini's father, Giovanni Antonio. See Antinori (1997), 130. Clement's instructions were as follows: "Imagines profanae circa organum depictae deleantur; eorumque loco aliae pingantur,

quae referant historiam aliquam veteris, aut novi testamenti huic loco convenientem" (ASV Misc. Arm. VII, vol. 3, f. 29r). Grimaldi (1972), 63, noted the organ's appearance in 1620, describing only sacred decorations, which he also attributed to Amico.

79 "Imagines profanae circa organum depictae deleantur; eorumque loco aliae pingantur, quae referant historiam aliquam veteris, aut novi testamenti huic loco convenientem" (ASV Misc. Arm. VII, vol 3, f. 29r).

80 Heideman (1982), 111–17.

81 "Ad Cap.a Assumpt.nis B.tae Mariae Marchionissae de Vallae ... Minerva Imago in sinistro parietes depicta ita permutetur, ut eadem sanctam aliquam repraesentit" (ASV Misc. Arm. VII, vol. 3, f. 86r).

82 As Erna Mandowsky (1939), 39, observed, Ripa's *Iconologia* consistently subjected pagan emblems to moral and religious criticism.

83 Ripa preferred to represent wisdom by the figure of a young woman, glossed in an explicitly Christan manner; see Ripa (1611), 467–68. Minerva appears as a subsidiary emblem of wisdom, but the text is at pains to historicize the emblem and make clear its fictive nature and pagan origins (469). Both emblems appear in the first and subsequent editions of the *Iconologia*.

84 This occurred on the visitation of St. Prassede (Carlo Borromeo's forme *titulus*) on 7 July 1596: "Haec cum multam diem sanctissimam detinuissent, ut temporis augustiis impeditus coeptum visitationis opus per se ipse minime posit, mandavit Praelatis Visitationi deputatis, utque vistanda supererant, ipsi visitarent, opportune decernerent, ac reliquum Visitationis munus absoluerunt" (ASV Misc. Arm. VII, vol. 3, 93r).

85 The end of Clement's involvement does not necessarily signal the end of the visitation. However, the Congregation's own records are largely lost. The surviving list of decrees record one more papal inspection in January 1598 (ASV Misc. Arm. VII, vol. 3, 96v). Thereafter, there are only sporadic reports in *avvisi*; see Von Pastor (1923–53), 24: 151.

86 Prodi (1959–67), 2: 554–55.

87 For the text of this letter, see Prodi (1984) 94–110. The episode is discussed further in Prodi (1959–67), 2: 551–62.

88 On the debates regarding the implementation of literary and textual censorship in these years, see Fragnito and Rozzo (1997).

89 Prodi (1984), 111–13.

90 Prodi (1959–67), 2: 511–15.

91 Prodi (1984), 111.

92 Alberti (1966), 74.

93 Zeri, (1957), 71–85.

94 Bellori (2005), 167.

PAINTING VIRTUOUSLY

THE COUNTER-REFORM AND THE REFORM OF ARTISTS' EDUCATION IN ROME BETWEEN GUILD AND ACADEMY

Peter M. Lukehart

On the first of May 1563, a full seven and a half months before the close of the third and final Council of Trent, Domenico Zaga da Siena, consul, presided over a meeting of the Università dei Pittori in Rome in which an important declaration was made: "Domenico [Zaga] ... admonished all of the forementioned participants on behalf of the [Cardinal] Vicar and Monsignor Cesarini that those who paint images of Christ and of the Madonna and of other male and female saints should do so virtuously (*honeste*), otherwise the [works] would be thrown out and destroyed and their makers would be punished, and that everyone should be on guard against misfortune."[1] This precious document, the only one yet found that explicitly links the Università dei Pittori (Guild of Painters) with the tenets of the Counter-Reform, offers only the most general outline for painters who were practicing at this salient moment both in the history of the Catholic Church and in the history of the reform of the fine arts. Not only were painters now subject to new levels of scrutiny by the Church – however vaguely defined through its mouthpiece, the cardinal vicar – they were themselves also advocating for their professional emancipation from the Università dei Pittori, which took place in a series of important moves and pronouncements over the course of the next thirty years until the Accademia di San Luca was officially established in 1593. The history of that transformation has received increasing attention in the past two decades and was the subject of a recent volume of essays published by the Center for Advanced Study in the Visual Arts; as such, it will not be addressed in this essay. What I would like to examine instead is a cluster of paradoxical issues related to the notion of *honestà*, "decorum" or "dignity," and the act of painting *honeste*, or "virtuously," within the framework of pedagogical and ecclesiastical institutions in Rome throughout the latter half of the Cinquecento. At the same time, I will address the anxiety and ambivalence that manifested themselves in the arts community with regard to the depiction of nude figures in sacred painting after the Council of Trent. More specifically, I will address the criticism and the expurgation of Michelangelo's *Last Judgment* and the ways in which later artists responded to these singular events.

The exhortation to the *pittori* of Rome to paint virtuously (or modestly) was issued, according to the notary's summary, by the cardinal vicar and Monsignor Cesarini. Although unnamed in the document, Giacomo Savelli (1523–87) held the position of cardinal vicar from 1560 until 1587, the critical period before and after the last session of the Council of Trent.[2] Savelli's intervention in the affairs of the Università must be explained within the juridical structure of Rome: as vicar he did not oversee the administration of the guilds. That role was played instead by the Senate and the Roman people, and guild affairs were adjudicated by the Conservatori.[3] Savelli was, however, the link between papal and lay Rome and responsible for promulgating the directives of the Camera Apostolica and the ecclesiastical councils, such as the Council of Trent.[4] In fact, beginning in June 1564 Cardinal Savelli "personally" organized the Visite Apostoliche to more than ninety churches in Rome in response to orders of the Council.[5] The document of 1563, dating to the transitional period of the painters' guild, offers rare testimony to the means by which the pronouncements of the Council of Trent were communicated to the lay professionals who created sacred images. Still, the personal intervention of the cardinal vicar in the affairs of the guilds and churches that were under his pastoral care but not his direct administrative supervision suggests that Savelli was a key player in effectuating reform in both the institutional and ecclesiastical life of late Cinquecento Rome. Not surprisingly, these years were marked, as Agostino Borromeo has indicated, by tensions between lay and ecclesiastical power.[6] It was not until 1624 that the Accademia di San Luca was brought fully under the jurisdiction of a cardinal protector, at which time the artists' institutional responsibility to Roman secular law waned and was directed instead to the cardinal vicar and the cardinal protector.[7]

There is less certainty about the identity of Monsignor Cesarini, though he undoubtedly belonged to the distinguished Roman family of the same name, several members of which became cardinals.[8] Whether Monsignor Cesarini was Cardinal Savelli's assistant or an independent agent of reform remains to be determined.[9]

At approximately the same moment as Zaga presented the cardinal vicar's mandate to the Università dei Pittori, the Council of Trent took up a subject that, for its summary nature, has posed no end of confusion and speculation among the scholars who for 450 years have tried to parse its meaning: a general pronouncement on the purpose and the expectation of the visual arts. In Session 25 the Council famously "proscribed any images that would inspire false doctrine, admonished artists to avoid all impurities, and exhorted the new art to delight, teach, and move the faithful through a simple, straightforward, and accurate representation of Christian doctrine and Church history."[10] John O'Malley's essay in this volume sheds new light on the overwhelming docket that faced the members of the Council, who were simultaneously rushing to complete their charge and facing the imminence of Pope Pius IV's death, which would, ipso facto, have brought the proceedings to an untimely conclusion.

O'Malley argues that, contrary to the recent contributions of Romeo de Maio, Fabrizio Mancinelli, and others, the Council had neither the time nor the inclination to address individual works of art either during the sessions or at the conclusion in its pronouncements.[11] Thus, even as it is now widely accepted that the Council itself reproached Michelangelo for errors of decorum and what I am here calling art that is *inhonesta* or *desonesta*, O'Malley corrects the timeline of events to demonstrate that all of the extant recorded discussion of Michelangelo's *Last Judgment* took place not in Trent, but back in Rome at the turn of the next calendar year during meetings of the *congregazione* called by Pius IV. I can also corroborate O'Malley's chronology based on a rereading of the decrees of the twenty-fifth meeting of the Council of Trent on 3–4 December 1563 and the subsequent action items undertaken by the *congregazione* assembled by Pius IV in January 1564. Indeed, all of the references to the deliberations over Michelangelo's *Last Judgment* during the ninth, or rather twenty-fifth, and final Council can now be attributed to a misunderstanding of the references to the sessions at Trent. The passage quoted in nearly all studies, from Ludwig von Pastor to Pier Luigi de Vecchi to Romeo de Maio, reads approximately as follows, though some omit the reference to the decrees of the twenty-fifth session: "Picturae in capella apostolica cooperiantur, in aliis autem ecclesiis deleantur, si quae aliquid obscoenum aut evidenter falsum ostendant, iuxta decretum secundum in sess. 9 [25] sub Pio."[12] Most art historians have assumed that the ninth (i.e., twenty-fifth) session of Trent was a literal discussion of Michelangelo's (in)famous fresco that occurred on 3 or 4 December 1563. Instead, if we look at decree 2 from the ninth session, we find a much more general – and quite well known – document entitled "De Invocatione, Veneratione et Reliquiis Sanctorum, et Sacris Imaginibus." The section concerning false or obscene art is not specific to any artist or work of art, but reads in part:

> If any abuses shall have found their way into these holy and salutary observances, the holy council desires earnestly that they be completely removed, so that no representation of false doctrines and such as might be the occasion of grave error to the uneducated be exhibited. And if at times it happens, when this is beneficial to the illiterate, that the stories and narratives of the Holy Scriptures are portrayed and exhibited, the people should be instructed that not for that reason is the divinity represented in the picture as if it can be seen with bodily eyes or expressed in colors or figures. Furthermore in ... the sacred use of images, all superstition shall be removed, all filthy quest for gain eliminated, and all lasciviousness avoided, so that images shall not be painted and adorned with a seductive charm.[13]

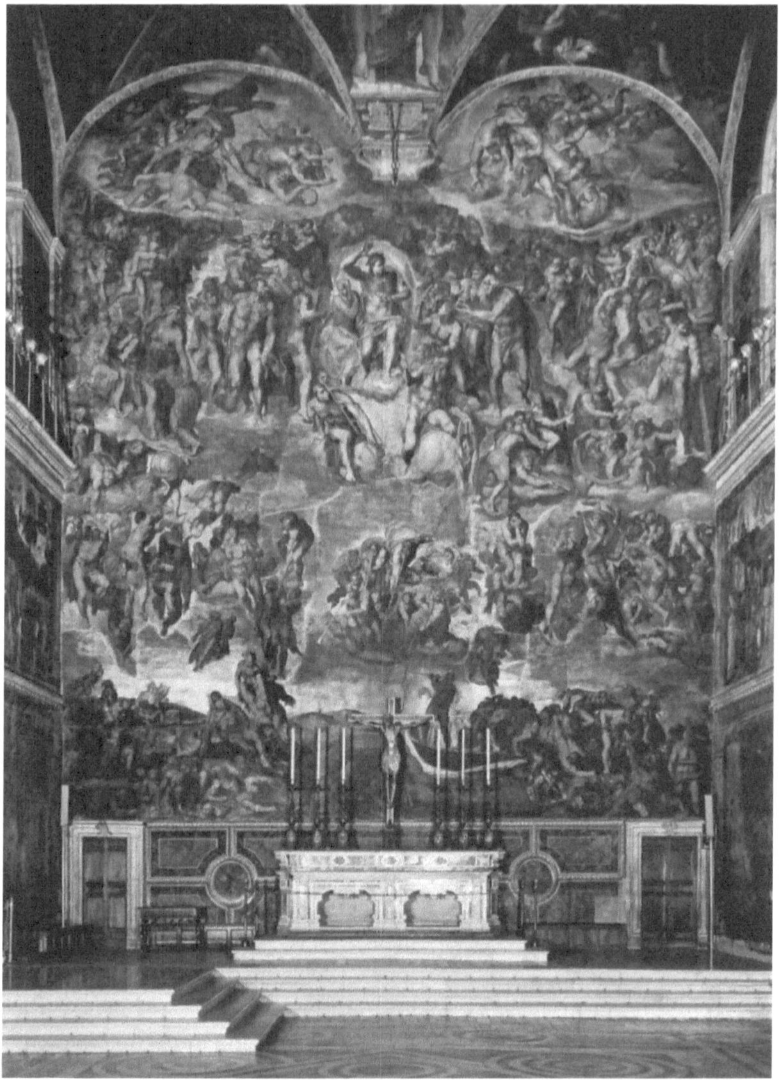

29. Michelangelo Buonarotti, *The Last Judgment*. Vatican City, Sistine Chapel. Photo: Erich Lessing / Art Resource, NY.

The subject of these discussions was a cause célèbre, as Michelangelo's *Last Judgment* was already one of the most controversial and complex paintings created in Christendom. On 21 January 1564, the *congregazione* decided that the objectionable parts of Michelangelo's *Last Judgment* (Illustration 29) – that is, the nude figures of the saved and damned souls – should be painted over.[14] They do not explain how or by whom, which we learn only subsequently with the hiring of the breeches painter, Daniele da Volterra. At the same time, the recent restoration of the *Last Judgment* has revealed that the originally nude figures of St. Blaise and St. Catherine of Alexandria were the most radically transformed: in addition to the heavy draperies placed on both of their bodies, Blaise's head was completely removed, a fresh *intonaco* laid down, and an entirely new head painted in its place, now directed toward Christ.[15] I contend that the first exhortation issued by the cardinal vicar in the summer of 1563 was a warning shot across the bow for the Università dei Pittori, before the Council of Trent concluded and before the *congregazione* of Pius IV had been organized. Nonetheless, the fate of the *Last Judgment* served as a pointed and timely message to any would-be pretender to Michelangelo's audacity. With the active campaign of bowdlerization, the *congregazione* of Pius IV proved it could and, more menacingly, would expurgate and/or destroy any work of art that it deemed to be *desonesta*. But what, precisely, did Savelli and others mean by painting virtuously?

During the mid–sixteenth century, *honestas/inhonestas* and their Italian equivalents, *onestà/desonestà*, were charged terms, appearing not only in the pronouncements of the Council of Trent ("nihil profanum nihilque inhonestum appareat cum domum Dei deceat sanctitudo") but also in treatises on art and poetry.[16] Robert Gaston's essay in this volume draws attention to the classical sources of *honestas*, meaning "propriety," and of its categorical opposite, *inhonestas*, or "profane," beginning with the writings of Cicero and Quintilian and tracing an arc through St. Ambrose to the Protestant and Catholic Reformers of the sixteenth century. Following on the prehistory of our previous example, in the period just before the final Council of Trent Michelangelo's *Last Judgment* came under severe attack, first by Aretino (letter to Michelangelo, 1545) and then by Aretino's close

30. Michelangelo Buonarotti, *The Last Judgment*, detail. Vatican City, Sistine Chapel. Photo: Scala / Art Resource, NY.

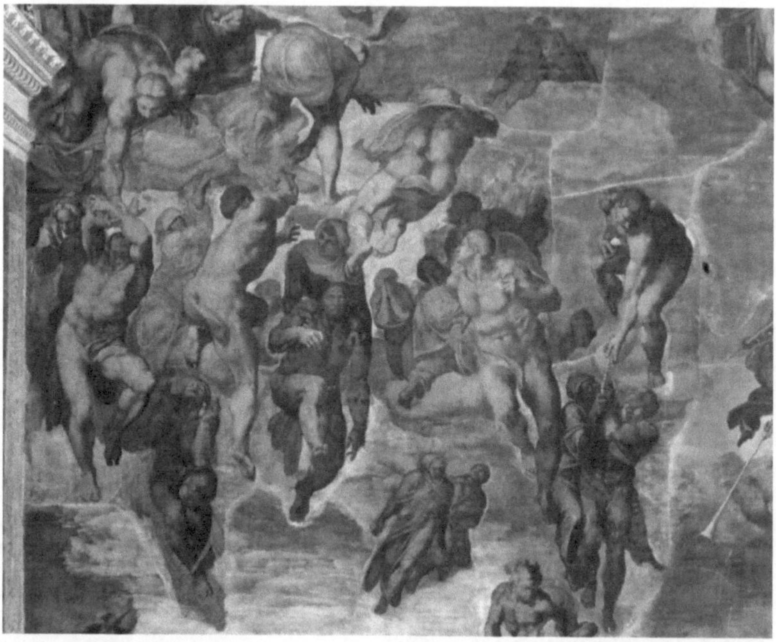

colleague and defender, Ludovico Dolce (*L'Aretino*, 1557), for lasciviousness and indecorousness. Dolce characterized the nudes in the *Last Judgment* as an affront to the prince of the Church (Peter) and to the numerous visitors to the papal chapel, leveling his strongest attack against the nudes that are shown "disonestamente dritti e riversi"[17] (Illustration 30). Anthony Blunt translated this passage as "shamelessly uncovered both before and behind."[18] As the expurgations by the breeches painter(s) demonstrate, Dolce's criticism was taken quite literally, as drapes were added to cover both the "before and the behind" of the figures. The priest Giovanni Andrea Gilio, similarly, called for painters to create sacred images "virtuously and devoutly, with those qualities that had been given to them by the ancients as betokens their holiness."[19]

Although the goals and purposes of these sixteenth-century authors might not always have aligned, the consistency of the appearance of *honestà*, as well as its adjectival and adverbial forms, in Latinate spelling with the "h" suggests that there was a good deal of cross-fertilization taking place. One of the most prominent of the figures in this discussion, as we have seen, was Gilio, a cleric by training and inclination and a commentator on the arts by circumstance. In his oft-cited *Dialogue on the Abuse of History by Painters*, as Charles Dempsey has shown, Gilio accused Michelangelo of error in the poetic ornamentation of sacred history painting.[20] Not fully acknowledged in this context of error and heresy is the complete passage, partially cited earlier, concerning the depiction of nudes, in which Gilio declared modern painting in general, and Michelangelo's *Last Judgment* in particular, to lack *onestà*. Gilio further stated: "Painting sacred images, honest and devout, with these signs that have been given to them by the ancients in accordance with their holiness, which has seemed to the moderns vile, clumsy, common, humble, outdated, and without ingeniousness or art; on that basis, they prefer art to virtuousness. Leaving [aside] the custom of making figures clothed, they have made or continue to make them nude; leaving behind the custom of making them devout, they have made them strained, as if it were a big deal to twist the head, the arms, and the legs, such that it seems that they represent someone performing a dance ('moresche') or a piece of theater rather than someone who is contemplating."[21] Later, in his treatise entitled *Topica Poetica* (1581), Gilio elaborated his conception of decorum as a correspondence between the style and the subject of the poem. He warned poets not to mistake "per le honeste, le rozzi" (virtuous [things] for coarse ones).[22]

Beyond this admittedly reductive focus on the term *honestà* looms the much larger conceptual and theoretical issue of decorum as it was understood in the sixteenth century. For this the reader is directed to discussions in the works of Robert Williams, Charles Dempsey, and Robert Gaston, each of whom has dissected the early modern notions of decorum with particular relation to the fine arts. Williams, for example, provides a useful tripartite model for qualifying the type of decorum referenced: "the relation of an image to its setting or function – conditions that affect the choice of subject matter and style ... the relation between things in a picture and the things that they represent ... [or] the relations among the parts of a picture to one another."[23] Of these, the type of decorum best exemplified in the censure of Michelangelo's fresco as well as in the cardinal vicar's and the Council of Trent's exhortation to the Università dei Pittori is the first, or the relation between the work of art and its setting or function. The Council was not proscribing the painting of nudes or lascivious scenes of any kind, rather those that included representations of Christ, the Virgin, or saints. Dempsey, by contrast, argues a more subtle point: that Gilio was spot on in his critique of the *Last Judgment*, attacking "the form chosen for setting forth themes of sacred history"; that is, Michelangelo used the heroic nude figures of ancient art to ornament his painting for the altar wall of the Sistine Chapel. Thus, Michelangelo "corrupted sacred [images]" by "wish[ing] to return art to the images of the ancients as found not only in the nudes but in the mixed modes of the epic employed by Raphael in the Vatican."[24] Robert Gaston's many publications on the concept of decorum, or "fitness," also lay out a proper frame of reference for understanding the twin attacks on artistic prerogative that occurred both before and after the Council of Trent; that is, following Dolce, "the religious justification of the nudes did not compensate for their lack of decency (*honestà*)."[25] His essay in this collection emphasizes the long history and "rhetorical embeddedness" of the notion of decorum.

At the same time that these literary and artistic debates raged, the terms that were bandied about had an even longer history within the Church itself. The notion of Christian virtue, for example, was indeed deeply embedded in the monastic orders. The rule of the Dominican Order urged its members "honeste vivere, discere et docere" (to live, learn, and teach virtuously).[26] In that sense there is a certain seamlessness in Gilio's thoughts that cuts across both painting and poetry, across both art and life, illuminating the critical terminology that likewise addresses both sacred and secular life, as well as artistic production.

In the few cases where there was both a consensus about what characterized a lack of virtuousness and a collective will to act on it, what recourse did Church or civic authorities have at their disposal? In other words, was the decision to repaint Michelangelo's *Last Judgment* strategically the only or the most appropriate option for the *congregazione* to have taken? In his study of Pietro da Cortona and Giovanni Domenico Ottonelli's *Trattato della pittura e della scultura, uso et abuso loro, composto da un theologo e da un pittore* (1652), Yvon le Gall recently attempted to divide post-Tridentine responses to lapses in decorum into four categories of censure that parallel Cardinal Savelli's exhortation: (1) moving the picture (most often suggested by Cortona and Ottonelli) to a private space; (2) hiding the pictures or covering them completely; (3) expurgating the offensive parts; (4) destroying the work completely.[27] Thus, by the middle of the seventeenth century, the Church's dicta had become codified, and although they postdate the discussions of the *Last Judgment* by nearly one hundred years, these recommendations illuminate the choices of both artist and censor in the early modern period. Since the first two options were clearly out of the question for such a large and architecturally fixed work, the authorities were faced, *faute de mieux*, with the latter two: expurgation or destruction of the fresco. By these standards the authorities opted for the lesser of two evils, choosing to cover the offending figures and confining their destruction to the small section with St. Catherine and St. Blaise that the *congregazione* apparently found most troubling of all.

The date of the decision to repaint the objectionable parts of Michelangelo's *Last Judgment* coincided almost exactly with Cardinal Savelli's announcement to the Guild of Painters. Thus, the threat of imminent destruction hung palpably in the air of Counter-Reform Rome, for even the work of the most renowned artist in the land could be altered or potentially destroyed if it breached the Church's standards of decorum, or *onestà* – just as in recent years bold actions of censorship or obliteration taken against prominent artists – whether Robert Mapplethorpe for his *X Portfolio* or Richard Serra for his *Tilted Arc* – had a chilling effect among their contemporaries.[28] The artists of the Guild, with far less grand reputations and far fewer well-placed champions than Michelangelo enjoyed, could not but have received the intended message: the cardinals, bishops, and priests were henceforth going to hold painters accountable for the *honestà* of their sacred works.

Little is known, however, about any legal action taken against *desonesti* painters beyond the very public censuring of Michelangelo's *Last Judgment*.[29] Much more widely known and circulated were the writings of Gabriele Paleotti, whose *Discorso intorno alle imagini sacre e profane* (1582) served as a treatise and dictionary of the fine points of sacred and secular art. The entirety of the unpublished book 3 was to have concerned "lascivious paintings that are not conducive to virtuousness." With chapters such as "What Is Indecency?," "How Much Indecency Is Abhorred by Nature, the Law, and God," one concerning the appropriate and inappropriate depiction of saints nude, and "Arguments by Painters Who Excuse Themselves for Painting Nude or Lascivious Images or with Actions That Are Hardly Decent," Paleotti planned to lay out the most complete case against the notion of *desonestà* yet undertaken.[30] But it was never written.

Despite the silence of Paleotti and other sources on confrontations between Roman painters and the Church in the decades following the repainting of the *Last Judgment*, it is clear that the matter of *oneste/desoneste* images continued to resonate among painters well into the foundation and early maturity of the Accademia di San Luca, the more independent institutional and pedagogical successor of the Università dei Pittori. Not least, Paleotti himself served as provisional cardinal protector of the Accademia from 1595 until his death in 1597; he was followed by Cardinal del Monte, both replacing Federico Borromeo, who was then serving as archbishop of Milan. Romano Alberti refers to these interim cardinal protectors as "educator[i] della riformanda."[31] In 1598, moreover, then-current *principe* Durante Alberti invited a Jesuit priest to address the Accademia. Like Savelli before him, the priest exhorted painters to create "virtuous [*oneste*] and praiseworthy things and to flee from any lascivious or indecent [things]."[32]

The question remains one of how and where artists in Rome learned the proper means of creating virtuous and praiseworthy things. In the founding documents for the Accademia di San Luca, penned on 7 March 1593, the six deputies declared their principal purposes for founding an academy to be "for the glory and honor of God and for all those who practice painting nobly." In addition, the academy was intended to be a place in which "to instruct the young and those engaged on the proper road of the study of painting." Further, the Accademia stated that painters should be of the type "who could paint – in churches and elsewhere – images that inspired piety and devotion as intended by the holy fathers who founded them."[33]

The late sixteenth century witnessed not only the professional and philosophical deliberations that brought the Accademia into existence, but also numerous ecclesiastical and educational institutions, such as the Oratorio di San Ignazio and the Collegio di Propaganda Fide. The will to educate – and inculcate – was thus firmly in place and everywhere in evidence. Of all the painters working in the late Cinquecento, perhaps the most sensitive to artistic education was Federico Zuccaro (1540/41–1609), who had witnessed firsthand the teaching and professional practices of the Accademia del Disegno during his stint as head of the decoration for the cupola of the Florentine cathedral after Vasari's death, from 1576 to 1579. Zuccaro subsequently played important roles in the direction of the Compagnia di San Giuseppe in Terra Santa, or Virtuosi, during the 1580s and in the foundation of the Accademia di San Luca in 1593.[34]

The backstory of Zuccaro's theoretical principles actually extended to his earliest training with his brother Taddeo in the 1560s (Illustration 31). Taddeo's autodidactic training and his misfortunes as a beleaguered apprentice make for a compelling artist's narrative that Federico captured in a remarkable series of drawings now housed at the J. Paul Getty Museum. It was under his autodidact brother's tutelage that Federico learned the importance of drawing after antiquity (Illustration 32) and after modern masters (Illustrations 33 and 34). One point to be made here is that not only was Taddeo's early career shown to be arduous, it was also peripatetic. The difficulty and the rewards of study are proportional to the physical exertion expended in the learning process: Taddeo literally walked the streets of Rome absorbing the art as much through labor as through artistic judgment and practice of hand. Thus, Taddeo apprehended the works of the ancient and modern masters through his combined senses of sight and

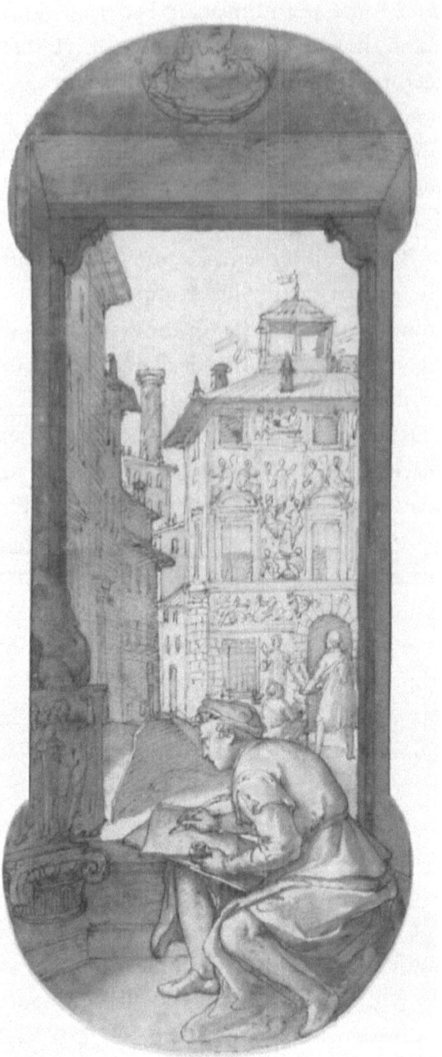

31 (right). Federico Zuccaro, *Taddeo Drawing after the Antique; In the Background Copying a Facade by Polidoro*, c. 1595. Pen and brown ink, brush with brown wash, over black chalk and touches of red chalk, 42.3 × 17.5 cm. Photo: J. Paul Getty Museum, Los Angeles.

32 (below). Federico Zuccaro, *Taddeo in the Belvedere Court in the Vatican Drawing the Laocoön*, c. 1595. Pen and brown ink, brush with brown wash, over black chalk and touches of red chalk, 17.5 × 42.5 cm. Photo: J. Paul Getty Museum, Los Angeles.

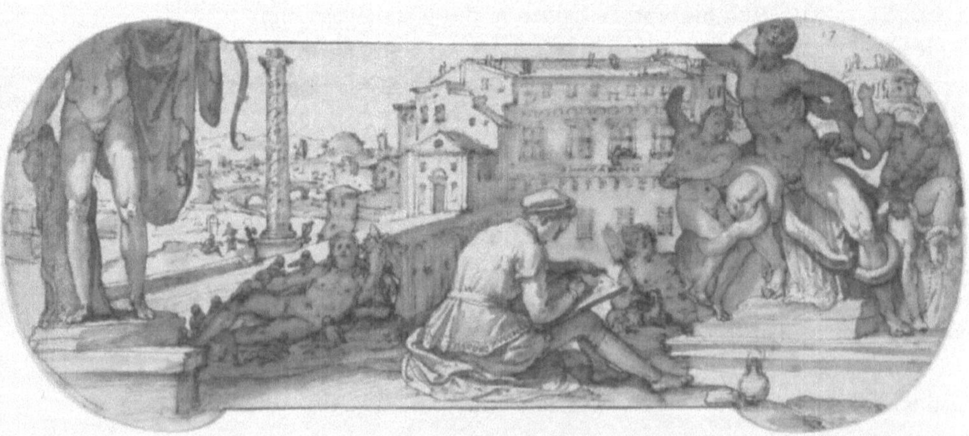

touch and his concomitant intellectual and bodily engagement with the works of art. His experience of copying and imitation were hence akin to muscular memories, fundamental to musical pedagogy and athletic training. Yet I want to be equally clear that as powerful as these images of "la vita agro-dolce of Taddeo Zuccaro" are,[35] Federico never advocated copying as the sole path for *giovani* to follow, as we learn in his later writings

33 (below, left). Federico Zuccaro, *Taddeo Copying Raphael's Frescoes in the Loggia of the Villa Farnesina, Where He Is Also Represented Asleep*, c. 1595. Pen and brown ink, brush with brown wash, over black chalk and touches of red chalk, 42.4 × 17.5 cm. Photo: J. Paul Getty Museum, Los Angeles.

34 (below, right). Federico Zuccaro, *Taddeo in the Sistine Chapel Drawing Michelangelo's Last Judgment*, c. 1595. Pen and brown ink, brush with brown wash, over black chalk and touches of red chalk, 41.9 × 17.7 cm. Photo: J. Paul Getty Museum, Los Angeles.

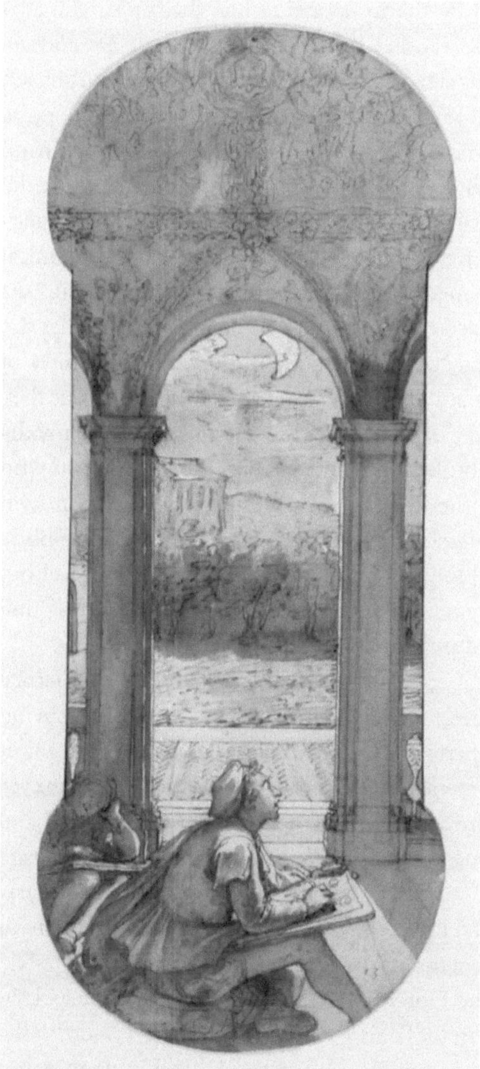

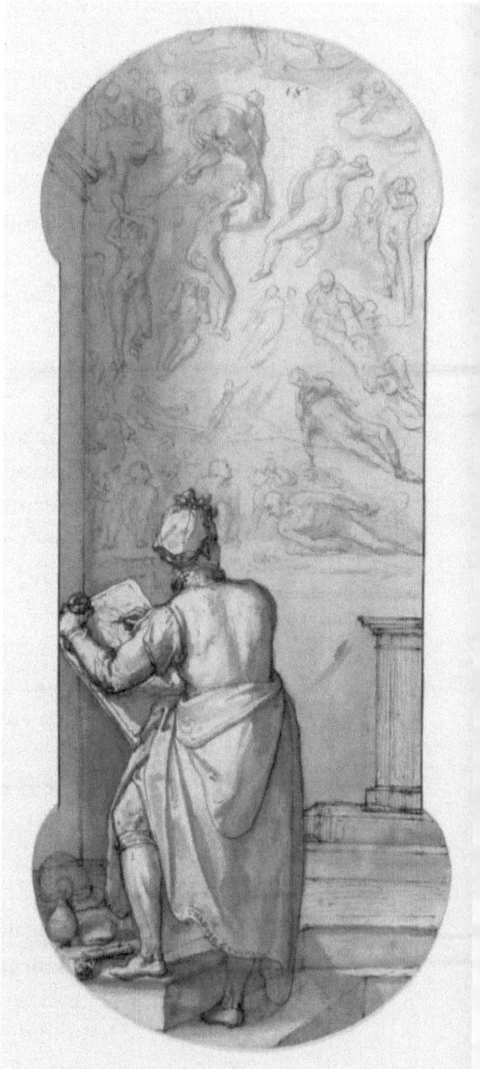

and in the narratives of the decorations of his two homes, one in Florence and the other in Rome.[36]

The Palazzo Zuccaro (or Casa Zuccari) on the Pincian Hill in Rome included a suite of rooms devoted to drawing as the father of all disciplines. Federico's fresco *Sic Salus Publica* (Illustration 35), for example, shows an allegorical figure, Public Health, enthroned in the center foreground of a complex space of work and study, including a library across the back wall; a work table, at left, with a skeletal model and an *écorchée*; a fully functioning alchemical laboratory directly behind Health; and at right an active anatomical theater. At the base of the plinth on which Health is seated lie three strategically placed books with their spines facing the viewer: those of Avicenna, Galen, and Hippocrates, all three fundamental texts for medical study. By the 1590s, when Zuccaro painted this scene, however, Andrea Vesalius and others had already demonstrated that anatomy could not be understood or apprehended by theory alone; rather, the aspiring anatomist had to participate in dissections. In the frontispiece for *De Humani Corporis*, for example, Vesalius steadies the arm of the corpse with his left hand and holds the exposed tendons of the corpse's hand with his right. As Claire Richter Sherman has argued, "The focus on Vesalius' own hand as writer and recorder shows his intellectual prowess as scholar, while the dissected hand demonstrates his manual skill as an anatomist."[37] The allegorical figure in Zuccaro's fresco holds what appears to be a botanical manuscript in his hands opened to a medicinal plant in an herbal.[38] At the worktable a scholar (or artist?) writes notes and apparently copies the study figures in front of him. Next to him the distillation apparatuses of the scientist or alchemist are at full boil. No one attends to them, but they are shown to be kinetic and not at rest. And, at far right, the men gathered around the corpse are broken into two groups: the two *garzoni* who assist with the dissection in the foreground and the two older men who supervise and witness the demonstration at the lower end of the body. The young men touch the bloody, partially flayed body as they go about presenting it to their colleagues. The older ones observe, thus preserving the separation of manual and intellectual effort.[39]

Two things are striking about Zuccaro's depiction of the laboratory. First, all of the men are actively drawing after, writing about, or copying from the dissection as they perform a variety of experiments or go about their research. Second, this interaction with tools, books, and notebooks is, like Taddeo's autodidactic process of artistic education, both physical and active. The process of learning is itself kinetic, and the participants engage in discourse or in recording – whether drawing or writing – their experiences. Further, this anatomical theater quite literally strips the body bare of all pretense and, with it, the sense of decorum that governed large public commissions like those of the Florentine cupola or the Sistine Chapel.[40]

Depicted behind the figure of Salus Publica (Illustration 35), or Public Welfare, is a scene of a dissection in a laboratory that brings together

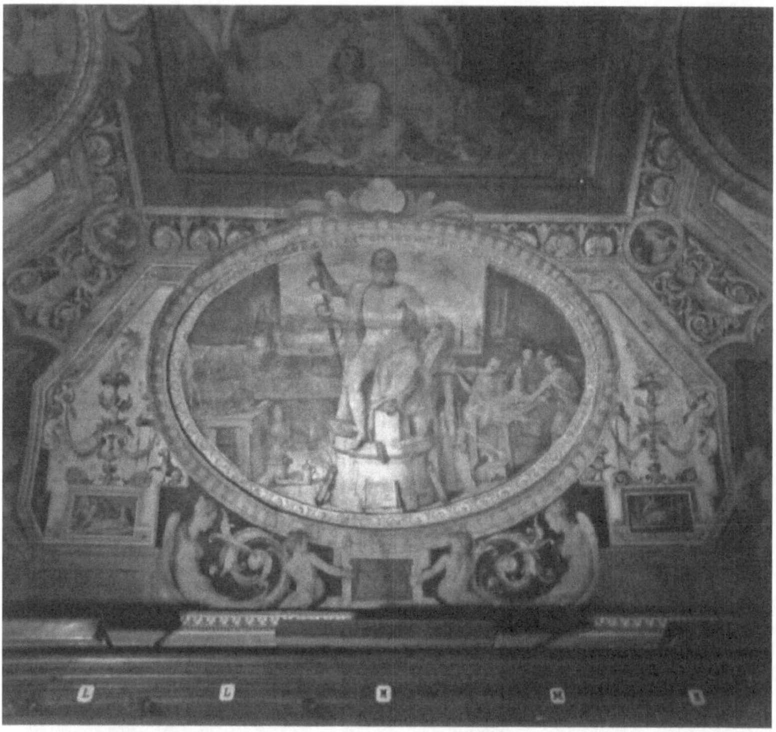

35. Federico Zuccaro, *Salus Publica*, detail. Rome, Casa Zuccari, vault of the Sala del Disegno. Photo: Bibliotheca Hertziana – Max-Planck-Institut für Kunstgeschichte, Rome.

the study of anatomy with the disciplines of natural philosophy, music, military arts, and medicine (Illustration 36). In the scenes contiguous to Salus/Medicine are those of Scientia, Militia, and Musica (Illustration 37). The allegorical figure Knowledge (Scientia) is adorned by the three levels of approbation: the juridical, the philosophical, and the theological, following, as we shall see, exactly Romano Alberti's model for the different types of nobility. In fact, the frame below Zuccaro's Scientia is inscribed, "Sic vera nobilitas."[41] Thus, even though Zuccaro did not himself write about the concept of the nobility of painting, he internalized the arguments made by Leon Battista Alberti and others to be used later for classroom teaching and for didactic narratives in the public rooms of his home.

It should be noted that precisely at this moment when Federico was designing and executing the decoration of his palace, he was also administering the Roman Accademia di San Luca. And we learn from the *Origine et progresso dell'Academia del Dissegno, de Pittori, Scultori, & Architetti di Roma* that in 1594 Zuccaro arranged for a dissection in the cold months of late January so that the members of the Accademia could make drawings after every part of the process, from layers of skin to muscles, bones, and veins.[42] Together, the Palazzo Zuccaro fresco and this description of a dissection in Alberti's *Origine* lend credence to Federico's commitment to mastering the internal structure and workings of the body.

One of the most important early champions of the Accademia was Romano Alberti – secretary of the institution, as well as poet and artist – who wrote the *Trattato della nobiltà della pittura* (1585), which remains a source for sixteenth-century art theory that has been overlooked for centuries.[43] The treatise was published eight years before the Accademia was officially founded and, according to the title page, at the behest of the burgeoning Accademia de[ll]i Pittori di Roma. This is a rather amazing claim, since the Accademia di San Luca, though sanctioned in 1577 by a brief from Pope Gregory XIII, had yet to complete its incorporation by 1585. By the mid-1580s, the Roman painters were still functioning as part of the Università dei Pittori and the Compagnia (Confraternity) di San Luca. Romano Alberti, a member of the acclaimed family of painters from Borgo San Sepolcro, dedicated his book to Cardinal Alfonso Gesualdo, first protector of the academy and cardinal of the Kingdom of Naples.[44] Alberti's treatise has a single

36. Federico Zuccaro, Vault of the Sala del Disegno. Rome, Casa Zuccari. Photo: Bibliotheca Hertziana – Max-Planck-Institut für Kunstgeschichte, Rome.

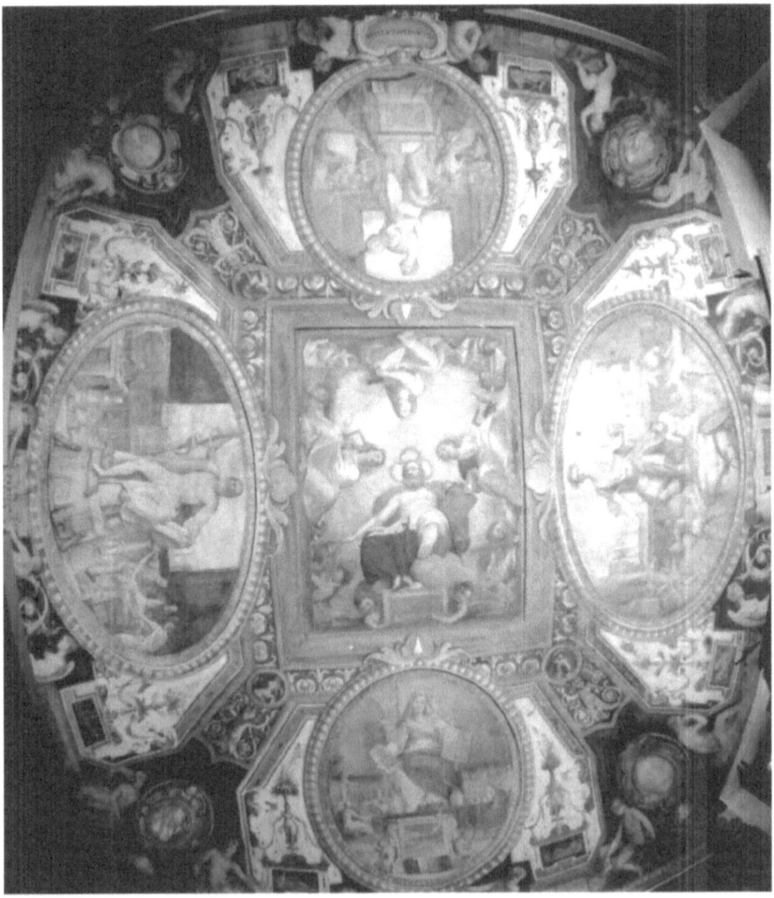

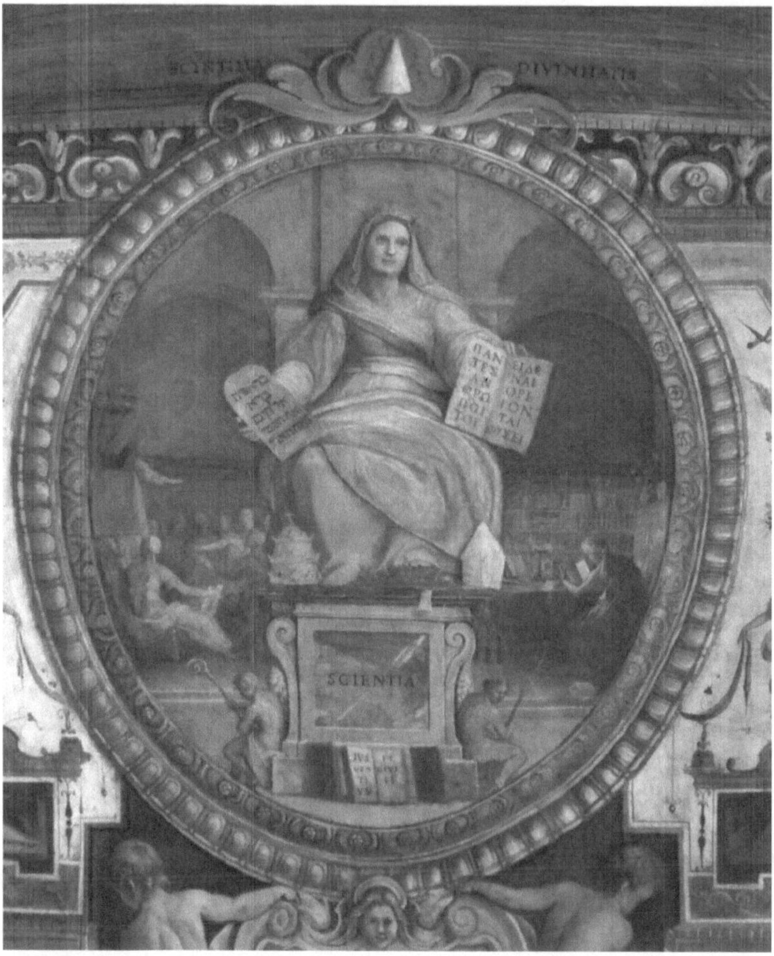

37. Federico Zuccaro, *Scientia*, detail. Rome, Casa Zuccari, vault of the Sala del Disegno. Photo: Bibliotheca Hertziana – Max-Planck-Institut für Kunstgeschichte, Rome.

theme and purpose: to elevate the status of painting from that of a vile and mechanical profession to that of noble and liberal art. The book addresses a skeptical audience and attempts to dismantle opposition to the liberality of painting in a series of arguments on the three types of nobility: (1) civil/political/extrinsic; (2) natural/philosophical/intrinsic; and (3) theological/spiritual/grace-given. And although Alberti cited well-worn references to the ancients from Aristotle and Plutarch to Pliny, Cicero, Horace, and Seneca, to more recent theorists like Leon Battista Alberti and Paolo Pino, he also drew on examples chosen from very contemporary documents and publications, including the Council of Trent and the writings of Cardinal Gabriele Paleotti. The relation of the texts can be observed in Alberti's carefully constructed argument that addresses several points: the emphasis on the purity of the motives for creation (i.e., not for vile profit), the avoidance of lasciviousness, and the lack of superstition. Alberti's treatise provides the clearest evidence of the response of the nascent Accademia to issues of the Counter-Reform – in this case blatantly self-serving ones. Toward the end of his treatise, Alberti deployed his most compelling theological reasoning, from which I would like to highlight the passage in which he advances the notion that painting is intrinsically ennobling and therefore its practitioners partake of divine nobility. Paraphrasing Paleotti's *De Imaginibus* (1582), Alberti cited the example of a criminal who was contemplating murder but, while visiting a church, viewed an image of the Crucifixion and was miraculously converted to Christianity and consequently abandoned his life of crime.[45] My point here is twofold. First, neither Paleotti nor Alberti made apotropaic claims for the painting; it is not presented as a miraculous image per se, like an ex voto[46] or an acheiropoieta.[47] Second, without the name of the artist or the church, the transformation of the soul of the criminal cannot be attributed to the divine manner of a particular painter or a specific sacred space. It is indeed the generic nature of the picture that gives this account weight and substance: the miraculous conversion is not occasioned by the sermon of a priest or by the reading of the Bible; rather, it is prompted entirely by contemplation of the Crucifixion as rendered by a painter. Thus, if a painting can prompt a conversion, the painter – its maker – shares in nothing less than the act of salvation. In a single stroke, then, the object of the painter's profession is ennobled and the painter, ipso facto, partakes of the highest form of nobility: the theological, or that bestowed by the grace of God.

In the same section of his treatise, Alberti pointed to St. Mary the Egyptian, who kept her eyes trained on representations of the Madonna and the cross. In this way, Alberti implied, she turned away from sin and was miraculously converted to Christianity.[48] Jacopo da Voragine's *Legenda Aurea* – Alberti's ostensible source – provides even more telling detail on the role of imagery in St. Mary the Egyptian's conversion: Despite many attempts to enter the church with the other pilgrims, she was always turned away. While she was bemoaning her fate in the inn, she looked upon an immured image of the Madonna, through which she received pardon from her sins, "which enabled me to enter the church and to adore the Cross."[49] Henceforth, St. Mary the Egyptian renounced her sinful past and became chaste. These two interventions of images in the conversion and worship practices of the saint speak doubly to Alberti's point that painting is intrinsically noble. The absolution of sin provided through the mediation of the image of the Virgin led Mary the Egyptian to a purified life of contemplation in which she was henceforth free to meditate on the images not only outside but inside the church.

Alberti continued his narrative with two further examples of the role of images in miraculous movements of souls: Bogore of Bulgaria and St. Anastasius the Persian. Bogore converted after seeing an image of the Last Judgment; Anastasius chose to be baptized after seeing many pictures of saints.[50] Together, Alberti reasoned, these miracles inextricably tied to images are not only indications of the call to remember the saints, but also points that link the efficacy of images as means of conversion, as promulgated at the Seventh Synod convened by Emperor Leo III in 754. This synod, where the veneration of images was declared idolatrous, preceded a period of iconoclasm. "Those who say that the use of images serves only the memory, but cannot be admitted for 'salvation' (that is, to be venerated), reveal themselves to be in a certain sense half-right and falsely truthful ... on one hand declaring the truth; on the other, acting perversely."[51] Instead, he argued, the Seventh Synod and St. Gregory maintained that images and objects of veneration in public spaces were inducements both to the memory of the acts of sacred personages and to pious discussions.[52] Further, painting "instruct[s] the intellect and mov[es] the will and refresh[es] the memory about divine things."[53]

Just as the Tridentine decrees stress the didactic function of art not only to instruct but also to move the spectator, so this crescendo of theological justifications in Alberti's treatise was meant not only to inform but also to convert the skeptic into a supporter of the nobility of painting. Remarkably, just twenty years later, in the *Origine et progresso dell'Academia dei pittori, scultori, et architetti* ... (1604), Alberti, now Zuccaro's *portavoce*, marginalized these same moral and spiritual arguments on painting for more technical and practical matters related to the education of the artist in the academy.

In the preamble to the *accademie* (lectures) given during his tenure as *principe* from 1593 to 1594, Zuccaro encouraged the *giovani*, or youths who had come to learn, to make drawings by their own hands; he would then respond by giving to the "best pupil" of the day one of his own. The "first things" every *giovane desideroso* was meant to learn included "the Alphabet of Drawing (such as it is called), the ABC, eyes, noses, mouths, ears, heads, hands, feet, arms, legs, bodies, backs, and other similar parts, whether of the human body or of animals, and figures, equally of the things of architecture, and works of relief in wax, clay, and similar exercises"[54] (Illustration 38). This is the only extant drawing from the first decades of the Accademia; it shows the *giovani* seated above around an altar, drawing a fragment, and Zuccaro sitting in the right lower foreground.[55] Thus, Zuccaro's message to neophyte artists is nothing if not consistent: drawing is the father of all the arts, and one must begin by mastering the fundamentals of the discipline, from the parts of the body to all aspects of art and nature. But for all its importance for the excellence of artists, Zuccaro's educational model did not begin and end with the practice of drawing; he also clearly advocated theoretical discussion, which he promoted through academic discourse and disputation.

Among the accoutrements of the Accademia, Zuccaro instituted a collection of drawings[56] and models for sculptors, as well as drawings, plans, and models of architecture, some of which were given away to the *giovani* as incentives.[57] From the beginning of March 1594, Zuccaro tapped members to speak about subjects ranging from the representation of movement

(Cavaliere d'Arpino), to decorum (Cherubino Alberti), grace and beauty, the ornamentation of figures in a history painting, and later to *spirito* and *vivezza*, painting in relief, how to compose a history painting well, how to achieve a *simile* or *verosimile concetto*, invention and capriccio, *morbidezza* and true expression, imitation from life, drapery and dressing figures, the nude and its musculature, perspective, and mathematics and its utility for painters.[58] The publication of the *Origine e progresso* was in fact intended to revive Zuccaro's pedagogical plan for the Accademia di San Luca, which had waned under subsequent *principi*. Whether he was successful or not in coercing his peers to lecture (many did not follow through), the point of this excursus is nonetheless significant: Zuccaro here outlined his conception for the complete training of the artist and pointed to the utility of the Accademia as an institution that could support and foster both the theoretical and the practical instruction of its members.[59] Further, this pedagogical model would satisfy the Counter-Reform tenets voiced by Savelli, Paleotti, and the unnamed Jesuit father who addressed the Accademia in 1598. In addition to learning the fundaments of the art of painting, they would be instructed in notions of decorum (presented in an *accademia* given by Cherubino Alberti) and virtuous representation.[60]

I conclude by returning to *The Life of Taddeo Zuccaro* created by his brother Federico, a series of drawings dated to about 1590 that has hitherto been viewed as evidence of the primacy of copying and imitation in the autodidactic education of Taddeo. Equally important, though rarely remarked, the monuments that Federico chose to highlight around Rome not only tell us which foundational works by the ancients and moderns attracted young artists to them like bees to floral nectar, but also serve as historical records of the appearance of Rome in the middle of the sixteenth century. Of special interest within the frame of the criticism of Michelangelo's *Last Judgment* is the image of Taddeo as a young man copying the lower left section of the fresco (Illustration 34). Here we find Federico struggling with several competing agendas. On one hand, he was charged with creating a temporal unity appropriate to the period during which Taddeo actually made his copies – that is, sometime during the late 1540s or early 1550s, before the *Last Judgment* was officially censured and physically altered by the addition of the breeches. It had, of course, been under fire for decades. As early as 1545, Aretino encouraged Michelangelo to turn " 'the indecent parts of the damned into flames and those of the blessed to sunbeams.' "[61] On the other hand, Zuccaro was nothing if not fully aware of the risks that a painter faced in challenging the Church's norms of decorum. The litany of Zuccaro's works that had been criticized or threatened with destruction included his dome of the Florentine cathedral (1576–79) – itself a *Last Judgment* whose audacious display of nudity (if only among the damned) and anachronisms drew fire from all fronts; the vitriolic response to critics of his failed altarpiece for Bologna in the painting for the facade of San Luca, the *Porta Virtutis* of 1581, for which

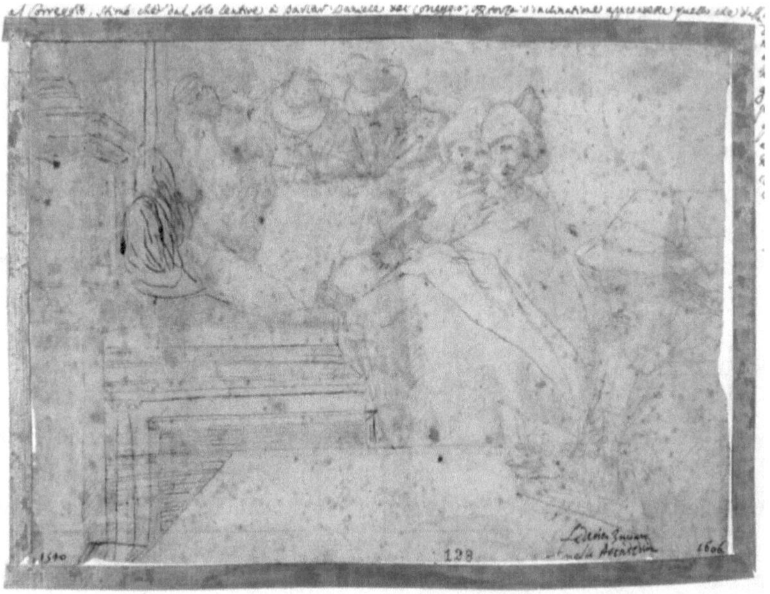

38. Circle of Federico Zuccaro, *Federico Zuccaro and Other Academicians Drawing at the First Site of the Accademia di San Luca*, c. 1590s. Pen, black and red chalk on prepared paper. Milan, Biblioteca Ambrosiana. Photo: Biblioteca Ambrosiana Auth. No. F 46/07.

Pope Gregory XIII banished him from Rome; and even his monumental decorative cycles for Philip II at the Escorial, which were completely repainted almost immediately after Zuccaro departed from Spain in late 1588. With these challenges to his artistic and religious integrity close to mind, Zuccaro created the *Life of Taddeo* in the 1590s, depicting nudes both sacred and secular. From Raphael's Olympian gods in the Loggia di Psiche at the Farnese Palace (Illustration 33) to the *Laocoön* and *Apollo* (Illustration 32) in the Belvedere Court of the Vatican, shown in all their original glory, to the now lost fresco cycles of Polidoro da Caravaggio (Illustration 38), we see the full range of work considered to be by artists in the Zuccaro brothers' pantheon of models worthy of study and imitation. It should be noted that all of these works were intended for secular contexts and fall, therefore, outside the scope of Cardinal Savelli's warning. In making his copy of the *Last Judgment*, a sacred painting in the holiest of spaces in Rome, however, Federico faced a potentially double-edged criticism: to show Michelangelo's nude saints as they appeared when Taddeo first saw them (as in his only known copy of a single figure now in the British Museum, T-11-78) and risk countermanding the Church's sense of painting *virtuously* or to add the (post-1564) breeches and risk breaching an equally compelling sense of historical decorum.[62] Unusual for the normally combative Zuccaro, he chose a diplomatic solution, a third way, if you will. Whereas one can see that the resurrected figures in Federico's drawing are nude, the offending genitalia and poses – shown, in Dolce's words, "disonestamente dritti e riversi" – are blurred, thus both visible and indistinct at once. With their pink flesh tones, the figures in Federico's copy of the *Last Judgment* are even more emphatically nude in the corresponding painting on leather (c. 1600, Rome, Galleria Nazionale d'Arte Antica, FN17130) made after the Getty drawing. Yet they, too, lack anatomical specificity, especially those depicted frontally.[63]

This indeterminacy of representation has repercussions for the study of the drapery campaigns that occurred after the Council of Trent ordered the censure of the *Last Judgment* on 21 January 1564.[64] The extraordinary restoration efforts and contemporaneous scientific and historic studies undertaken in the 1980s revealed that these censorious interventions probably took place over the course of centuries and that, even as late as 1762, workers were covering "offensive" passages of the fresco. For our purposes the first campaign is the most significant for the early history of the Counter-Reformation and for the role of painters under the aegis of the Università dei Pittori when the cardinal vicar (Savelli) exhorted them to paint virtuously or modestly. Those who have studied the documents for the scaffolding have concluded that the first breeches were probably added between August 1564 and December 1565. Fabrizio Mancinelli has further determined that the dimensions of the scaffolding during the first campaign suggest that the workers could have reached as high as the figures of St. Blaise and St. Catherine (which, as indicated, were chiseled out and completely repainted in fresco). The scaffolding was also broad enough that the breeches painters – Daniele da Volterra, followed by Girolamo da Fano – would have had access to the entire width of the fresco.[65] Thus, the detail of the lower left quadrant that Federico Zuccaro included in his drawing of Taddeo copying Michelangelo's *Last Judgment* could and probably would have already been retouched in the mid-1560s. The assumed documentary nature of Federico's drawing has always in fact been said to depict a post-restoration fresco. Consequently, many scholars claim that Zuccaro's drawing proves that the lower left corner of the *Last Judgment* had not been touched in the 1560s.[66] I would argue, instead, that Zuccaro expressly showed the fresco in its pre-restoration state, since that is how Taddeo would have known it. He would have had any number of prints to consult (such as those by Giulio Bonasone, c. 1546–50, and Giorgio Ghisi, c. 1564–69), as well as Marcello Venturi's 1545 painted version (Naples, Museo di Capodimonte) and, most likely, his own early drawings.[67] This line of reasoning does not definitively settle the question of when certain passages were retouched; however, it does call into question the overly simplified explanation of the order of the breeches campaigns with reference to prints and drawings. One should not, therefore, assume that the figures on the lower left were not covered with breeches until after 1590.[68]

Indeed, Federico Zuccaro's drawings for the *Life of Taddeo*, whether completed in the late 1570s or around 1595 – as most scholars now believe – shed new light on the history and interpretation of the interventions to the *Last Judgment*. If Zuccaro's calculated response to contemporary notions of *honestà* enabled him to satisfy both standards of decorum and his critics, his novel solution also illuminates a fascinating moment in the history of the reforming Church, the newly established Accademia di San Luca, and the place of the sensuous body within their respective religious and pedagogical agendas.

Notes

I would like to thank Tracy Cooper and Marcia Hall for their important suggestions and their encouragement. I am also beholden to John O'Malley for a series of very illuminating conversations about the transactions of the Council of Trent. In addition, I am grateful to Jill Pederson and Daniel McReynolds for their assistance with the bibliography and photography. Lorenzo Pericolo made wise suggestions about the translation and meaning of Italian and Latin passages in the text. All translations in the text are mine, except where indicated, and I accept responsibility for any errors that remain.

1 Leproux (1991), 330. The documents republished as transcriptions by Leproux can be found in ASR, *Collegio dei Notai Capitolini*, buste 26–40. The original passage reads: "Item il predicto Domenico consule ha admonito tutti li sopradetti presenti da parte del signor Vicario et Monsignor Cesarini che quelli che depingono le imagine del Signore et della Madonna et de alteri sancti et sancte, le habbino a dipingere honeste, altramente le si butteranno et guasteranno et loro Serrano gastigati, et che ognun se guardi della mala ventura." Zaga served as consul of the Università dei Pittori in Rome for the year 1563; Melchiorre Missirini also reports that Zaga served as *camerlengo* (treasurer) in 1568. See Missirini (1823), 16; also see Salvagni (2009), 69–121, esp. 78. The third session of the Council of Trent was held between 18 January 1562 and 4 December 1563. Ercole Gonzaga presided until his death and was replaced by Giovanni Morone. Neither the cardinal vicar of Rome nor Cardinal Cesarini was in attendance as far as I can determine; however, they were clearly charged with communicating reform policies to the guilds of Rome, perhaps at the behest of Pope Pius IV (1559–65). See Salvador Miranda, *Cardinals of the Holy Roman Church*, www2.fiu.edu/~mirandas/bios1539.htm, under the name of Cardinal Savelli. The term *honeste* when applied to paintings and painters carried a moral charge, and it is found in all the literature concerning the controversy over Michelangelo's *Last Judgment*. According to the dictionary of the Accademia della Crusca, *honeste* is taken as an adverb directly from the Latin, i.e., either with "honesty" or "virtue" or with "honestly" or "virtuously." See Nencioni and Barocchi, *Vocabolario della Crusca* (1612), vocabolario.signum.sns.it/, under the term [*h*]*oneste*/*onesta.*

2 Cardella (1792–97), 4: 232–33.

3 See Nussdorfer (1987), 176, esp. n. 12; and Nussdorfer (2009), 58–59.

4 See Lukehart (2009b).

5 A. Borromeo (1997), 61–62. Borromeo's larger point is that the cardinals, bishops, and priests played important, if unequal roles in promulgating and enacting reform within the churches in their care. What is fascinating about Savelli is that he began instituting Tridentine policies even before the Council ended; further, he made a massive sweep of some ninety-three churches where he conducted the *visite apostoliche.*

6 A. Borromeo (1997), 27–104. For the distribution of offices and responsibilities of bishops, see Fragnito (1997), 13–25, where there is mention of the new powers assigned to bishops and nuncios with regard to inquisitorial activities, apostolic visits, benefices and fiscal issues, absolution, etc.

7 Nussdorfer (2009), 57–59. What the new document published by Leproux (1991), 329–30, establishes is that the cardinal vicar already had some authority over the Università dei Pittori by 1563 – i.e., more than a decade before Pope Gregory XIII penned the brief that established an Accademia dei Pittori e Scultori – at least in the realm of sacred imagery.

8 Lucantoni (2004). Throughout the second half of the sixteenth century there was a flurry of activity involving the decoration and renovation of the Palazzo Cesarini in Rome. For later members of the Cesarini family, see Nussdorfer (1987), 184–85, citing Gigli (1958), 254.

9 Lucantoni (2004), 194. The Cesarini were very much in favor during the early 1560s when the cardinal vicar made his pronouncements known to the Università and began organizing his *visite apostoliche*, though they lost their palace and possessions between 1568 and 1571 when the family's financial fortunes changed. I want to leave open the possibility that the notary misunderstood or mistranscribed the monsignore's name, as Cardinal Cesi was directly involved in the proceedings of the Council of Trent and had worked with Savelli with the poor and vagabonds; see Miranda, *Cardinals of the Holy Roman Church*, www2.fiu.edu/~mirandas/bios1539.htm.

10 Hsia (1997), 152.

11 The dates of the discussions of the *Last Judgment* at the Council of Trent and the subsequent engagement of the "breeches painter" were quite imprecise before the late twentieth century. In *Geschichte der Päpste* (1886–1928) Ludwig von Pastor published some of the earliest documentation on the chronology of events, from the final session of the Council of Trent to the decision to alter some of Michelangelo's offending figures in the *Last Judgment*, properly situating the bowdlerization to January 1564. See Von Pastor (1938–61), 12: 618. It also appears in the nearly contemporary work of Ehses in *Concilium Tridentinum* (1901–2001), 9: 1148–49, under "Tertia congregatione die 21 ianuarii [1564]." Nonetheless, Mâle (1932), 2, dated the Council's deliberations to the 1550s, under the aegis of Paul IV, and the first drapery campaigns to 1559. De Vecchi (1984), 168, n. 40, was the first to republish the document either from Pastor or from the *Concilium Tridentinum* – without citing his source – of 21 January 1564, in which the decision was made to add drapes to the figures in the *Last Judgment*. De Maio (1978), 39–40, apparently first stated that the discussion of the *Last Judgment* took place during the twenty-fifth and last session of the Council of Trent between 11 November and 3 December 1563. De Maio cites Jedin (1935), 134–88; 277–91. On the basis of the passage in De Maio and especially Mancinelli's republication of the document in Pastor (Mancinelli [1998], 155–86, esp. 171), almost all subsequent scholars have tended to reassert and conflate these accounts of the discussions of the *Last Judgment* during the last Council in late 1563 and the ultimate decision to censure in 1564. See John O'Malley's important revisions in his essay in this volume.

12 See, e.g., Ehses in *Concilium Tridentinum* (1901–2001), 9: 1148. Most twentieth-century authors quote a version of this text in which a few words or adverbs may be slightly different but the meaning is essentially the same. In addition, they usually make reference to Decree 2, Session 9, of the Council of Trent under Pius IV.

13 Schroeder (1950), 216–17. The translation is his. The original Latin text appears in many compilations of the canons and decrees, with a few variations in punctuation and paragraphs. See, e.g., Ehses in *Concilium Tridentinum* (1901–2001), 9: 10.

14 Barnes (1997), 77. I looked through the lists of participants at the meetings of the Università dei Pittori for the years 1563–65 and could not find the name of Daniele da Volterra, "il Braghettone," among the members who attended meetings. He did participate in meetings relatively regularly between 1548 and 1550 and again briefly around 1560. See Leproux (1991), 302–26.

15 Barnes (1997), 1, based on her observations of the restoration reports and photographs in Mancinelli, Colalucci, and Gabrieli (1994), 236–55.

16 From the second decree, "De Invocatione, Veneratione et Reliquiis Sanctorum, et Sanctis Imaginibus," documented on 3 December 1564 and republished many times since the nineteenth century. See, e.g., Ehses in *Concilium Tridentinum* (1901–2001), 9: 1078. The passage is translated in Schroeder (1950), 217, as "nothing that is profane, nothing disrespectful [may appear], since holiness becometh the house of God."

17 "Chi ardirà di affermar che stia bene nella chiesa di San Pietro prencipe degli apostoli ... si veggano dipinti tanti ignudi che dimostrano disonestamente dritti e riversi?" Dolce (1960), 1: 188.

18 Blunt (1962), 124.

19 The translation is mine; for the original text, see Gilio (1961), 111.

20 Dempsey (1982), 66–70. For an excellent précis of the last Council of Trent's decree of 21 January 1564, see Schlitt (2005), 113–49, esp. 115–16, 145, n. 10.

21 Giovanni Andrea Gilio's *Dialogo nel quale si ragiona degli errori e degli abusi de' pittori circa l'istorie* appeared within a year after the conclusion of the Council of Trent. D. Freedberg (1971), 229–45; this passage cited 239, n. 7. Freedberg contends that Johannes Molanus's *De Picturis et Imaginibus Sacris, liber unus, tractans de vitandis circa eas abusibus ac de earundem significationibus* (1570) is rather the first treatise to take on the issue of nudity in the arts in a substantive manner. Freedberg (1971), 238, translates Molanus's passage that includes the word *honeste* as "modestly."

22 Gilio da Fabriano (1580), 10. This passage is quoted in Jansen (2001), 287, n. 11. See also Preti's *Discorso intorno all'onestà della poesia* (www.edres.it/preti.pdf): "Che a dirne il vero, egli è cosa malagevole il esser cose male e operar cose buone, l'andar vagando fra poesie inoneste ed esser vago d'onestà."

23 Williams (1997), 85.

24 Dempsey (1982), 70.

25 Gaston (1996), 8: 612–14; quote on 612. See also Gaston (2001), 136–62. Of particular interest is his notion of the "rhetoric of decorum" (139) in prayer, and by extension in art, that governs the relation of human communication with the divine.

26 *Honeste* as a desirable quality for the monastic community is found in the Rule of the Friars Preachers of Saint Dominic: "et hec est eorum regula, honeste vivere, discere et docere." De Frachet (1896), 138.

27 Le Gall (2000), 71–93, esp. 87. See also the discussion of Ottonelli and Cortona's treatise in Maria Loh's essay in this volume.

28 In the aftermath of the Robert Mapplethorpe exhibition and the removal of Richard Serra's *Tilted Arc* in the late 1980s, a spate of books and articles appeared on censorship and iconoclasm. Among them were two issues of the

Art Journal 50/3–4 (September–December 1991). See also LaMarche (1991), 56–58, and Senie and Webster (1992), esp. their introduction, xi–xvii.

29 Christopher Witcombe presented a paper at the first meeting of the Accademia di San Luca Seminar in December 2004 in which he argued that the Accademia must have been founded partly in response to the reformist intentions of Pope Gregory XIII and the Curia.

30 Paleotti (1582), 2: 504–506, reprints the chapter headings for book 3.

31 R. Alberti (1604), "Dedica," n.p.

32 R. Alberti (1604) recounted the history of the Accademia di San Luca from 1593 to 1599. See also the discussion in Lukehart (2009b).

33 Archivio di Stato di Roma, 30 Notai Capitolini, Ufficio 11, 1593, pt. I, vol. 25, fols. 426r–v. These and all the other Accademia documents from the years 1589–1635 are published in an online reference database: Lukehart (2010), www.nga.gov/casva/accademia.

34 See Lukehart (2009b), esp. 171–76.

35 I am here glossing the title of the important seminar organized by Gail Feigenbaum – "La vita agro-dolce di Taddeo Zuccaro" – that took place at the Getty Research Institute in October 2007, in conjunction with the exhibition of the drawings (see notes 36 and 62, this chapter).

36 See Lukehart (2007), 105–12.

37 Sherman and Lukehart (2000), 72, cat. no. 5. The same entry indicates that the choice of the flexor muscles of the fingers was deliberate because they "are considered the anatomically complex feature associated with human identity and intelligence."

38 Tongiorgi Tomasi and Willis (2009), xxvii. Tongiorgi Tomasi argues that the herbal that Galen points to in Zuccaro's fresco is meant to reinforce the scene's connection to the discipline of medicine.

39 Sherman and Lukehart (2000), 72, cat. no. 5; see also the foreword, 7. In conversations with the author, we found it striking that the printmaker – evidently with the author's consent or even at his behest – emphasized the manual nature of the anatomist's practice. As Sherman and Lukehart point out, tradition has it that barber-surgeons or demonstrators carried out the most gruesome aspects of dissection in the early modern period; physicians typically lectured on what was being shown. Zuccaro, unlike Vesalius, therefore wanted to emphasize the intellectual and noble processes of the acquisition of knowledge, even as he represented the "hands-on" nature of experiential learning.

40 Cunningham (2010), 1–15, 18–82, provides a useful history of the study of anatomy from antiquity through the eighteenth century.

41 For a discussion of the Sala del Disegno, see Strunck (2007), 115, 120–21.

42 R. Alberti (1604), 28. For additional information and bibliography concerning anatomical study in Rome, see De Renzi (1999), 107–109. De Renzi points out that "[p]ublic dissections were regularly performed not only at the Sapienza, but also in various hospitals of the city, like S. Maria della Consolazione and S. Giacomo."

43 The oversight was due, in part, to its earlier misattribution to the Genoese painter Giovanni Battista Paggi and often dated to the 1590s.

44 R. Alberti (1585), 1.

45 R. Alberti (1585), 44, links this episode to similar examples in Cedren and Thomas Aquinas in which miscreants and pagans become believers after viewing Christian images. None of these examples concerns an ex-voto

that provides miraculous curative or intercessory powers, but rather salvationist ones.

46 See the important new work by Fredrika H. Jacobs, summarized in Jacobs (2008), 113–15.

47 On the definition of the acheiropoieta, see the publications of Hans Belting, such as Belting (1994) and Belting (1998), 1–11.

48 R. Alberti (1585), 43, says that he found this example in the life of the saint but does not give a specific source.

49 Da Varagine (1990), 1: 263.

50 R. Alberti (1585), 44.

51 R. Alberti (1585), 44–45. Seventh Synod, act. 6.

52 R. Alberti (1585), 45, citing St. Gregory, bk. 7, letter 53.

53 R. Alberti (1585), 45.

54 R. Alberti (1604), 5 (quoting Federico Zuccaro in his "Ordini da osservarsi"). Herwarth Roettgen presented a paper on this topic at the Accademia di San Luca seminar held in Rome, June 2005.

55 Zuccaro (1607), 2: ch. 4.

56 Julian Brooks (personal communication) reminded me that among Zuccaro's possessions at the time of his death was a collection of more than three hundred drawings by *giovani*. This fact provides testimony to the practice described in R. Alberti (1604), 5: every other Sunday when the young artists met at the Accademia di San Luca, they would first make drawings for the prince, and he would respond by giving the best practitioner an example by his own hand. See the 1609 inventory in Körte (1935), 82–84.

57 R. Alberti (1604), 30–31.

58 R. Alberti (1604), 53–56. I have rearranged the topics a bit according to subject and disciplines.

59 The most complete formulation of the training of artists in the Accademia di San Luca is Pietro Roccasecca's (2009), 123–59.

60 R. Alberti (1604), 53: "A M. Cherubino Alberti dal Borgo San Sepolchro, toccò di ragionare e discorrere, che sia, & s'intenda decoro nella Pittura, & che vaglia il rappresentarle bene & che imperfettione dia il mancare d'esso."

61 Klein and Zerner (1966), 123.

62 J. Brooks (2007), fig. 31; discussed 84. Proving my point, this figure is shown completely nude and anatomically correct.

63 J. Brooks (2007), 42, cat. no. 30.

64 Mancinelli, Colalucci, and Gabrieli (1994), 236–37.

65 Mancinelli (1998), 172.

66 Mancinelli (1998), 174; Mancinelli, Colalucci, and Gabrieli (1994), 237. Interestingly, in his very useful study of the contemporary copies after Michelangelo's *Last Judgment*, Julian Brooks reads Federico's drawing as showing Michelangelo's figures with draperies, the only scholar to suggest this; see J. Brooks (2007), 79–85, cat. no. 18. A comparison of Federico's drawing with the reconstruction of the censorious interventions published in Mancinelli, Colalucci, and Gabrieli (1994), 241 – or with Venusti's copy – shows instead that Federico eschews the drapery additions on all the figures of the lower left register except perhaps for the reaching man directly below the bending one, whom Michelangelo himself covered with a loincloth at upper left. My point is that Federico deliberately obscured the genitalia, which may account for Brooks's assumption that they are covered with drapery.

67 That such drawings exist and more likely existed, see J. Brooks (2007), 84, cat. no. 70. For example, in *Demon Carrying a Man* (Paris, Musée du Louvre, Cabinet des Dessins, 740), dated to the 1550s, Federico explicitly shows the genitalia of the devil. Later (c. 1564–65), this figure would have a drapery added, as indeed it does today.

68 Some scholars believe that the drawings were made for the Casa Zuccaro in Florence and would thus date to about 1576–79. See, e.g., Wazbinski (1985): 275–346. At the study day hosted at the Getty Research Institute in October 2007, I raised the possibility that the painted leather version of the *Life of Taddeo* series might allow for the transportability of the decoration. Thus, the same decorations could have graced the home in Florence and later the Palazzo Zuccari in Rome after Federico moved there.

CARLO BORROMEO AND THE DANGERS OF LAYWOMEN IN CHURCH

Richard Schofield

MANY PRELATES OF the Cinquecento knew the boundless ocean of primaeval, misogynistic literature originating in the Old Testament as well as Carlo Borromeo, but very few were as powerful or as determined as he was to enforce what it suggested about how to deal with the dangers presented by laywomen in church.[1]

The edicts of the Third Provincial Council in Milan of 1573 requiring the use of the veil in church – adapted from Paul (1 Cor. 11:5–10) and enunciated in the 70s of the first century by Pope Linus, according to the *Liber pontificalis* 2, 1, are crystal clear and the sources cited impeccable.[2] They left no way out, not even for Milanese noblewomen with powerful husbands. Twenty-one noblewomen, including Anna Borromeo, wife of Giacomo Antonio Arconate, Ottavia Trivulzia, wife of Conte Gian Giacomo Trivulzio, and Leonora Gonzaga, wife of Conte Ercole Gonzaga, received an unsettling letter from Gian Giacomo Panico, Carlo Borromeo's *vicario generale*. The letter of 24 January 1575 said that the ladies would be excluded from the churches in Milan unless they presented themselves at the Curia Arcivescovile before 29 January to explain their actions.

What had they done? Panico, writing to Borromeo, related that they had arrived in church "without a veil, showing off their hair piled-up and decorated with little gold and silver flowers, and, as far as I understand it, some with little eagles, others with *cori* and yet others with *eufridi* on top";[3] and this shameful behaviour had been repeated frequently by women entering churches bareheaded with their hair immodestly coiffeured, causing the maximum scandal and spiritual damage to the faithful. It was not just that the veil had to be worn to indicate submission, but that hair, like jewellery, make-up, and especially women's eyes, held insidious perils for male onlookers.

Despite the rapid reactions of some of the husbands who appealed to the Spanish governor, Don Antonio de Guzman, the result was that representatives of at least three of the women (the documentation is lacunose) had to present themselves at the Curia to ask for forgiveness: Sforza Speciano, the representative of Lucia Mazenta, said that she was away from Milan and therefore knew nothing of the decree. Pietro Aluisio Vimercate interceded for Leonora Gonzaga and Paolo Alessandro Trivulzio for Ottavia Trivulzio. The women promised to obey and all three were absolved. Borromeo therefore had won; the governor was well aware that he was powerless because the matter was purely ecclesiastical.[4]

In an undated "Supplica" to the governor provoked by Borromeo's edicts, a number of noblemen and noblewomen declared their "disgust" and "profound dissatisfaction" with the letters sent to the wives threatening exclusion from the churches of the diocese, particularly since such regulations did not exist elsewhere and implied that the women of Milan were less modest, less religious, and less observant of the divine cult than those elsewhere. The noblemen found these regulations unheard of, pointless, and utterly detestable (*perodiossissime*).[5] On 7 March 1575 Borromeo reported to Nicolò Ormaneto that he had sent the letters to twenty to twenty-five women to induce "un poco di terrore," since some of them went to church not only without veils but even with those elaborate hairdos introduced by Genoese women decorated with little cupids, hearts pierced with arrows, and other immodest adornments. Some promised to obey immediately, but six or seven lamented through their husbands to the *marchese*, who handed the matter to Doctor Landriani, his *vicario di provisione*, with the idea of writing a letter of protest to the pope. Carlo observes that that is absurd, as though the bishop cannot control women's behaviour in church and, indeed, outside church, where the prospects of sinning are greater, as all theologians and canon law experts agree. It is absurd to say that the order about veils gives good women a bad name; that would be like saying that the civil authorities cannot pass laws against crimes because that would give the city a bad name.

Carlo then mentions his own edict at the Third Provincial Council and its sources (referred to earlier), saying that the *marchese* and the *gran cancelliere* had in fact commended it, most people approved of it, and indeed some of the husbands had jokingly remarked to the *vicario* that it was a good idea because it stopped their wives from spending their money. Carlo reports that he sent people to churches to observe whether women wore veils, and in fact four of his informants say that the custom was an ancient one in Milan; and the order pleased the pope.[6]

But the battle of the veils went on. There survives another letter of 26 March 1583 from Eleonora Vignarca, who had gone to church a number of times without a veil, and had even been banned by the priest at S. Babila; but she had committed these misdemeanours only because she was preoccupied with her pregnancy and not because she was in revolt against the decrees of Carlo Borromeo.

Nobody explains the paradox that women must be veiled but that men's hair should remain visible better than Federico Borromeo in his long-forgotten *Trattato sopra il gesto*; citing Tertullian, Federico tells us (as do many other authors starting from 1 Cor. 11:5, 7) that women must cover their heads as a sign of reverence, sorrow, and submission and to avoid licentious gazes and jealousy, as stated by innumerable writers and decrees of the Church. But men should not cover their heads, because the male head is the highest and most noble member of the body, the seat of the intellect, where one shows one's emotions and where the greatest part of human feelings are housed. Obviously soldiers cover their heads when the enemy approaches to show hatred, anger, and readiness for battle; but uncovering the male head in church signals obedience, love, and a desire to humble oneself.[7]

In an ideal Borromean world, women should be separated from men in church even after death; in S. Maria Podone, of which the *ius patronatus* belonged to the Borromeos, tombs for men and women were kept apart.[8] But in the land of the living, difficulties caused by women in church could be avoided in other ways, and various ancient authors, cited in Borromeo's decrees, had mentioned the physical division of churches or the use of separate churches by men and women.[9] In 1579 it was announced that men and women should go separately to certain churches at certain times. Borromeo states that his decree of 8 March 1578 should be observed: this said that only women could attend certain churches in the morning from the sound of the bell till midday and only men from midday to evening.[10]

Where such a separation by time and place was not possible, the division of the sexes within churches would be effected by means of sheets hung longitudinally down the nave or by means of a wooden dividing wall.[11] Giambattista Casale, writing in his diary on 13 March 1573, tells us that they began to put such divisions down the naves of churches to separate the men from the women to create a greater sense of devotion and sexual modesty; they began, he says, with S. Stefano in Brolio and wanted to include the other *chiese stazionali* of Milan.[12]

In his *Instructiones* of 1577 Borromeo decreed that churches should be provided with more than one door in the facade because Roman basilicas had multiple doors for various reasons, one of which was to provide separate entrances for men and women.[13] According to Casale, Milanese churches with facades with just one door should be provided with three, and lateral doors should be closed; he reports that this process began with the Duomo, then at S. Ambrogio, S. Francesco, S. Nazaro, S. Stefano, S. Maria alla Scala, S. Marco, and S. Lorenzo, followed by all the others.[14]

One of Carlo's hagiographers, Giovanni Battista Possevino, assures us that after the closure of the doors of the transepts of the Duomo, Borromeo, doubtless bearing in mind the strictures of the *Constitutiones apostolicae*, ensured that two priests stood at the doors of the facade to make sure that women did not go into the men's half, and vice versa, and that the women wore veils; if any man, young or old, dared to go into the women's half with bad intentions, the officials would arrest him and put him in the archbishop's jail in the Arcivescovado.[15]

In the *Instructiones* Carlo ordered the construction of wooden partitions in churches because, according to ancient custom reported by Chrysostom and ancient practice in the Diocese of Milan, men must be separated from women; the partition should be supported on stout wooden posts, 5 cubits (2.1 m: 1 ecclesiastical cubit = 0.426 m) apart, running down the nave from the presbytery to the principal door; grooves set in the sides of the posts would allow the slats or boards to be removed from the partition when necessary.[16] There should be small doors in the partitions for those occasions when people needed to pass from one side of the nave to the other, which should otherwise remain closed with bolts. When parts of the mass were being celebrated on one side of the partition, it would sometimes be necessary for people on the other side to see the ceremony, so there should be a series of hinges with which to lower sections of the partition. One set of hinges should be at least 2 cubits (0.85 m) from the pavement so that even kneeling worshippers could see the priest on the other side; the second set of hinges should be about 3 cubits (1.27 m) from the pavement in case standing worshippers on the wrong side needed to see the priest on the other (Illustration 39).

So on 30 January 1576, the *deputati* of the Duomo ordered the construction of such a partition extending from the presbytery to the main door, and Casale records on 12 February 1576 that they had completed it for the Jubilee; he adds that just outside the doors there was another wooden barrier ensuring that men entered the right side of the church towards the Arcivescovado, and women went to the left side, where the Altar of the Madonna dell'Albero was, in order to generate "magior devozione."[17]

Borromeo insisted that men should go to the right (south) and women to the left in churches orientated to the east, as had been recommended by many mediaeval authors whose writings he knew well: for example, Micrologus,[18] Durandus,[19] and Honorius of Autun (d. 1151), who is fascinating on the subject; he reports that the deacon used to turn to the south while reading from the Gospel because those to whom he must speak about *spiritualia* are gathered there; men are spiritual, and the south signifies the Holy Spirit. Now, however, the custom is that he turns to the north, where women, who are carnal, stand, so that the Gospel can summon them to *spiritualia*. Pagans and the devil, at whom the Gospel is directed to convert them to Christ, are signified by the north.[20]

In the *Instructiones*, Borromeo does not say whether the partition – which would have impeded both sexes from going to chapels on the opposite side of the church from their own – was to be permanent or temporary. Already in 1574 it was specified that the *chiese stazionali* would be so divided on indulgence days, feast days, and any other occasions that produced great influxes of the faithful.[21] Possevino even tells us that Carlo partitioned *all* churches in the diocese, thus imitating Basil the Great, who

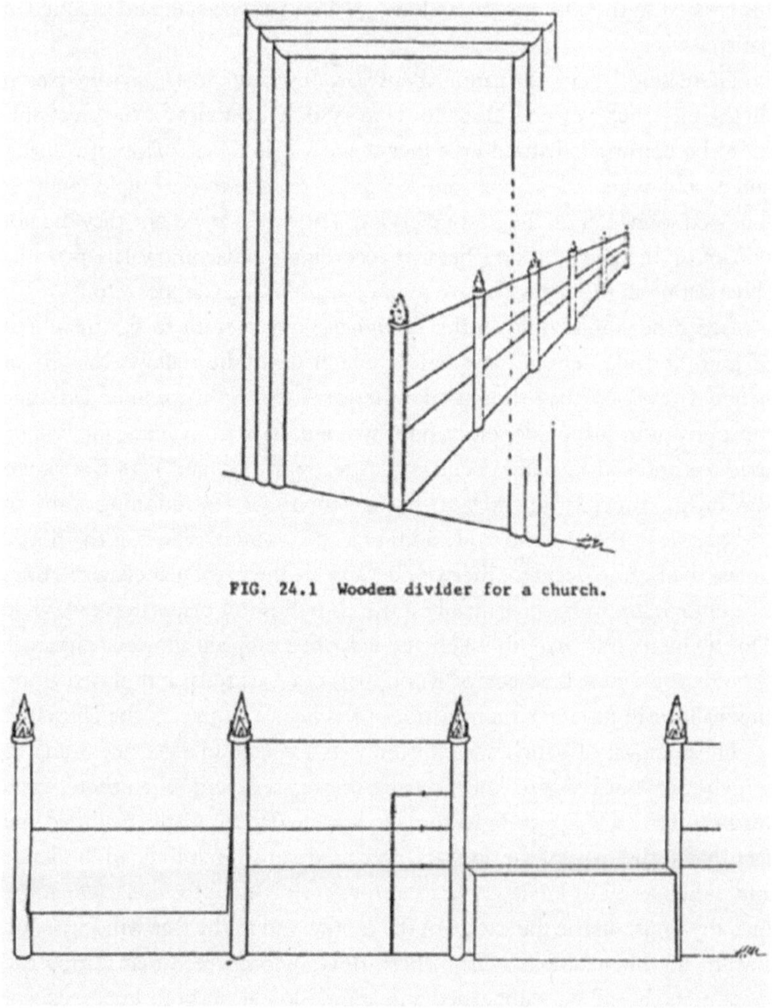

39. Borromean wooden partition. After Voelker (1977), p. 322.

put up veils or cloths in church to prevent men and women from looking at each other during mass.[22]

A curious and spectacular result of the separation of the sexes in the nave of the Duomo is described by Casale. In April 1581 Borromeo had the statue of Adam by Cristoforo Solari, once in the Camposanto, put on the pier at the entrance of the choir at the left ("su il pirone nel entrare nel coro del Domo da man sinistra") and the Eve by Angelo Marini on the other pier.[23] Casale seems to state that the Adam was placed at the left, or north, of the choir for anybody looking from the main door. But presumably the statues were placed on the appropriate piers to signal the different sides of the nave allocated to men and women, and therefore the Adam must have been on the right (south) of the choir. Evidently Casale was referring, on this occasion, to the right and left of the bishop and his throne in the presbytery, as in fact Borromeo himself did when he made his *visitatio* to the Duomo on 25 June 1566 and as was standard practice in pastoral visits.[24]

There is no other information about how or where the statues were placed on the piers; but we know that already in 1580 the contract for the great pulpit to be constructed around the pier at the left, in *cornu evangeli*, was made, and exactly where the statues were located in relation to the pulpits (another followed soon after on the north pier) is unknown. In any event, they did not remain on the piers for long, because according to Giacomo Valeri, presumably writing in the 1630s, they were once again in the Camposanto.[25]

Two other injunctions in the *Instructiones* are relevant to the treatment of men and women: in churches in which the bishop allows the use of benches (*bradelle*), they should take the form that he recommended; they must be put in at the side reserved for women, away from altars, and will be used for both sitting and kneeling on. Already in 1577 and 1578 Borromeo was busy removing (in order to replace them) or repositioning some of the *bradelle* in the Duomo.[26] He adds that the women's side is at the north, unless the bishop decides otherwise because of the particular characteristics of a church, meaning, presumably, if the church is not orientated east/west. On the men's side there should be no *bradelle*; if they are allowed seats at all, though, they must be made of wood, without backrests, and placed along the walls or in the intercolumniations so as not to clutter up the church.[27]

The removal of benches is explained in a decree of 1574, according to which everybody was to kneel during the mass, except when there was a reading from the Epistle.[28] In the *De Septem Basilicis* Carlo recorded the fact that at the time of the apostles, everybody in church listened in silence and either stood or knelt, citing Psalms 5:8 (7): "But as for me, I will come into thy house in the multitude of thy mercy: and in thy fear will I worship toward thy holy temple."[29] Elsewhere Borromeo decreed that during the mass men should be bareheaded and should kneel on both knees, except for when the Epistle is being read, when they must stand up; then, nobody is permitted to sit. Antoniano, one of Borromeo's closest associates, expands on the theme in 1584 by reporting that it was ancient custom to stand during the mass on Sundays throughout the year and between Resurrection and Pentecost in honour of the Resurrection and the Triumph of the Saviour, but that now this custom is not observed; considering the ease with which we are distracted, he thinks that it is better to kneel all the time since that humiliates the body and concentrates the mind.[30]

With regard to holy water stoops, Borromeo says that they should be placed inside, not outside, churches, in clear sight of those who enter and if possible on the right, presumably referring to small churches. But with respect to larger churches, they will be placed at both the men's and women's entrances, a rule adopted soon by the Council of Constance in 1579, for example.[31]

The last element of our discussion of women and ecclesiastical architecture is the confessional. It is not surprising that, given the maniacal

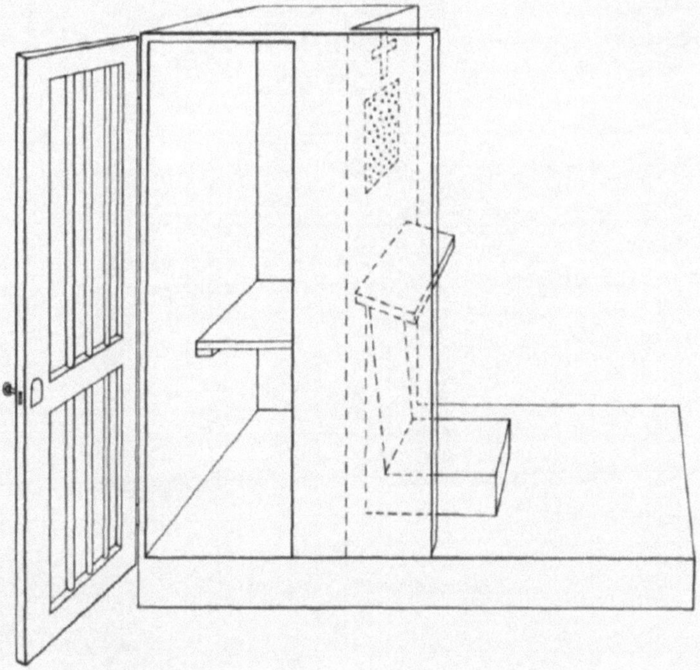

40. Borromean confessional. After de Boer (2001), p. 92, fig. 2.

obsession of this generation of Reformers with the visual and physical separation of the sexes, we find in the *Instructiones* what is evidently the first reference in the history of the Italian church to the closed confessional.

Borromeo and many other prelates of the period were preoccupied about priests being incited to lust by women during confession, and vice versa.[32] The main advantage of the closed confessional described by Borromeo was that the confessor and the penitent could not see or touch each other; and since the act of confession was a sacrament, it should be seen to be carried out in some location visible to everybody in the church. According to the *Instructiones*, there should be two confessionals in every parish church so that, to avoid irreverence and offending the pious, men should not be crowded together with women when gathering for confession, and men and women should confess in separate confessionals, as happens in most of the churches in the diocese.[33]

Borromeo required that the confessional have two compartments, both open at the front, with that for the confessor enclosed on three sides and on top, and supplied with a door if required to keep out laypersons, tramps, and smelly people. The seat of the confessor should be separated from the kneeling penitent by a wooden partition allowing communication only via a small perforated metal window; the penitent and confessor, therefore, could not see or touch, but only hear, each other (Illustration 40). In 1581

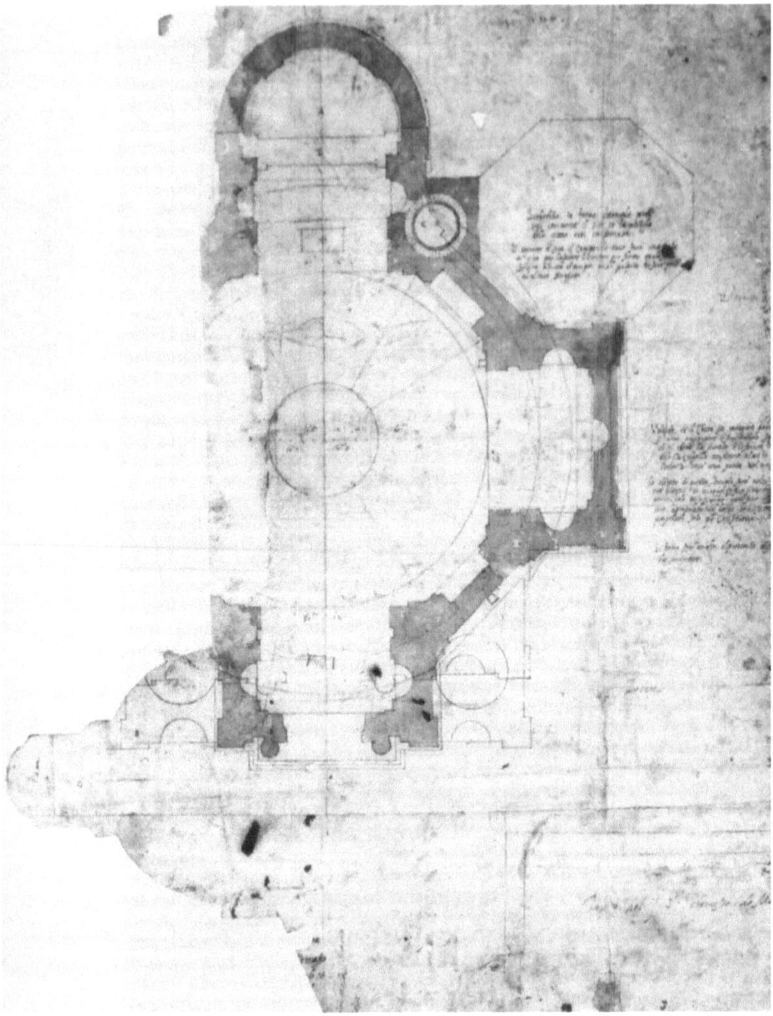

41. Pellegrino Tibaldi, first project for S. Fedele, Milan (1567), showing the niches in the walls for confessionals. After Della Torre and Schofield (1994), p. 115.

the English Catholic Gregory Martin described perfectly the new type, which had already arrived in Rome: "Their seate is so made of joyned bordes, that on the one side is a seate for the ghostly father, on the other a place for the penitent to kneele, and betwene them bothe a partition with a grate in the middes, having litle holes like a skimmer [sieve], so that the voice only may passe through, and the partie is not discerned. So are al the seates made (I thincke) through Italie and I wish it in other places."[34]

The driving principles were (1) that the penitent should kneel to the west of the confessor and (2) that the confessor should sit at a right angle to the penitent; so when the confessional was located at the left of the church, the confessor would be seated at a right angle to the wall facing south in the direction of the nave, with the penitent kneeling to the right facing in the direction of the main altar. When the confessional was at the right of the church, the penitent would kneel at the left of the confessor, in the direction of the high altar. Therefore, in theory, mirror-image confessionals should have been constructed for the left and right sides of the church, a consequence not considered explicitly by Borromeo.

42. Milan, S. Fedele, confessional. Photo: R.V. Schofield.

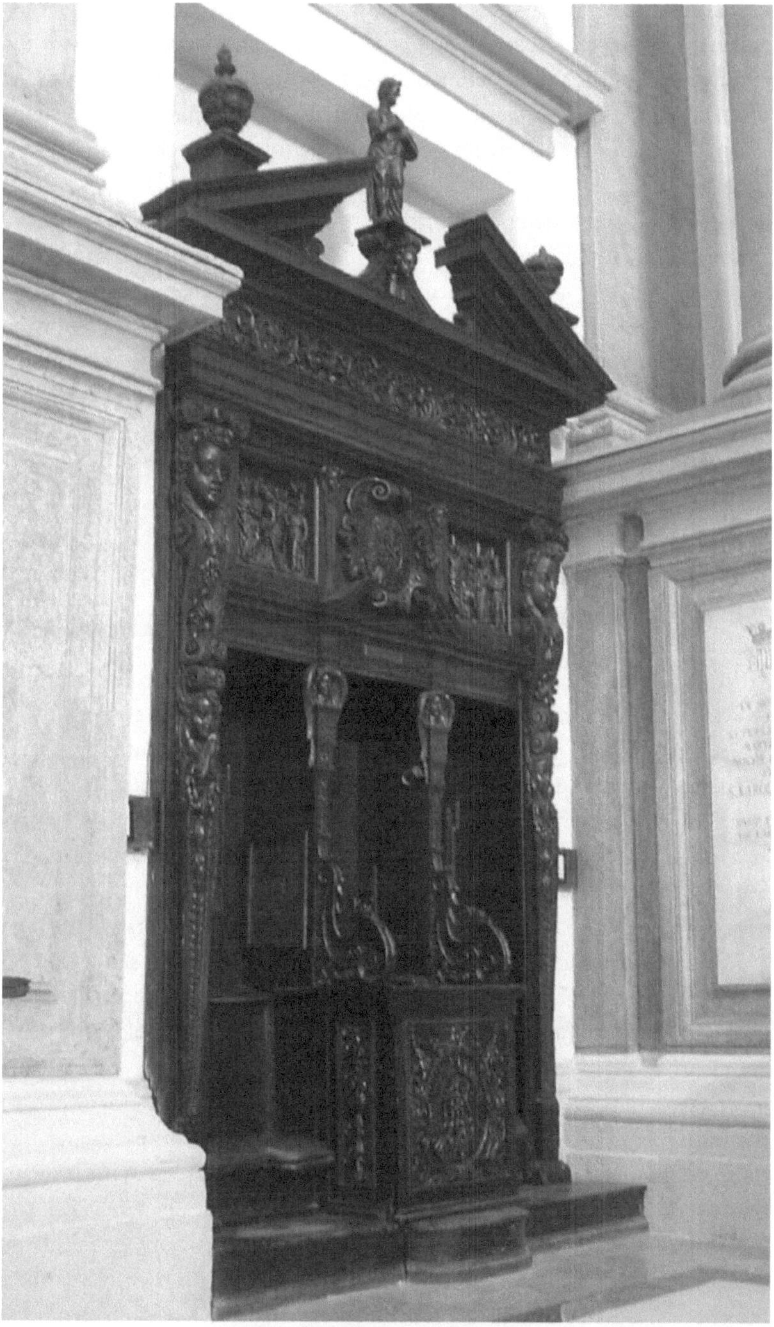

Although the closed confessional is first described in the *Instructiones* of 1577, we may ask whether the type was invented by Borromeo and his advisors in 1576–77 or had been devised before, and by others. Pellegrino Pellegrini's extraordinary initial octagonal design for S. Fedele in Milan, developed before December 1567, includes niches specially constructed to house confessionals and identified with the caption "appropriate for confessionals only" – apparently the first niches with this function in the history of Italian ecclesiastical architecture (Illustration 41).[35] In 1568, after the abandonment of the centralized design project, Pellegrino went ahead with the construction of the present church. In 1579, just after the publication of the *Instructiones*, the Taurini family began constructing the splendid confessionals for the niches in the present building, which Pellegrino had carried over from his initial project (Illustration 42). But the confessionals in S. Fedele do not match those described in the *Instructiones* of 1577; instead they have two *bradelle* facing the wall to the right and left of the central compartment occupied by the confessor, ignoring the rule implied in the *Instructiones* that the penitent should be at the west, or left, of the confessor. We know, in fact, that Borromeo – ingeniously prurient as he always was – did not like the confessionals at S. Fedele, not because they had two kneeling stools but because, we are told, the presumably more athletic confessors could touch the women's feet with his; Borromeo made a particular fuss about this, as though lust could enter through people's shoes, whereas he did not complain about the fact that in the confessionals at S. Fedele the mouth of the woman was placed right next to the ear of the confessor, though separated from it by a metal grill, which the Jesuit *preposito* of S. Fedele, our source for the incident, clearly found much more suggestive.[36]

In the 1580s, then, the Jesuits ignored the Borromean rule according to which the penitent should always be to the west of the confessor in a closed confessional provided with two compartments; instead they clearly liked the fact that their three-compartment confessionals could be placed indifferently to the right or left of the nave, with the confessor always at a right angle to the wall, but the penitents kneeling to the north or south.[37]

Confessionals in niches, then, were designed for the first version of S. Fedele in 1567 and in the great rectangular church we see today. So the question now becomes: Were the niches in the first plan designed by Pellegrino intended to house (1) confessionals of the old type with a table, two chairs, and a division in the middle of the table, or (2) confessionals with two compartments of the type required by Borromeo in the *Instructiones* of 1577, or (3) confessionals with three compartments like those constructed in the present church by the Taurini from 1579? It seems that we do not have any way of resolving the problem decisively. But the presence of the niches proves that in 1567 the Jesuits bore in mind the desideratum that confession should take place in a location visible to all in the church, as many archbishops' decrees and mediaeval councils required,

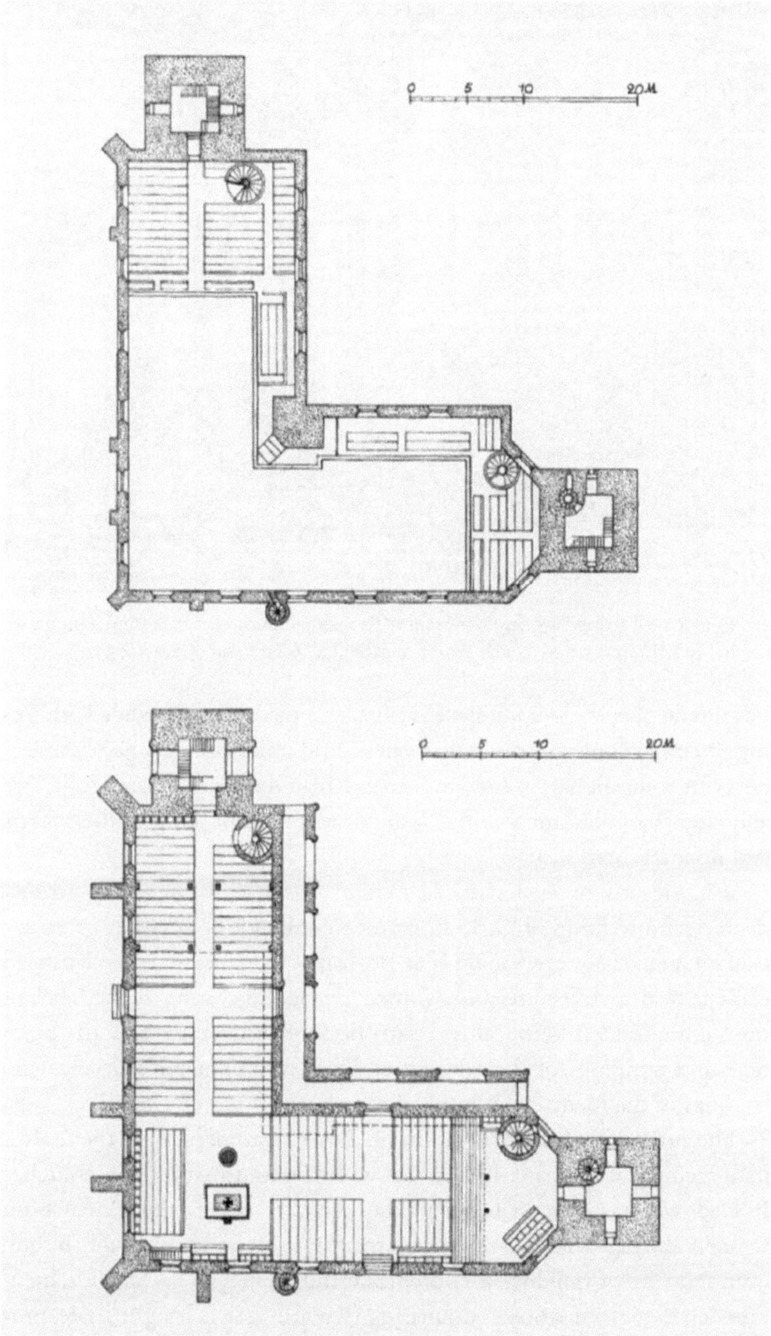

43. Freudenstadt, Evangelische Stadtkirche, 1601–1608.

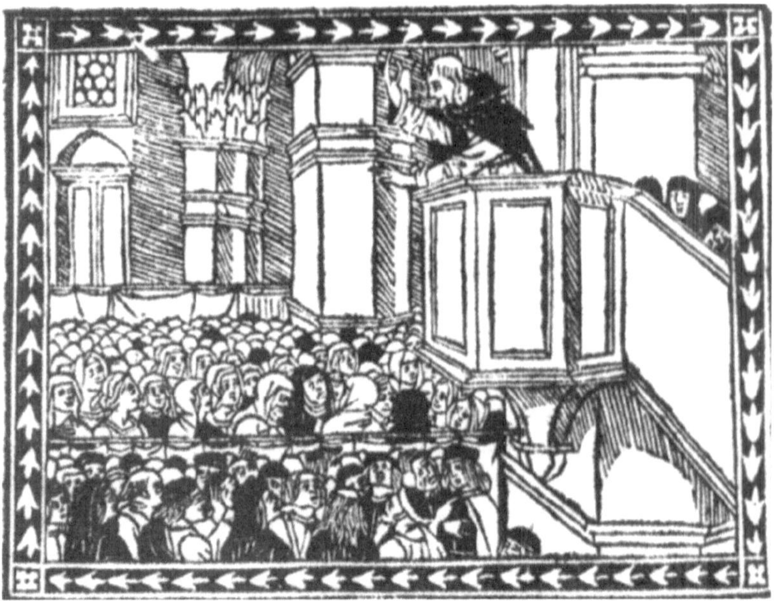

44. Woodcut showing Savonarola preaching to a semicircular audience from a pulpit to the left (north) of the nave of the Florence cathedral. After Villari (1888), p. 307.

but this fact per se does not necessarily prove that they were already thinking of closed confessionals at that date.[38] And unfortunately the few references to confessionals in the Duomo at Milan that can be dated to before and after the publication of the *Instructiones* tell us nothing of their form, and none of them survive.[39]

With regard to ecclesiastical architecture and women, the actions, decrees, and writings of Carlo Borromeo could not be anything but reactionary; practically everything that Borromeo said and did in relation to ecclesiastical architecture and women revived and strengthened beliefs from a multitude of biblical and patristic sources but also from the practices and traditions of the Church codified in innumerable decrees and writings of the mediaeval Church.[40]

The orthodox of the generation of Carlo Borromeo found themselves in agreement with many Protestants with respect to women in church.[41] Indeed, whilst sharing a belief in the necessity of separating men from women during services, not even the most rigorous Catholic bishop ever thought of building a church like the Evangelische Stadtkirche at Freudenstadt (1601–1608), comprising two arms set at a right angle, presumably one for the men, the other for the women, with the altar at the angle (Illustration 43).[42]

Borromeo and many other ecclesiastical patrons of the Cinquecento changed the interiors of churches in various ways, particularly by transferring the old *scuole cantorum* or *cori bassi* to the apses behind the high altar; in Milan, for example, this happened in S. Francesco (1571),[43] S. Maria alla Scala (1560),[44] S. Nazaro (1578),[45] and S. Simpliciano (1571).[46] Mediaeval and Renaissance sources mention, and artists occasionally illustrate, the separation of the sexes inside and outside churches by means of partitions or suspended sheets.[47] The practice must have been widespread in mediaeval churches, and revivals of it are recorded in the 1530s in Naples[48] and Verona,[49] then at S. Stefano in Venice (1571),[50] and in Jesuit churches (1573 and afterwards).[51] In Milan, before and after Trent, the pulpits in many churches were to the left of the nave – at S. Ambrogio, S. Fedele, S. Francesco Grande,[52] S. Simpliciano, and the Duomo at Monza. When the pulpit was in the nave, the congregation arranged itself in a transverse semicircle around it for sermons, as in the celebrated woodcut of Savonarola preaching from a pulpit to the north of the nave of the Duomo in Florence to an audience with the men to the west and women to the east divided by a clothesline (Illustration 44). In 1580 Borromeo began to build the first of the two spectacular pulpits, one for the archbishop, the other for other preachers, attached to the great piers to the left and right of the opening of the choir in the Duomo (Illustration 45). After the pulpits' construction, all sermons would have been delivered immediately in front of the high altar and the Eucharistic tabernacle; in this way Borromeo and Pellegrino concentrated the high altar, the tabernacle, and pulpits together, and they therefore became more visible and the preachers more audible to the clergy seated in the presbytery behind the altar, and particularly to the congregation, than they were in churches supplied with the transverse rood screens (or a *tornacoro*, as in the Duomo in Verona) or pulpits in the nave.

Now, in the case of the Duomo, the use of a pulpit in the nave with the congregation arranged in a semicircle around it north/south was precluded when the wooden partition was present; but on great occasions the longitudinal partition was not an insuperable obstacle during

45. Milan, Duomo, the presbytery with the two pulpits and tabernacle in the centre. Photo: R.V. Schofield.

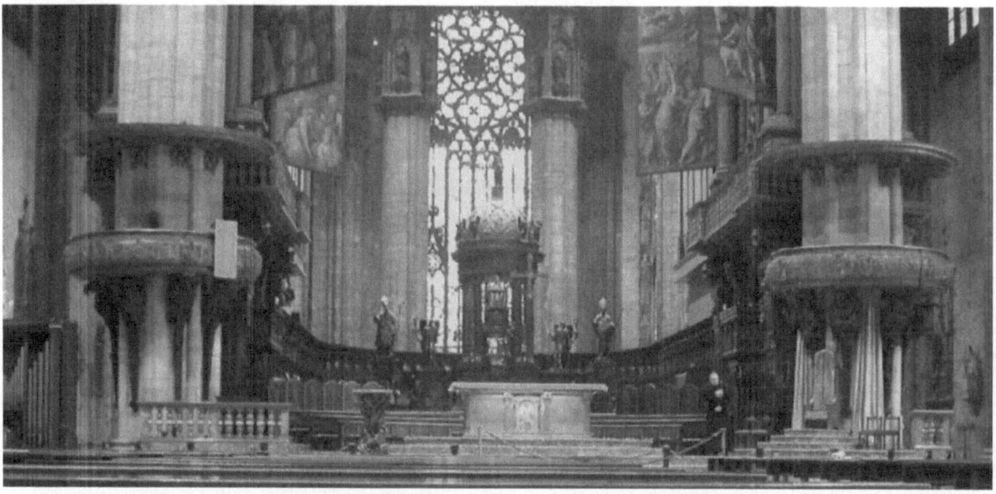

mass, because it was supplied with panels that could be lowered.[53] And it seems fair to deduce that the idea of constructing longitudinal wooden partitions expressed in the *Instructiones* of 1577 tells us that Borromeo had already decided to build twin pulpits at the mouth of the choir by that date.[54]

Clearly the presence of a *permanent* wooden partition and the presence of pulpits in the nave of the Duomo would have been mutually exclusive: a permanent partition, if such it was, would have been reserved for the Duomo alone, seeing that in the majority of other Milanese churches, double pulpits at the mouth of the choir were not built and the pulpits stayed in their original positions in the nave.[55] This is why, only apparently contradicting himself, Borromeo is able to speak of the longitudinal partition in the *Instructiones* but also to say that in large churches two *ambos* should be provided, one at the right and the other at the left, "in gremio ecclesiae," evidently meaning in the nave rather than in the crossing,[56] and that in small churches one was sufficient and should be located to the north (left) of orientated churches. The deacon reading the Epistle could direct himself to the south of the church when no partition was present.[57] Overall, then, it seems likely that even in the case of the Duomo with its double pulpits, Borromeo has in mind a temporary wooden partition only for great occasions.

Such, then, were the results of Carlo Borromeo's determination to ensure that his great church had two fundamental characteristics: (1) a concentration of all the essential functions immediately in front of the high altar, more visible and audible than ever to as many people as possible, (2) and a means of preventing men on specially crowded occasions from casting longing glances at those sirens bent on enticing them to perdition with their beautiful eyes, piled-up hair, revealing clothes, and alluring make-up – all castigated so violently by our powerful prelate and the venerable fathers of the church.

Notes

1 Some of this material derives from Della Torre and Schofield (1994), 234–35, and from the last section of Schofield (2006), 282–352, where the sources read by Borromeo concerning women are collected. Though bizarrely ignored by scholars, the essay by Franca Mellano (1986), 2: 1073–1134, presents a rich collection of passages concerning nuns and laywomen from the decrees of the Milanese church and Borromeo's homilies; De Filippi (2006), 155–84.

2 *Acta ecclesiae mediolanensis* (1890–96) (hereafter AEM), 2, col. 266; see also AEM, 2, col. 1170 (*sine die*); Duchesne (1955), 1: 121.

3 Unfortunately I have not discovered what the words *cori* and *eufridi* mean.

4 Marcora (1962b), 316–18, using MSS F 49 inf., 1–6 e P 12 inf., fol. 33 (Milan, Biblioteca Ambrosiana); see also Archivio Storico Diocesano of Milan, XIV, 139, fol. 118r–119, for another copy of the list of noblewomen; de Boer (2001), 119, n. 90, for a document from the 1570s, according to which failure to wear a veil in church was considered a *mortal* sin.

5 *Memorie Storiche della Diocesi di Milano* (1954–64; hereafter *MSDMi*), XIV, 139, fol. 120r, letter of Eleonora Vignarcha; 122r fol. 123r for the "Supplica."
6 Bonomelli (2008), 149–50.
7 Milan, Biblioteca Ambrosiana, F 5 inf. *Gesto, azione dello stato contemplativo, cioè Trattato sopra il gesto, la voce, il luogo e le vestimenta del corpo umano in ordine al culto divino composto dal Card. Federico Borromeo*, cap. 4, 20v, citing Tertullian, *Apologeticus adversus gentiles*, in Migne (1841–61) (hereafter PL), vol. 1, cols. 503–504, and *De velandis virginibus*, in PL, I, cols. 935–62 passim.
8 At least according to Gualdo Priorato (1666), 81.
9 AEM, 2, col. 7 (Con. Prov. I, 1566) and col. 1122 (*Editto per il conversar con riverenza, e divotione nelle chiese*); cf. G. B. Fossano in Marcora (1962a), 616.
10 AEM, 3, cols. 573–79 of 3 February 1582, the *Indulgentiae stationales viris separatim constitutae e foeminis*; Bascapé (1983), 259.
11 AEM, 2, col. 896; Sinodo IV, 1574, decree 36; see Bascapé (1983), 802, for the *tabulati interpositi.*
12 Marcora (1965), 263. The other six *chiese stazionali* were the Duomo, S. Ambrogio, S. Lorenzo, S. Nazaro, S. Simpliciano, and S. Vittore.
13 Borromeo 2000, 23 (see also the review by Schofield [2001]); Bascapé (1983), 424, 804.
14 Borromeo (2000), 23; Marcora (1965), 318.
15 G. B. Possevino (1591), 55, 90. Domenico Tibaldi, Pellegrino's brother, refers to the separation of men from women in his discussion of church porticoes (Pigozzi [1989], 315–33, app. I, for the *Discorso del modo da tenere nel disegnare et modificare le chiese*).
16 Borromeo (2000), 119–21. Carlo refers to passages such as Chrisostom's *Homilia 74 in Mathaeum* or the *Ecloga de non contemnando ecclesiam*, cited in his own *De Septem basilicis* (AEM, 3, col. 544). Fascinating too is an unpublished letter of Borromeo to Cesare Speciano of March 1579 in which he observes that, within his own memory, churches were divided *transversely* with walls (*sic*: "muri") but that it was decided that for "maggiore decoro," for the greater convenience of those listening to the mass and particularly so that men and women could see the service taking place separately, it was better to divide churches *longitudinally*, as had been the practice since the Anno Santo (1576) (Milano, Biblioteca Ambrosiana, F 55 inf., 36v ff.).
17 *Annali della Fabbrica del Duomo di Milano* (1877–85), 4: 139 and Marcora (1965), 281.
18 Borromeo (2000), 108–109, 120–21 (in his discussion of the *bradella* Borromeo speaks of the north as the women's side). Micrologus, *De ecclesiasticis observationibus opusculum ...*, in *De divinis catholicae ecclesiae officiis ac ministeriis, varii vetustorum aliquot ecclesiae patrum scriptorum libri ...*, Cologne 1568, 439; Borromeo mentions both Micrologus and Alcuin in his *Lettera sopra la prima domenica di quadragesima* (AEM, 3, col. 502; 1 March 1576) as great liturgical authorities; he was referring to Alcuin's, *De divinis officiis*, cap. 12, *De quadragesima* in PL, vol. 101, cols. 1190–91.
19 Davril and Thibodeau (1995–2000), *Corpus christianorum continuatio mediaevalis*, vol. 140, in particular lib. 4, cap. 16, 24.
20 Honorius, *Gemma animae sive de divinis officiis et antiquo ritu missarum*, I, 22 (PL, vol. 172, col. 551).
21 AEM, 2, col. 896, Synod IV, 1574: Bascapé (1983), 802.

22 G. B. Possevino (1591), 55; Bascapé (1983), 289–91.

23 Marcora (1965), 349; *Annali*, 4, 52, 57–58, for Angelo Marini's Eve, which another contemporary witness, Urbano Monti, also mentions (Marcora [1965], 234). Cristoforo Solari was busy with an Adam and an Eve in 1502; but we encounter a strange problem since the relevant document says they will be "figures 24 *braccia* in magnitude or as (large as) they could be" (*Annali*, 3, 120: "figure magne ... brach. 24 vel ut fieri poterunt"): however, 24 Milanese *braccia*, if it refers to the height, is enormous – 14.16 m; and the statues that we have today of Adam and Eve are in fact 183 and 182 cm, respectively (3.1 br).

24 For example, Palestra (1977), 163, no. 8: "On the right hand side, 'in *evangeli* parte,' the Altar called S. Mary of the Tree," referring to the chapel then in the left (north) transept.

25 Giacomo Valeri, *Cose degne d'essere vedute et considerate nella grande città di Milano* ... (Milan, Biblioteca Ambrosiana, MS S. 117 supp., 251r): cf. Rovetta (1999), 307–15.

26 Borromeo (2000), 120; Borromeo had removed some benches from the church in 1566 and put others behind the choir (Palestra [1977], 188, no. 178 and 189, no. 191); in 1577 he decreed that the *scabelle* of both sexes should be like those described in the *Instructiones* (ibid., 217, no. 345; AEM, 3, col. 547); in Sinod V of 1578, however, it was decreed that the women's *bradelle* should be removed immediately (AEM, 2, col. 939).

27 Borromeo (2000), 120 ff.

28 *Editto per il conversar con riverenza e divotione nelle chiese* of 13 November 1574 (AEM, 2, col. 1122).

29 Sassi (1747–48), 2: 175–76, for *Homilia* no. 59, of 1583 on the necessity of kneeling in church, citing many biblical passages.

30 Antoniano (1926), lib. 2, 61, 167.

31 Borromeo 2000, 105; Mansi (1759–98), 35, col. 932 ff.

32 AEM, 2, coll. 1870–93 (*Avvertenze ... ai confessori nella città et diocese sua*); see the remarkable articles of de Boer (1991), 553 ff.; (1997), 105–14; (2001), 84–125; excellent too is Onida (2002), 150–59; Prospero (1996), 508–42. That mine of information, Lea (1911–15), 1: 415–90, remains indispensable; he notes that the first reference to a closed confessional dates back to a letter written by the Archbishop of Toledo to Charles V of 1547, which, unfortunately, I have not been able to check.

33 Borromeo (2000), 111 ff.

34 Parks (1969), 65. The Borromean type was in part anticipated at Ravenna in May 1568 when the decision was made to use confessionals, apparently with two seats, separated by a vertical wooden board with a metal or wooden grill, which seems very close in form to Borromeo's, except that it is not clear whether the priest was enclosed (Council of Ravenna, *De poenitentia*, cap. 2 in Mansi [1759–98], 35, col. 619). An undated decree issued by Borromeo is important in this context – the *Istruzione generale ... per le cose materiali pertinenti alle chiese* – which says that the confessional should be made of wood and should include a *bradella* for the penitent to kneel on with a wooden partition between them and the usual grill or perforations through which to communicate: the confessional must be in a location in the church visible to all; women's confessions can be heard only in church, nowhere else, especially not at night, and at home only if a woman is ill (AEM, 2, col. 1967; undated). de Boer (2001), 94, n. 25,

dates the document to between 1566 and 1569, preferably to 1567, without saying why; if he is right about the date, then Borromeo's invention of the type came some ten years before its description in the *Instructiones*. The text is not in the other editions of the Acts of the Milanese church (*Constitutiones et decreta condita in provinciali synodo mediolanensi*, Padova, 1566; *Decreta provincialia mediolanensis sub Carolo Borrhomeo card. Archiepiscopo ... edita*, ed. Cesare Speciano, Cremona, 1595; *Acta ecclesiae mediolanensis Federici Borromeaei iussu ...*, Brescia, 1603 and Milan, 1619); and I have been unable to trace the copy mentioned by Saba (1936), 94 with press-mark S *B* M I 11 n. 1 in the Biblioteca Ambrosiana.

35 Della Torre and Schofield (1994), 117 ff., 234 ff., 323. The word *confesionario* of itself does not tell us that the confessional was closed and had therefore already been invented by 1567, since the word was often used from at least the time of Giberti, and no doubt innumerable times before him, to describe the old type, with a table with a division across it, e.g., at the Council of Siracuse in 1553 and at the Council of Naples in 1567; see de Boer (2001), 94, n. 26.

36 Rurale (1992), 275, n. 152. The confessionals in S. Fedele are now equipped with little gates at the front of the central compartment, which are presumably additions to the original design caused by San Carlo's complaints; a "portina" is explicitly mentioned as one of the works done on the confessionals in 1596.

37 I confess to be being entirely in the dark about the use of three-compartment confessionals at S. Fedele. It was surely impossible that two penitents were heard simultaneously; what then was the point of having two *bradelle*? Was one compartment for men, the other for women? If so, why would neither group look to the high altar as recommended by Borromeo, and how is it that there are now confessionals on the back wall of the facade at S. Fedele, with the confessor looking at the high altar, the penitents to the west? It is noteworthy that Ammanati's S. Giovannino in Florence, the next church to include niches for confessionals, includes confessionals with both two and three compartments.

38 The same conclusion emerges from the fact that in October and November 1565 at the First Provincial Council (AEM, 2, col. 52) a decree was issued saying that the confessor and the penitent, both seated, would be separated by a board of wood – referring to the old type of confessional, described by Giberti of Verona in the 1540s, rather than the closed confessional; see de Boer (1991), 543–72.

39 In June 1566, Carlo decreed that a confessional should be made for the Chapel of S. Caterina of Siena (Palestra [1977], 187, no. 174; and "Nella sacristia meridionale si facia un oratorio per confessare," 178, no. 79. Presumably the twenty-four confessionals ordered by the *deputati* in January 1576, simultaneously with the construction of the wooden partition, were closed; so too were those mentioned by Casale, then by Ragazzoni and Borromeo during their visits to the Duomo (*Annali*, 4, 139; Marcora [1965], 281). In May 1576 it was decreed that the confessional should follow the form envisaged in the *Instructiones* (Conc. prov, IV, AEM, 2, col. 356); for Ragazzoni, AEM, 2, cols. 1187–88. The Duomo did not have suitable locations for them, and Borromeo asked the *deputati* to decide where to place them in February 1577 (Palestra [1977], 207, no. 302 and 217, no. 343). In 1592, according to Casale, a large walnut confessional with relief decoration

was to be placed behind the choir, and again in 1593 he mentions two of them in that location (Marcora [1965], 401).

40 Some of the rules issued by Borromeo regarding the clothing permitted in church for laymen and laywomen were in fact versions of sumptuary laws issued by the civil authorities in Milan and elsewhere in the Quattrocento and Cinquecento, but reinforced by the authority of Clement, Chrisostom, and St. Jerome; see, e.g., a long, spectacular decree of the Marchese del Guasto of 6 February 1539 about the "abusi" of "costumi": Formentini (1881), 321–33; Venturelli (1999); Bulzoni (1999); de Boer (2001), 115–18; see also the essays by Laughran (2003) and Muzzarelli (2003), 185–220.

41 The great Protestant ecclesiastical historians cite all the sources about women used by Borromeo and Baronio and for the same purpose; see, e.g., Flacius et al. (1559–74), vol. 1, cols. 535–38, 581–82, for the usual citations from Chrisostom, *De verginitate* and a long diatribe against make-up. Cf. Hospinianus (1603), 86 ff., for Chrisostom, *Hom 74 in Matt.* (separation of the sexes in church); Philo, *De Vita Contemplativa* (the Essenes); the *Constitutiones Apostolicae*, lib. 2, cap. 61 (reissued by Surius [1567], 1: 33–124); Gregorius nazianzenus, *In somnium Anastasiae*, and the life of Chrisostom by Symeon Metaphrastes; Ambroge, *De lapsu virginis*, etc.

42 Hamberg (2002), 52 ff.

43 Marcora (1965), 256–57; Caciali (1997), 144.

44 Gualdo Priorato, (1666), 95–97.

45 Baronio (1968), 146, doc. 596; Marcora (1965), 327–28; Bascapé (1983), 467; Fiorio (1985), 279.

46 Schofield (2004), 96.

47 See, e.g., Aston (1990), 237–93; Rainey (1991), 217–38; Randolph (1997), 17–41.

48 Gaetano Thiene at S. Paolo Maggiore in Napoli in 1538 and in SS. Apostoli (Capello [1880], 477–78). See Silos (1672), 111–12, for the removal of the choir to behind the high altar and the separation of men from women in the nave. For Thiene's friendship with Giberti see Paschini (1926).

49 Writing about Giberti activities in the 1530s, Zini (1556; written in 1542–43), c. 18v, reports that at Easter a wooden partition was set up in church so that during sermons the women and men could not look at each other.

50 Paola Modesti very kindly brought a document about S. Stefano to my attention; in 1571 there was introduced the practice of building a "recinto" (enclosure or partition?) made of wood and canvas by which the women, separated from the men for greater devotion and modesty, could listen to sermons and concentrate on the service (Biblioteca del Museo Correr, Cod. Cic. 1877, *Memorie MS sopra la Chiesa e Monistero di Santo Stefano in Venezia*).

51 Pirri (1955), 268, no. 7; Foschi (1988), 41–42. On separate baptisteries for men and women see Leclerq (1910), cols. 398–99 (s.v. Baptistère); Pracchi (1996), 185–86.

52 Caciali (1997), 146.

53 Presumably without lowering some of the boards of the partition, some men at the right could not properly see the pulpit used by the archbishop to the left of the choir, nor could all the women at the left see that to the right.

54 On the two pulpits see Stabenow (2006), 227–80; Repishti (2006), 265–72.

55 So when G. B. Possevino (1591), 55, and others say that Carlo equipped all the churches in the dioceses with high wooden partitions ("tramezzò Carlo *tutte* le chiese della sua diocese con tavole alte"), he was either speaking only of special occasions or simply exaggerating Carlo's piety and rigour.

56 See Du Cange (1938), 109; but the point is not clear-cut. Even if we accept that *gremium* does not mean "presbytery," it may refer to the crossing, and the double pulpits at Milan were indeed attached to the piers of the crossing, in which case there would be no contradiction between the pulpits or *ambones in gremio* and the presence of a longitudinal partition.

57 Borromeo (2000), 119–21.

"TO BE IN HEAVEN"

ST. PHILIP NERI BETWEEN AESTHETIC EMOTION AND MYSTICAL ECSTASY

Costanza Barbieri

AFFECTIVE, EMOTIONAL INVOLVEMENT in the visual arts and sacred imagery, a crucial feature of the development of the baroque, has a fundamental source of inspiration in the life and teaching of St. Philip Neri, born in Florence but active in Rome from 1533, the founder of the Congregation of the Oratory. His reactions before various works of art involved the senses to the highest degree: fainting in front of Barocci's *Visitation of the Virgin*, tears caused by a particularly moving crucifix, tremors experienced before a painting of St. John the Baptist. These responses to sacred images were known to his contemporaries and were reported in detail in the process for Neri's canonization, started in 1595, just after his death, and completed in 1622, when he was proclaimed a saint.[1] They deserve analysis for two reasons: first, they present a vivid, early document of an ideal mode of viewing religious images that was developed in the baroque; second, Neri's responses to images led to the creation of an Oratorian aesthetic that flourished for two hundred years.

The iconography of St. Philip Neri, developed shortly after his death in 1595 by Pomarancio and Guido Reni, presents touching images of the saint in ecstasy before the Virgin Mary – the touchstone of his spiritual life.[2] As we shall see from his biographical data, his fervor and joy suggest that the sublime, heavenly apparition overlaps or transcends the actual representation of the Madonna before him. This leap from the material to the immaterial is the key to understanding Neri's spiritual response to art.

Philip's approach to sacred imagery is not completely new in the history of devotion, but his stance toward sculptural and painted figures takes on a new meaning given the historical conditions in Catholic Reformation Rome in the late sixteenth century. His is a precise response to Protestant criticism of the Catholic use of religious images;[3] his reactions were closely allied to the pronouncements on images given at the final session of the Council of Trent and to the elaboration of those ideas by other key ecclesiastical figures involved in the debate on images, including Carlo and Federico Borromeo, Gabriele Paleotti, Silvio Antoniano, Onofrio Panvino, and Antonio Possevino – all men who knew Neri and his life.

Contemplation of paintings and sculptures depicting sacred subjects was not an end in itself. On the contrary, Neri was keenly aware of the dangers of venerating works of art rather than the subjects depicted in them.[4] But for Neri, these works served as a catalyst to move the *affetti*, the "passions of the soul," to ascend to the spiritual via visual pleasure. In this process, the senses lead the viewer from mundane beauty to divine glory, passing through various stages of intellectual and spiritual enlightenment. Philip's affective bond with sacred images, as we shall see, represented a poignant and positive example in the controversy on the arts during the Counter-Reformation. His example was followed by his pupils, including the historian Baronius, who were responsible for disseminating Philip's approach to sacred images.

LOST IN RAPTURE: PHILIP AND VISUAL PASSIONS

Although Neri's ideas on the value of sacred art were not conveyed to us through autobiographical sources, they can be understood by the way others recorded his predilection for visual stimuli. The saint's biography is full of episodes in which heavenly visions, divine manifestations, and sudden apparitions were triggered by concrete images that shook Philip deeply. The first testimony of his strong feelings in front of a sacred image goes back to when he was still a young layman and "attended some lectures on philosophy and theology at the Dominican convent of S. Marco. His devoutness at the sight of a crucifix hanging there was so deep that he was not able to pay attention to the lectures but was shedding tears time and time again."[5]

Several times during his life Philip was overcome by emotion when contemplating the Virgin or the crucifix, as testified by his biographers with full details. Philip's ecstasy in front of Barocci's altarpiece in the Roman church of the Oratorians, the Chiesa Nuova, representing the visitation of the Virgin Mary to Saint Elizabeth (Illustration 46), is among the best-known episodes. A witness to the canonization process testified that "one morning I entered the chapel of the Visitation (with the painting by Federico Barocci) to receive Philip's blessing; he was seated in a small chair, reclining, as if out of himself; it seemed he could not feel anything; I shook him so much that he eventually recovered, and he called brother Gallonio."[6] Pietro Giacomo Bacci, his contemporary biographer, reported the same episode, explaining that "another time he was in the chapel of the Visitation, where he liked to stay since he loved Barocci's painting, and when seated, as he was used to, in a small chair, he was overcome by rapturous ecstasy.... Some penitents were there, and shook him in order

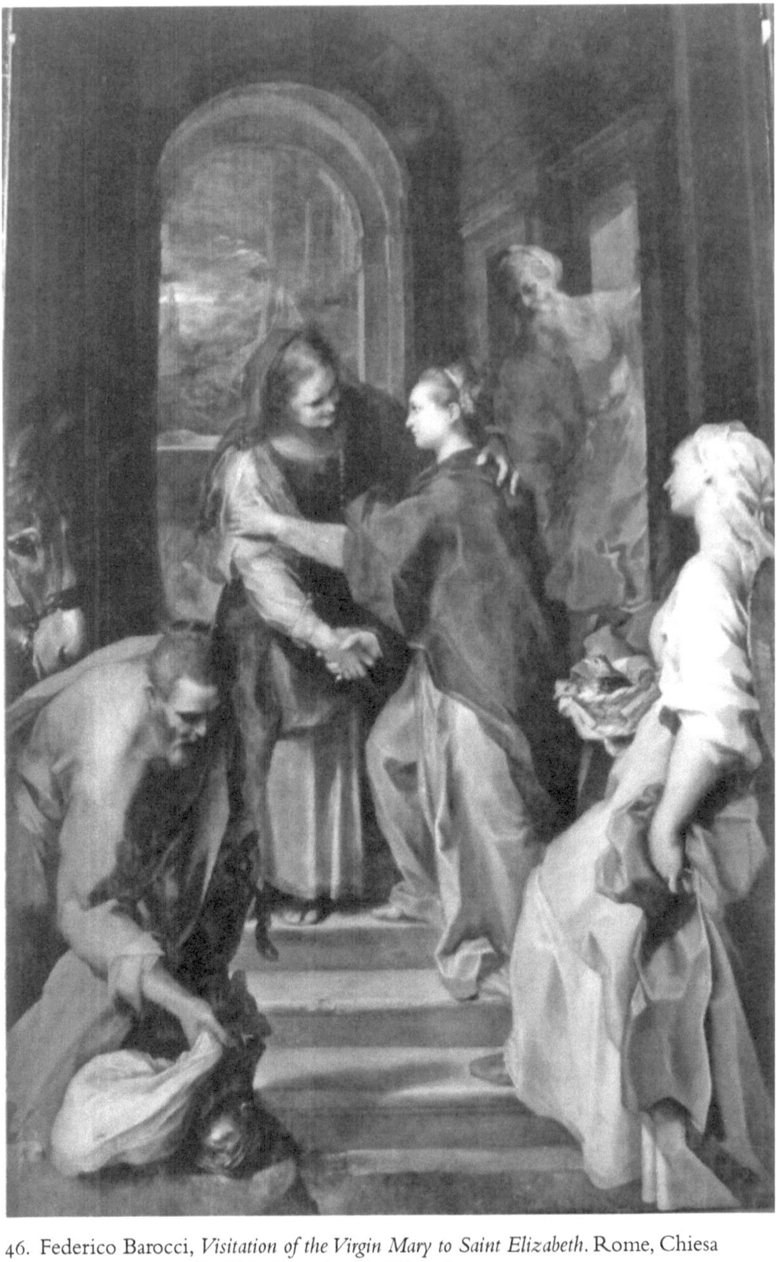

46. Federico Barocci, *Visitation of the Virgin Mary to Saint Elizabeth*. Rome, Chiesa Nuova (S. Maria in Vallicella), Chapel of the Visitation.

to wake him up .... Philip grew angry at them and started to scream and called Gallonio to send away those women because they did not leave him alone and let him relax.... He did so in order to discourage the idea that they could bear witness he was in ecstasy."[7] Philip's unwillingness to admit to ecstatic transports witnessed by others was interpreted by the Oratorians as a sign of modesty; however, his companions recognized that Neri's contemplation of the beauty and simplicity of the story of the

Virgin painted by Federico Barocci prompted a mystical ascent to divine revelation as well.

While Philip searched for inspiration in front of images in his church, he also described to his disciples miraculous apparitions that seemed to be related to smaller private devotional objects in his rooms – objects that made his heavenly visions more real and concrete. One example is his vision of the Virgin Mary, who healed him in May 1594, an episode portrayed by Niccolò Tornioli in the vault of the "Sala Rossa" in the saint's rooms (Illustration 47), as well as in Luca Ciamberlano's engraving in the *Vita di San Filippo* by his biographer, Pietro Bacci. According to Francesco Zazzara, one of Philip's most faithful disciples, he recovered from gallstones when he beheld his beloved painting of the Madonna. Although he had been sick in bed for several days, he arose with uplifted arms and exclaimed repeatedly, "Our Lady, Our Lady!" Zazzara reports further that he added, "I am not worthy of Your visit – and continuously cried, and he said to Gallonio – give me my Madonna, my little Madonna! – and he added – My Madonna! How beautiful you are!"[8]

The identification of a salvific apparition with a familiar image also occurred on another occasion, when Philip revealed to Cardinal Alessandro de' Medici that a bronze Madonna kept in his room protected him from nighttime fears.[9] This bronze Madonna could be that listed in the inventory of his private collection of artworks compiled after Philip's death (most of them gifts, now lost, from disciples and followers).[10]

A marble bas-relief, the *Man of Sorrows* (probably similar to the one by Donatello for the St. Anthony altar in Padua), was placed on the altar

47. Niccolò Tornioli, *The Virgin Appears to Saint Philip.* Rome, Chiesa Nuova (S. Maria in Vallicella), vault of the "Sala Rossa," Camere di San Filippo.

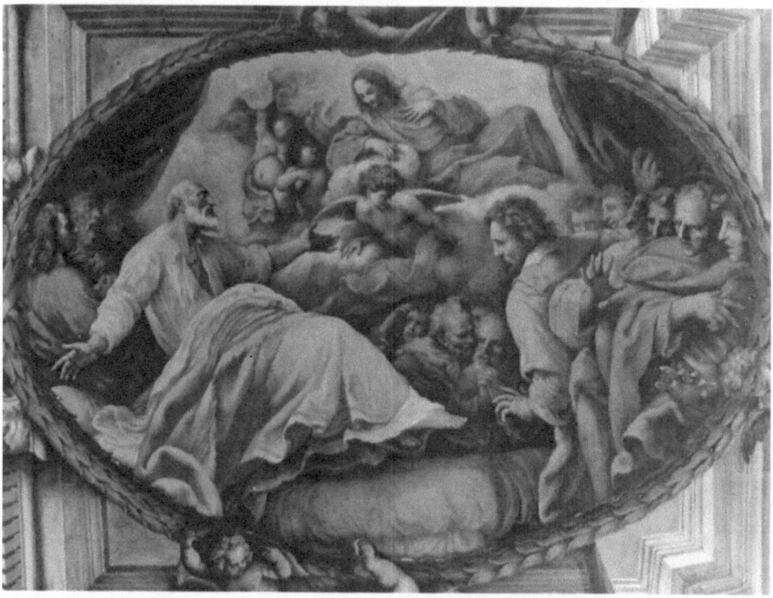

of Philip's small chapel and recorded in the inventory. It is mentioned in two similar miraculous episodes. In the first, Francesco Zazzara recalls that Neri, while celebrating mass, asked him if he saw blood coming from the wound of the image of Christ exposed over the altar; it seemed that the blood was more copious than on other occasions, although it was seen only by Neri as if in a vision in which the supernatural image overlapped the material one.[11] On the second occasion, the *Man of Sorrows* inspired a vision that revealed to Neri the positive result of the commission investigating the orthodoxy of Girolamo Savonarola's works. In 1559, due to the threat of condemnation of Savonarola by the Inquisition, theologians and Dominicans were assembled in prayer at S. Maria sopra Minerva, the Dominican church of Rome. Philip participated in the prayers because he was very devoted to the Ferrarese friar, who had preached in his home city of Florence. During the prayers, Philip went into ecstasy and fainted,

48 (below). Luca Ciamberlano, *Estasi di S. Filippo all'Oratione delle quarant'hore nel Convento de' frati della Minerva.* Engraving. From Bacci (1625).

49 (right). Pomarancio, *Saint John the Baptist Appears to Philip.* Rome, Chiesa Nuova (S. Maria in Vallicella), Chapel of Saint Philip.

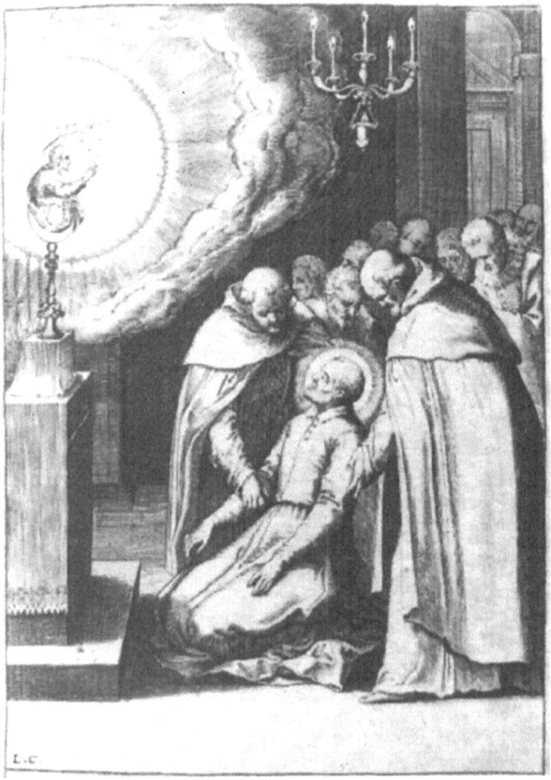

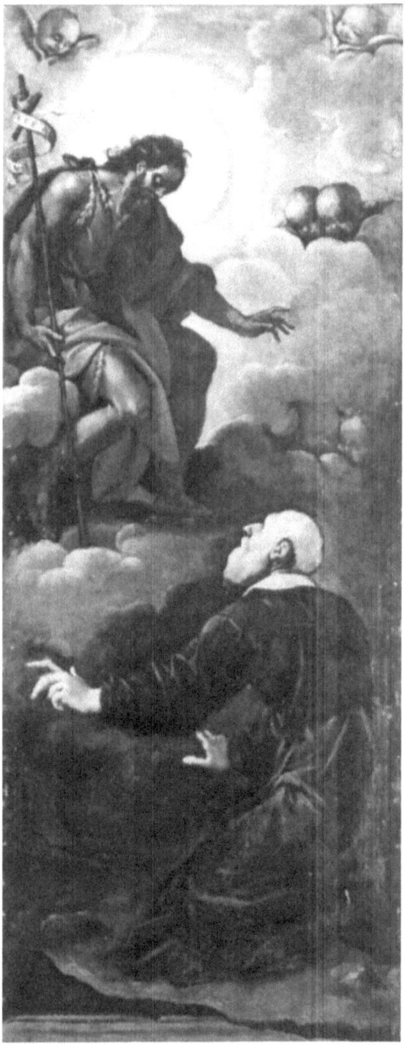

and the friars became extremely concerned. When he eventually recovered, he cheerfully informed the Dominicans that the risk of Savonarola's books being placed on the Index had vanished, and the author of the revelation was Christ himself, "who had appeared to Philip half-length (as in the bas-relief he owned), and had blessed them."[12] Marcello Ferro, one of the eyewitnesses whose deposition was reported in the process of canonization, testified that Neri "saw in the holy Sacrament, the bust of ... Christ pronouncing a benediction over them."[13] The scene is shown in the engraving by Luca Ciamberlano, entitled *Estasi di S. Filippo all'Oratione delle quarant'hore nel Convento de' frati della Minerva*, in Bacci's *Vita di San Filippo Neri* (Illustration 48).[14]

Another episode documents this association of supernatural images with figurative arts in an even more detailed and revealing manner. This time Philip had a particularly vivid dream during which the will of God was made manifest to him. The episode is narrated by Cardinal Federico Borromeo: "[L]ying in his bed a person appeared to him – similar as he told me – to the common paintings of Saint John the Baptist; he was seized with tremors and a vehement spirit. The image disappeared and he understood what God wanted."[15] The episode is represented in the painted series devoted to the life of Neri by Pomarancio, decorating his funerary chapel in the Chiesa Nuova. St. John the Baptist sitting on a cloud appears to the kneeling Philip, who contemplates him ecstatically (Illustration 49).[16] Thus, concrete images, identified by Philip in familiar paintings, like St. John the Baptist, the patron saint of his native Florence, played an essential role in provoking the emotions that led to heavenly visions.[17]

The relationship between religious images and spiritual enlightenment has long been discussed by Catholic theologians. Starting with the argument of Pseudo-Dionysius, as discussed by Abbot Suger in the twelfth century, material objects may represent the beginning of anagogical ascent.[18] Thomas Aquinas, in the *Summa Theologica*, argues that the divine cult is both exterior and interior because man is made of body and soul. The exterior worship is regulated by liturgy and ceremony, which fully integrate devotional images and devotion.[19] Alvise (Luigi) Lippomano, writing against the Protestants in 1555 on the utility of the exterior cult, stated that "all the faithful in this life see God as in a shadow and in a mirror and from the visible are led to the invisible. Not only are they obliged to give God interior, invisible worship, but also the exterior cult. Everybody needs ceremonies."[20] His texts are present in Philip's library.[21] This tradition goes back to the church fathers, such as St. Jerome, whose mystical raptures – according to the canonical iconography – usually occur in front of the crucifix.[22]

During the fifteenth century, there was a diffusion of practical devotional manuals to instruct the faithful on the practice of interior visualization to better memorize sacred stories. Painters and the faithful referred to the same sources: sermons and devotional texts. Among the latter, the most popular were the *Giardino de Oratione*, owned by Philip,[23] the *Meditationi de la Vita et Passione de Nostro Signore Misser Iesu Christo*, and the *Libro de l'occhio morale et spirituale vulgare.* The purpose of these devotional manuals was to teach through contemplation of the mysteries of Christ's life with the eyes of the mind. Artists were to comply with the same sources in order to meet the requirements of correct representation attentive to the scriptural canons, appropriate both for altarpieces and for images intended for private worship.[24]

Girolamo Savonarola's sermons on the same subject are also relevant, given the devotion and admiration that Philip developed for the Ferrarese friar during his youth in Florence, when he was acquainted with the Dominicans of S. Marco.[25] According to Ronald Steinberg, Savonarola believed that the ability to produce verbal and visual images with the aim of understanding God's will was to be considered a gift from God himself. The arts could play an important role in the lives of Christians and enhance spiritual and intellectual comprehension of sacred mysteries.[26] Savonarola's treatise *Il trionfo della Croce* is a passionate apology for the power of images, in which the friar effectively compares the synthetic and intuitive dimension of a visual discourse to the complexities of a doctrinal argument, often too abstract for ordinary people. Images convey several levels of meaning at once and help the viewer contemplate Christian mysteries. According to Savonarola, "Love is like a painter; a good painter, if he paints well, greatly delights men with his paintings. In contemplation of the painting men remain suspended, and at times they may appear to be in ecstasy and outside themselves and seem to forget themselves [as corporeal beings]."[27] He also believed that the contemplation of harmonious compositions could promote the viewer's proximity to God.[28] Savonarola's exposition seems to be performed almost literally by Philip in the presence of a work of art.

THE DEBATE ON IMAGES

Philip's association of concrete images and heavenly visions – fully experienced through the senses – plays a major historical role when it is considered in relation to the debate on sacred images, the subject of heated discussions for Catholic theologians and clergymen in answer to the Protestant critique of church art. Philip's attitude toward figurative arts, as we have seen, is characterized by an essentially devotional interest (yet not lacking aesthetic judgment), an interest shared by the leading Catholic writers of the sixteenth century, who wrote in defense of images. It should be stressed that many of them had a direct relationship with the Florentine saint and substantially shared his point of view. These apologists for the figurative arts argued that images were a necessary component of the "exterior cult," and this theory was put into practice at the Chiesa

Nuova.[29] While it is impossible to prove that Philip had a direct influence on writings in defense of sacred images, there are strong affinities between the works of Charles and Federico Borromeo, Gabriele Paleotti, Silvio Antoniano, Antonio Possevino, and the spirituality of the founder of the Oratorio. Indeed, as we shall see, they were all acquainted with Neri and often attended services in the Chiesa Nuova.

Regarding the theme of figurative arts, all Catholic Reformers, whether theorists or engaged in apostolic activities, were united in their rejection of the Protestant campaign, which demonized images and led to their destruction.[30] The first generation of supporters of the Catholic cult of images, including Alberto Pio and Ambrogio Catarino, who published *De Certa Gloria Invocatione ac Veneratione Sanctorum Disputationes* in 1542, met the Protestant attacks with arguments that remained fundamental to the Counter-Reformation treatises of the second half of the century.[31] Their efforts were aimed at finding scriptural and historical traditions and testimonies to justify recourse to images. According to the tradition, Christ himself had wished to leave a testimony of his image on the road to Calvary, and Veronica's veil was one of the four most venerated relics of the Catholic world.[32] For Luther, on the other hand, the veil was nothing but a sensational forgery.[33] By the mid–sixteenth century, the debate on images reached a climax unknown in the Christian world since the iconoclastic controversy of the eighth century.

Image veneration was considered heretical and idolatrous by Calvin, while Erasmus's less radical approach derided its merely superstitious character.[34] For Protestants, the cult of images made Catholics appear similar to pagans, with all the dangers associated with the shift of interest from spiritual values to material artifacts. Paintings and statues were considered the devil's work because they became venerated objects, replacing the idea that they signified.[35] Protestants were also scandalized by the value attributed to miraculous images, and it was only a short step to accusations of idolatry.[36] Catholics then increased their defense of the extraordinary power of icons, insisting on the long tradition of innumerable miracles worked by sacred images.

This argument is of the utmost importance in the deliberations of Trent and in the policies of the Counter-Reformation, as stressed by Scavizzi: "Two of the most debated issues in the 1560s concerned miracles and idolatry. A miracle was the free intervention of God in human affairs; tradition maintained ... that it was an important element by which God manifested his will and invited the veneration of the people. Both the miracle and veneration could take place through certain objects, one of which was the *simulachrum* or image."[37] Catholic writers of treatises often focused on the miracles worked by images. For example, Giulio Castellani, author of the *De Imaginibus et Miraculis Sanctorum* (Bologna, 1568), argues that the worship of sacred images is approved by God, who rewards such devotion with an abundance of miracles. In listing a series of miracles performed by an image, *Madonna with Child*, in Faenza, Castellani dares to state that images are an essential component of God's action.[38] Onofrio Panvinio, church historian and archaeologist, who was friendly with the Oratorians as well as with St. Charles Borromeo, promoted belief in the extraordinary powers of early medieval icons depicting Mary and the infant Christ, located in Roman churches; he catalogued with enthusiasm their miraculous effects in his treatise *Le sette chiese di Roma* (Rome, 1570).[39]

One of the key elements of Catholic Reform was a return to Rome's early Christian roots, and devotion to early Marian icons played an essential role in Church renewal. The Oratorians, under Philip's guidance, were leaders in this radical reform, which was codified in the *Annales Ecclesiastici* of Baronius, the great Oratorian historian, in 1588–1607.[40] The modern Church received authoritative confirmation from the primitive Church because the two were linked by the tradition of extant ancient images with miraculous powers that stemmed from the prototype. Baronius discussed in the first volume of the *Annales* the validity of miraculous images such as the Madonna painted by St. Luke, the image of Christ sent to Abgar, king of Edessa, and the statue of Christ and the sick woman in Caesarea.[41] For the Oratorians and other Reformers, such as Paleotti, the extraordinary power of such images and their association with miracles was not due to their diabolic powers, as Protestants claimed, but depended on the sanctity of the prototype of which they were *umbrae*, that is, "shadows."[42]

The value of images is based on their four main uses for the faithful. According to Alberto Pio, images prove themselves useful in terms of *memory*, in recalling the saintly models of the past; as *Biblia pauperum*, in teaching the illiterate; as *excitatio* (excitement, in stirring the senses and the soul), and *gaudium* (joy, that is the pleasure of ascending to sublime things, a concept that Pio derives from Neoplatonism).[43] A painted image represents sacred history at a glance and allows for the recollection of all the implications associated with this subject. This was also a fundamental aspect of Oratorian thought.

The concept of *excitatio* (excitement), which involved both the senses and the emotions, was particularly useful in explaining the anagogical virtues of the arts. "Paintings and images, according to Ambrogio Catarino, a Dominican from Siena who combated Erasmus's attacks, stimulate senses and fancy, thought and meditation, and finally the contemplation of the mind is aroused."[44] This idea is not new, as we have already encountered it, for instance, in Savonarola's sermons; however, its importance is thoroughly reconsidered and systematized in the sixteenth century in response to Protestant attacks.

According to Pio, *gaudium* (joy) is closely related to sight (and images): "[I]t lets us see many things in one instant ... and the things happen easily, with delight: this the other senses are not able to do." Thus, the ease and pleasure of sight – the most spiritual and refined of all the senses – leads to *gaudium*, a word closely associated with Philip Neri's spirituality. It was much discussed in relation to church ceremonies as *honesta voluptas*, an "honest pleasure."[45] When the soul through the aesthetic experience is raised to the contemplation of heavenly things, it experiences an intuitive participation in the divine, accompanied by a sense of joy. For Pio and Catarino the contemplation of images leads us straight to *gaudium* and puts us in direct contact with the prototype.[46] The image is the meeting point with the divine.

Among the major authors on this topic in the second half of the century, we find some of Philip's close friends, such as Federico Borromeo, Antonio Possevino, and Gabriele Paleotti, habitual visitors of the Chiesa Nuova.[47] Paleotti was a member of the Oratory from the time it was housed in S. Girolamo della Carità, in 1569, and Philip was his confessor.[48] In his fundamental text of the Counter-Reformation, the *Discorso intorno alle immagini sacre e profane*, published in Bologna in 1582, Paleotti sustains the concept of *honesta voluptas*, that is, the honest pleasure achieved through the contemplation of sacred images: "It is no wonder if Christian law ... received images in order to honour true God and the saints.... Images are part of the external cult ... through which we experience immense pleasure in having in front of our eyes the representation of His Majesty.... As to the delight, nothing else is, so to speak, so pleasing to our eyes and motive of the sweetest recreation as a well-done painting."[49]

Federico Borromeo, Philip's penitent, takes the visual language as the most effective way of arousing the viewer: "Piety towards God and the Saints, praise, imitation, fear, pain and hope are just the soul's feelings aroused by the sacred images, which could be said to be alive and inspiring when they will excite our minds and they will shake us almost like a vital blow..... In fact, painting is a language painters speak not to men's ears but rather to men's souls."[50]

Finally, it is not without reason that in 1591 the cardinal Agostino Valier, another participant in the Oratorian circle, entitled his dialogue, dedicated to Neri, *Philippus, sive de Christiana Laetitia Dialogus* (*Philip, or the Dialogue of the Christian Joy*); in the dialogue, he lets Borromeo say that joy consists in contemplation: "No other part of the body but the eye offers a greater and nobler help. This is the reason why I believe that those who are devoted to contemplation not only lead a pleasant life for themselves but also of much advantage to others because of meditations and prayers."[51]

The authoritative model of Philip's ecstasies, his spiritual as well as bodily experiences, provides a moving example of the *honesta voluptas* as a mean for the ascent to the divine. When he is transported by the crucifix, or prays at the Visitation Chapel in front of Barocci's altarpiece, or associates the heavenly visions with concrete images of his private devotion, he is stressing the fundamental role of sacred art as an instrument of ascent to God through the senses. Visual arts speak the language of beauty, which leads to the Neoplatonic archetype of divine revelation, which is perceived first by the senses and second by the ecstatic mind. This attitude is a powerful response to Protestant criticism that disparaged images as well as relics. Philip takes a stand in this controversy with several actions. Most public was his veneration of early Christian icons such as the *Salus Populi Romani* of S. Maria Maggiore and the Marian icons in S. Agnese in Agone and in S. Maria in Trastevere.[52] Also, the chapel of Veronica's veil in St. Peter's was one of his preferred destinations for prayer and meditation in front of the holy face.[53] In order to supply the Chiesa Nuova with a similar powerful icon, a miracle-working Quattrocento fresco, *Madonna with the Infant Christ*, was detached from a street wall in order to be preserved and placed on the main altar of the church, becoming a central image for Oratorian spirituality (Illustration 50).[54]

In addition to the themes of *gaudium* and *excitatio*, Philip was familiar with the value of images as historical testimony and *exemplum*. The portrait as "memory" was very dear to Philip: on the death of one of his acquaintances, Marco Antonio Corteselli, Neri asked a painter to accompany him to portray the effigy of the deceased in order to preserve his memory.[55] The same wish led Philip to ask Cavalier d'Arpino for an image of his friend Brother Felice da Cantalice; since the brother was very reluctant, the painter had to attempt a trick by sketching unseen the portrait of the Capuchin. The drawing, almost a snapshot of the saint of Cantalice – is valuable as evidence of Philip's love for the visual substantiality of memory. St. Antoninus's portrait, which appears in Neri's collection, meets the same criterion of image conservation, not of the friend but of his spiritual model. The fifteenth-century archbishop of Florence, a Dominican at S. Marco, was a great source of inspiration to Neri.[56]

The Counter-Reformation treatises of the second half of the sixteenth century amplify the relationship between image, memory, and history. Baronius, Neri's disciple who, upon Neri's request, wrote the monumental *Annales*, thoroughly analyzed the theme of sacred images from the historiographical point of view. Paleotti enlarged this argument in his *Discorso intorno alle immagini sacre e profane* and maintained that images, rather than text, could claim historical priority. Paleotti explains: "We consider ... it is possible to say that the introduction of images ... preceded the written word.... Whoever ... honours images with this priority in terms of time ..., affirms that images represent ideas directly, without other means ... as signs of interior concepts, according to Aristotle."[57]

Furthermore, the antiquity and naturalness of the figurative arts honor God by mirroring his creation and recalling sacred history. Indeed, Paleotti shares Philip's enthusiasm for sacred images when he praises the priority and dignity of painting in relation to its aim, that is, to unite humans with God, which is the purpose of divine love and charity.[58] As Alessandro Zuccari pointed out, Paleotti's *Discorso intorno alle immagini sacre e profane*

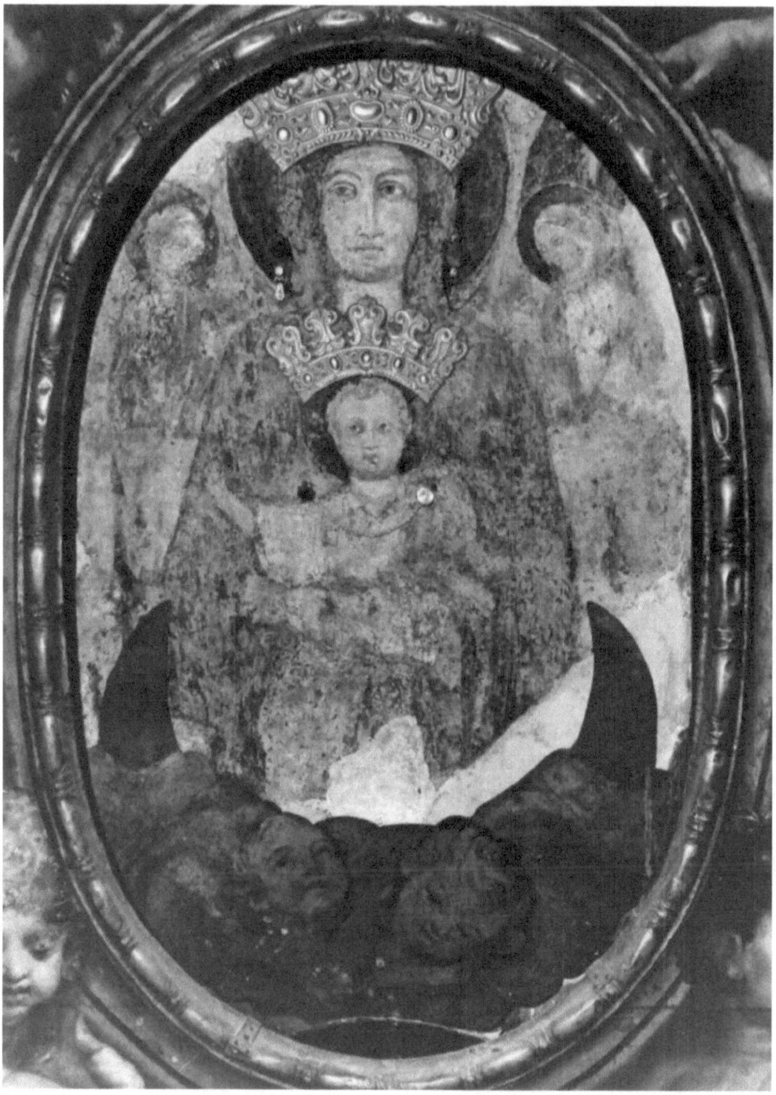

50. *Madonna with the Infant Christ* (*Madonna della Vallicella*). Rome, Chiesa Nuova (S. Maria in Vallicella), detached fresco, high altar of the church.

was officially approved by the Congregazione Oratoriana, almost as an imprimatur, when Baronius published an enthusiastic review of it in his *Annales*.[59]

The emotion and rapture felt by Philip before the image of the crucifix or Barocci's altarpiece are a clear testimony to the ideal passage from the visible to the invisible, described by theologians and writers in the treatises of the Counter-Reformation. A concrete image in front of the eye allows one to preserve God effectively in one's heart. In this sense Philip's spirituality is different from that of Ignatius of Loyola, founder of the Jesuits, who builds his *Spiritual Exercises* on interior images and the method of the *compositio loci*. As Alessandro Zuccari explained, whereas Ignatius valued interior visions as simple instruments to mark chronologically the narration of Christ's life independent of exterior representations, those exterior manifestations are, for Philip, the necessary, most intuitive, and immediate means of bringing human and divine into contact.[60] As testified by Philip's experience, a double process takes place in contemplating sacred images. On the one hand, through physical forms the divine appears to men and women; on the other hand, through contemplation, they raise themselves to God. This concept influenced the most authoritative ecclesiastical writers of the Counter-Reformation.[61]

"PAINTERS SPEAK TO MEN'S SOULS:" VISUAL MYSTERIES IN THE CHIESA NUOVA

Philip Neri's spirituality is rooted in the belief that the ultimate purpose of art is to lead the viewer to the contemplation of divine mysteries.[62] Indeed, the decorative program of the Roman Oratorian church, the Chiesa Nuova, also known as S. Maria in Vallicella, was conceived as a visualization of the mysteries of the life of Christ and of the Virgin depicted in the altarpieces on each altar. According to Philip's last will, "[E]ach of them had to depict a mystery of the Saviour where the holy Madonna should also be painted."[63] Philip also heeded Savonarola's warning that painting and decoration could become too lavish, leading to distraction rather than contemplation.[64] During the completion of his church, his fellow Oratorians suggested stucco decorations for the chapels, but Philip refused, citing financial problems, an answer that left the fathers astonished because it was clearly a pretext.[65] The same attack against ostentation and rich ornamentation had also been launched by Philip's intimate friend, Charles Borromeo, who published in 1577 his *Instructiones Fabricae et Suppellectilis Eccleasiasticae*.[66]

Though enriched by gilded stucco decorations in the seventeenth century, the Chiesa Nuova was originally more modest and had been designed to offer people a homogeneous iconographic program focused on the mysteries of the life of the Virgin. The primary (but not exclusive) source of the program was Alberto da Castello's *Rosario de la gloriosa Vergine Maria*, a popular devotional manual intended to teach pious men and women a model of prayer through the Rosary and contemplation.[67]

Philip originally intended to have Federico Barocci paint the nativity of the Virgin for the high altar, but after his death in 1595 the Oratorians transferred the commission to Peter Paul Rubens, who was charged to create the *Madonna and Child in Glory* to surround and protect the miraculous Quattrocento image of the Virgin housed in the church (Illustration 51).[68] However, Neri's beloved Barocci was commissioned in 1603 to paint the altarpiece of the left transept, the magnificent *Presentation of the Virgin to the Temple* (Illustration 52).[69]

The program, according to Philip's will, continued with the stories of the Virgin and Christ in the ten side chapels of the nave. On the left, the first chapel presents the *Annunciation*, painted by Domenico Cresti called Passignano in 1590–91,[70] followed by the famous *Visitation* by Barocci dated 1586;[71] the third chapel, patronized by Silvio Antoniano, shows the *Adoration of the Shepherds* by Durante Alberti (before 1590),[72] while the fourth chapel depicts the *Adoration of the Magi*, by Cesare Nebbia, realized around 1578.[73] The fifth chapel of the left nave is dedicated to the purification of the Virgin, whose altarpiece was painted by Cavalier d'Arpino in 1627.[74] The first chapel of the right nave, close to the entrance, is decorated with Scipione Pulzone's *Crucifixion*, a painting greatly admired by the Oratorians, dated 1586 (Illustration 53);[75] in the second chapel was originally the famous Caravaggio *Deposition*, now in the Vatican Museum.[76] The following chapel presents the *Ascension* by Girolamo Muziano, which includes – as do all the others – the image of Mary as expressly requested by the Congregation in 1581.[77] Wensel Coebergher originally painted the altarpiece of the fourth chapel, the *Descent of the Holy Spirit upon the Apostles and the Virgin*,[78] while the image of the last chapel of the right nave is the *Assumption of the Virgin*, painted by Aurelio Lomi in 1587 (now replaced by a similar painting by Domenico Cerrini).[79] The final image of the cycle devoted to the Mother of God, in the right transept, is the altarpiece of the *Coronation of the Virgin* by Cavalier d'Arpino (Illustration 54). The latter took twenty-five years to finish, but it did not satisfy d'Arpino's patrons. In 1617 he had to repaint the figure of Mary, who was originally conceived with her head in profile, covered by a veil, and with her hands joined in prayer. Apparently the Congregation considered this iconographic solution unsuitable to the dignity of Mary and asked the artist to uncover the head, to repaint her face and expression, and to move the hands toward her heart, in a more affectionate gesture.[80]

In the seventeenth century the Congregation continued to elaborate their idea of devotion to the Virgin: she is the focus of the decoration of their church, especially in the mid-Seicento frescoes of the ceiling, the dome, and the apse painted by Pietro da Cortona. A well-known episode of Philip's life is represented in the ceiling of the nave.[81] During the construction of the Chiesa Nuova, Mary appears to Philip in a dream and supports a timber that miraculously remains suspended, avoiding a tragic collapse of the new building. It is always the Virgin who dispenses innumerable graces toward Philip; in her honor, Philip composed a prayer teaching his disciples the cult of "Maria Mediatrice."[82] His insistence on the glory of the Mother of God explains his stance against the Protestant desire to demote Mary and reduce her role. Thus, the iconography of S. Maria in Vallicella[83] reflected Philip's devotion to the Virgin, especially her role as mediator between humanity and divinity, one of the salient points of Philip's spirituality.[84]

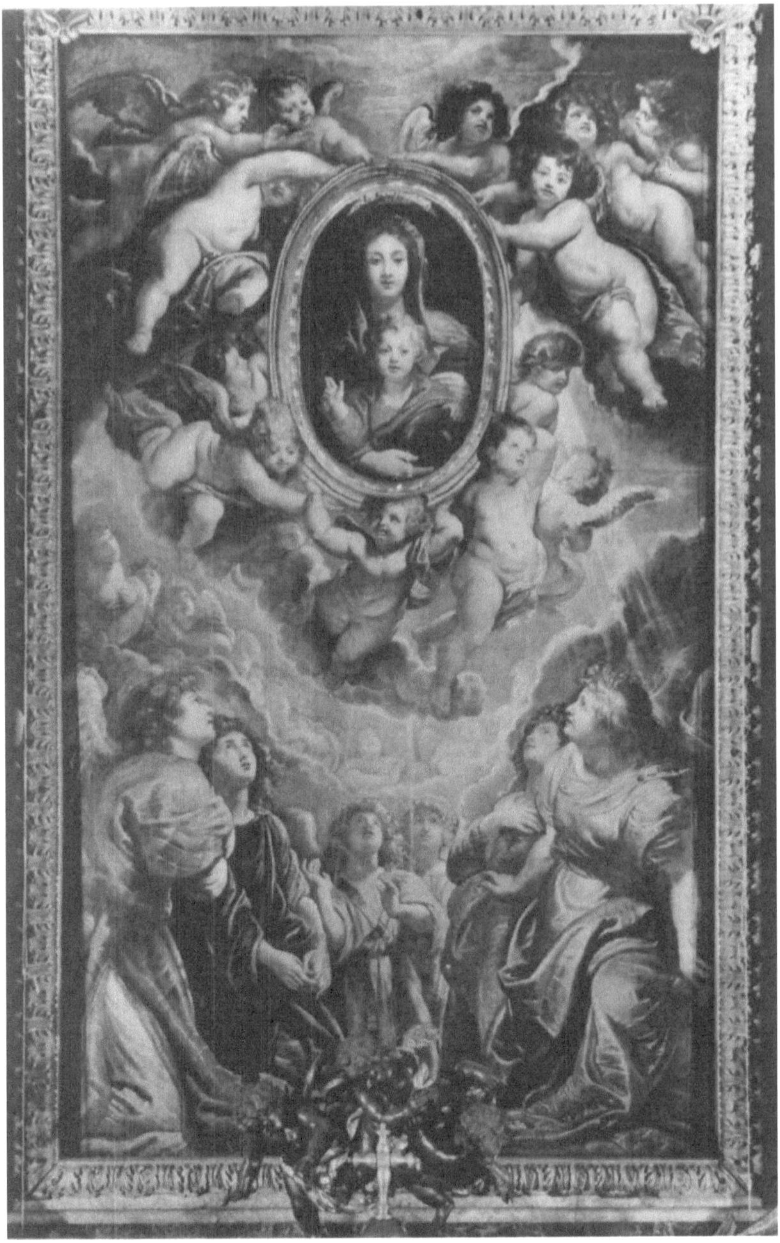

51. Peter Paul Rubens, *Madonna and Child in Glory.* Rome, Chiesa Nuova (S. Maria in Vallicella), high altar of the church.

Among all the altarpieces commissioned to decorate the altars of the Chiesa Nuova, we saw that Philip preferred the image of Federico Barocci's *Visitation of the Virgin to Saint Elizabeth*, in front of which he frequently prayed and experienced rapturous ecstasies. Philip reacted not only to the subject, but to the aesthetic merits of the work. In fact, Barocci was at the height of his career and was much sought after by important patrons, including Federico Borromeo.[85] The artist's style apparently met perfectly the expectations both of Counter-Reformation theorists and of laypeople.[86]

In studying the relationship between Barocci and the Oratorians, Ian Verstegen pointed out that the style of the *Visitation* is characterized by "bright, shimmering masses of draperies ..., and idealized faces ... paired with details painted with skillful illusionism ... creating ... plausibility of the image ... and new means to appeal to the viewer."[87] His images are indeed intensely appealing to the viewer: the controlled feelings of his characters contrasted with rich, explosive colors, a device intended to stimulate and

52. Federico Barocci, *Presentation of the Virgin to the Temple.* Rome, Chiesa Nuova (S. Maria in Vallicella), left transept.

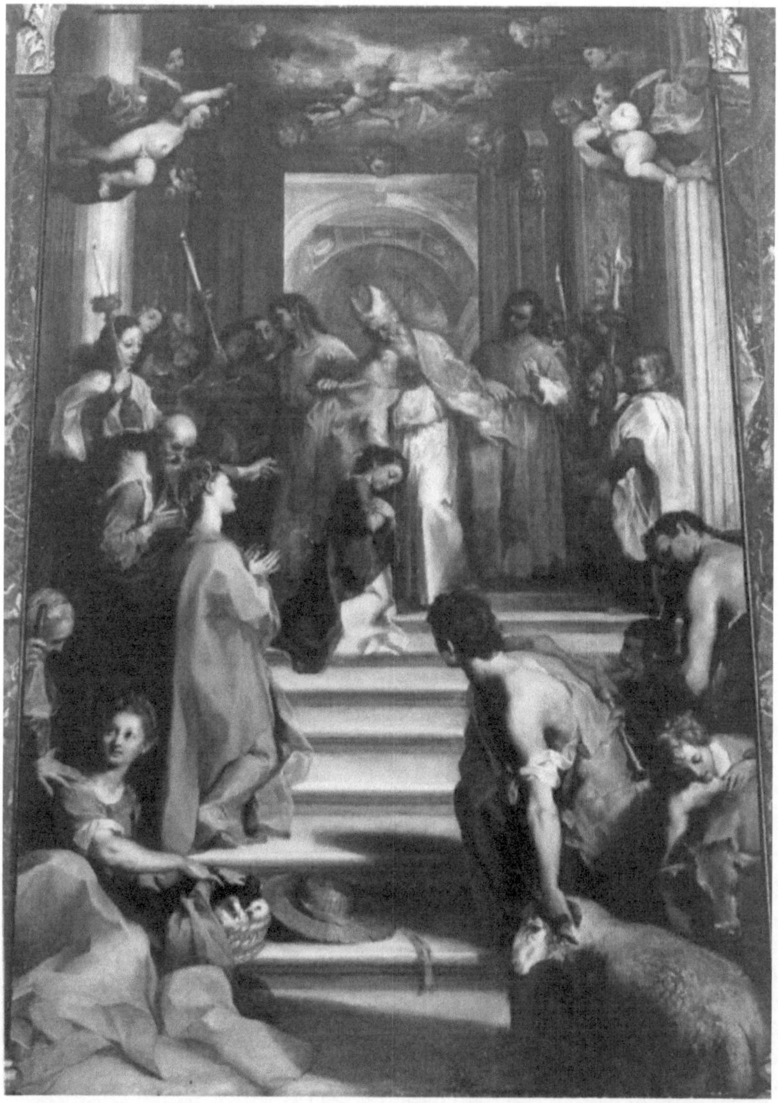

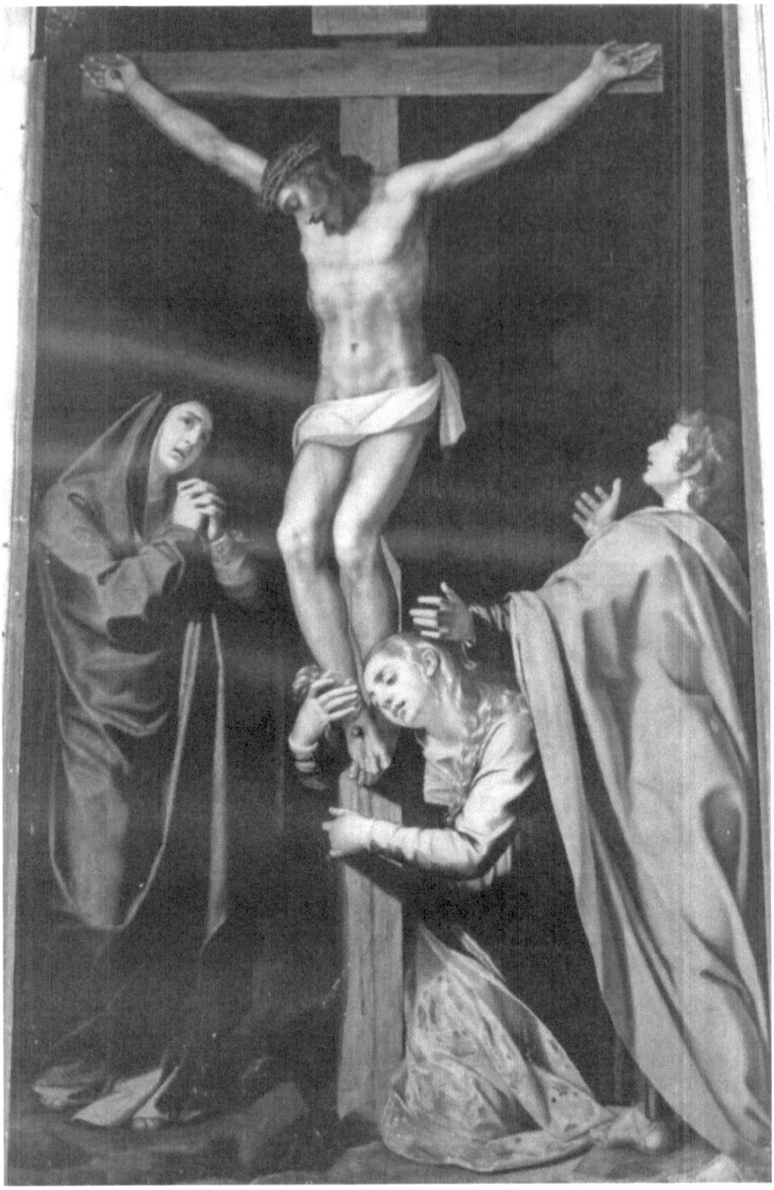

53. Scipione Pulzone, *Crucifixion*. Rome, Chiesa Nuova (S. Maria in Vallicella), Chapel of the Crucifixion.

involve the beholder. Modesty of demeanor and convincing naturalism are played against stunning, spectacular hues, combining everyday life with a hint of the beauty of the supernatural world. Sublime, magnificent colors (as in Rothko), alluding to transcending passions, are coupled with an apparently simple composition, perfectly befitting the subject: Mary's ardent charity and humility in visiting St. Elizabeth.

A simple, spontaneous language – at least to be perceived as such – was exactly what Gabriele Paleotti, Philip's intimate friend, hoped for in sacred

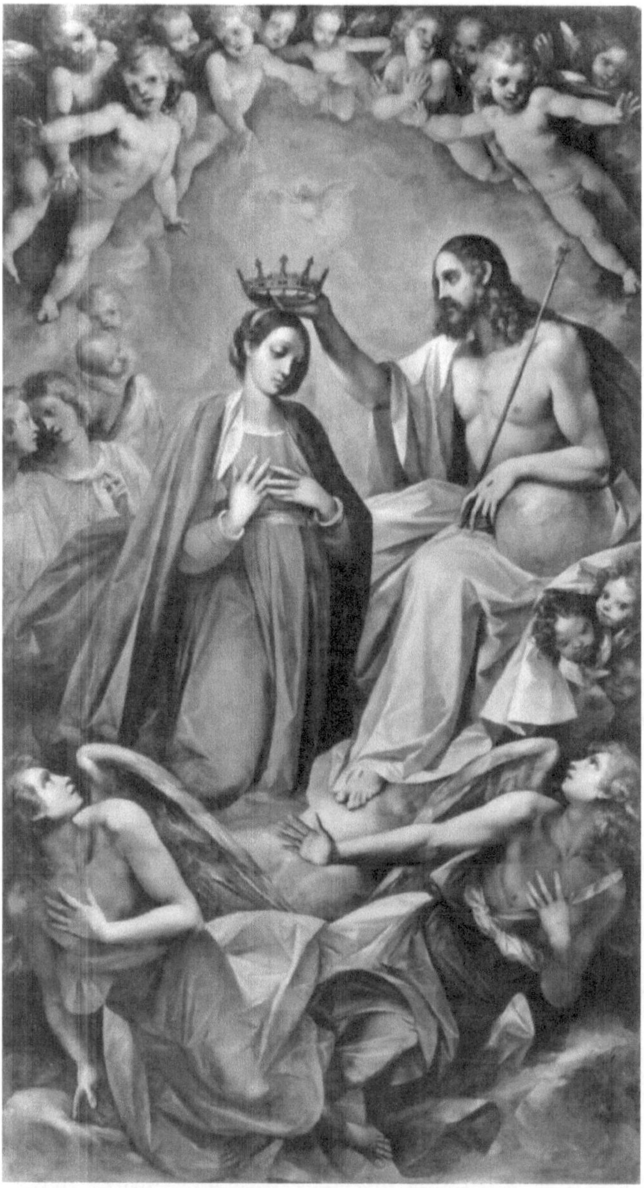

54. Cavalier d'Arpino (Giuseppe Cesari), *Coronation of the Virgin*. Rome, Chiesa Nuova (S. Maria in Vallicella), right transept.

images: the painter had to avoid artificiality, choosing instead the "best clarity in defining the arrangement of the figures, in a way that the onlookers were able to recognize, at first glance, the story represented."[88] Concerning the *affetti,* or "emotions of the soul," Paleotti said that "a sacred image has to perform two things: one is to move the senses, the other is to excite the soul and devotion."[89] Desire for simplicity paired with spirituality motivated Philip in the decoration of his church. Again it is significant to record a convergence of ideas with those of Savonarola, quoted by Steinberg: "Ask the painter what pleases more, a figure that is affected and unnatural or one that is without such affectation. They will reply that the natural figure is better and more pleasing. Thus, rhetoric pleases more when it is hidden"[90] – an interesting analogy to Castiglione's *sprezzatura.*

Guido Reni achieved such a painting of clarity and simplicity in his altarpiece of 1614 representing Philip lost in rapture as if transported to heaven (Illustration 55). The work, commissioned by the Oratorians for Neri's titular chapel in the Chiesa Nuova,[91] became the canonical image of the saint because it synthesizes vision and ecstasy. Philip is represented kneeling, with his head turned aside, dominated on the left by the apparition of the Virgin Mary with the Christ Child in her arms. He is possibly in the same position of confident abandonment that he assumed while contemplating his beloved image of the Madonna, a scene that must have been familiar to his fellow Oratorians. We can easily recognize that the apparition is not in front of Philip – his eyes are not truly looking at it; rather, it is an inner vision, seen with the eyes of the mind.[92] Pomarancio and then Reni arrived at this simple yet effective composition, promoted by the Oratorians and documented by Philip's biographer, Bacci.

The frequency of subjects involving Mary in Philip's own collection perfectly reflects his devotion and finds a significant parallel with the printed texts of his library, many of which are still kept at the Biblioteca Vallicelliana: the *Rosario della Gloriosa Vergine Maria* by Alberto da Castello, the *Mariae Virginis Miraculorum libri tres* by Silvano Razzi, the *De partu Virginis* by Sannazzaro, not to mention innumerable sermons – by Savonarola, Ambrogio Spiera, Le Fevre d'Etaples – devoted to the Virgin.[93] She is the core of Philip's spirituality and an essential part of his iconography.[94]

Instead of writing treatises, Neri conveyed his love for the figurative arts through the images in his church. His disciples correctly interpreted his delight in images as an effective means to achieve spiritual visions. The Oratorian culture and Philip's example acquired a definitive meaning in relation to the debate about sacred art, in stressing the role of visual pleasure as a progression to the divine, an aesthetic and edifying value, a parallel to the rhetorical tools of *delectando docere.* For Philip, as for Paleotti, a painter is a silent theologian or an orator who has to teach, to delight, and to move the senses.[95] Neri also responds to Protestant criticism about images with the concrete arguments offered by his spiritual life: with his vision of the Virgin, who intervenes to heal him when he prays before her likeness, or when the *Man of Sorrows* appears to him to reveal that his prayers have been answered.

In favoring the figurative arts as indispensable stimuli to his visions, Neri reasserts the authority and dignity of images and of the exterior cult. Furthermore, using the visible, Philip suggests a mixture of interior images, apparitions, visions, and exterior images, where the figurative arts are fully

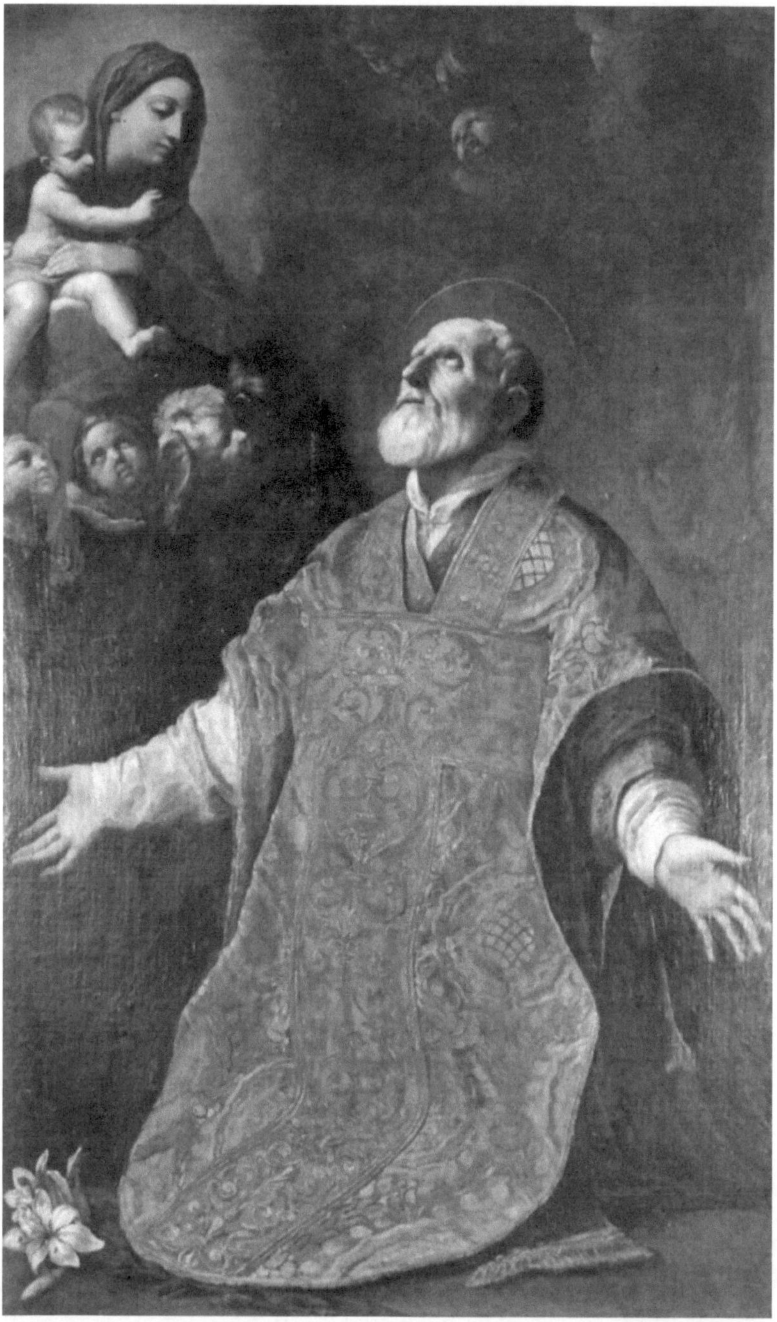

55. Guido Reni, *Saint Philip in Ecstasy Contemplating the Virgin*. Rome, Chiesa Nuova (S. Maria in Vallicella), Camere di San Filippo.

experienced by the senses. The interior cult is bound to the exterior cult; the boundaries between interior experience and exterior representation become more frail. In this way Neri lays the foundations for the transition to the baroque culture of the image par excellence.

Notes

For this essay, I have drawn on material presented in Barbieri (1995), resulting from research promoted by the Soprintendenza ai Beni Storico Artistici di Roma – Polo Museale di Roma and by the Congregazione dell'Oratorio, finalized in the exhibition dedicated to St. Philip Neri, *La Regola e la Fama*. I give special thanks to the Oratorians, attentive keepers of – and responsive to – the treasures of their church (especially father Vladimiro Tyka, exceptional parish priest of the Chiesa Nuova). I am also grateful to Alba Costamagna and Claudio Strinati from the Soprintendenza of Rome for their generous support and stimulating suggestions. The study of the extensive archives of the Vallicella was possible thanks to the collaboration of my friends and colleagues Sofia Barchiesi and Daniele Ferrara, with whom I shared endless discussions and enthusiastic discoveries. The impetus to look back at the Oratorian culture and the visual arts with a new perspective came from Marcia Hall, to whom I am very grateful. Also, I am deeply indebted to Carolyn Valone, for her knowledge, intuition, and patience in editing my text and for the many suggestions in improving it. The mistakes are entirely mine.

1 For the life of the saint and his circle see *Processo* (1957–63) (henceforth cited as *Processo*, with volume and page number); Ponnelle and Bordet (1928); Cistellini (1989); Prodi (1995); Russo and del Re (2000). For St. Philip Neri's influence on the arts, see the fundamental studies by Zuccari. See also Strinati and Costamagna (1995) and Turks (1995). For the first Oratorian Church and its decoration see Barbieri, Barchiesi, and Ferrara (1995). On the works of art possessed by Philip and his concept of sacred art, see Barbieri (1995).

2 On the iconography of St. Philip Neri see Melasecchi (1995); Melasecchi and Pepper (1998); Pampalone (2000); Gerken (2004).

3 The main contributions to the debate on figurative arts between the Reformation and Counter-Reformation are by Scavizzi (1981, 1992).

4 Perhaps it is useful to remember that Philip was aware of the negative as well as the positive power of images when he warned his disciples about looking at something too much, giving the following example: "[T]he blessed Father advised his spiritual sons that when he was orating they should not stare at an image or a crucifix obsessively, that could create its own risks to the mind." He felt he had to maintain a careful, balanced attitude toward such revelations: "[H]e said that visions occur but it is important to know how to receive them because it was necessary to be detached and humble." See Cistellini (1994), 161–66.

5 Testimony by Giacomo Crescenzi of 7 July 1598: *Processo*, 2: 207. Cf. Bacci (1837), 10. For Baronio, as for Philip before him, the crucifix inspires tears in the viewer who looks at it attentively: this teaching was immediately understood by his disciples. On this theme, see Zuccari (1995a), 340–54; Zuccari (1995b), 82.

6 *Processo*, 4: 117; my translation.

7 Bacci (1837), 192; my translation. Cf. Emiliani (1985), 2: 228.

8 *Processo*, 1: 64. Cf. the depositions by Angelo Vettori (*Processo*, 1: 152) and Ridolfo Silvestro, the medical doctor according to whom Philip's emotion in front of the Virgin's image was even stronger: "He raised from his bed saying loudly, my blessed Madonna how beautiful you are!" (*Processo*, 4: 95; my translation). See also Gallonio (1600), 207–209, and Incisa della Rocchetta (1972), 90–91.

9 *Processo*, 1: 174.
10 Barbieri (1995), 68.
11 *Processo*, 1: 61. This *pietà* is identified with a "marble Madonna" sent in 1596 by Baronio to the Oratorians of Naples in memory of Philip (1: 61, n. 208). However, this identification does not seem acceptable, because Father Zazzara describes clearly the bas-relief as "our Lord with the bust naked" in the absence of the Virgin in the traditional iconography of the *Vesperbild* such as the *Pietà* by Michelangelo in St. Peter's.
12 *Processo*, 1: 82: "Aveva veduto Cristo dal mezzo in su, che dava loro la benedizione." Indeed, Savonarola's textbooks were not listed in the Index in spite of Pope Paolo IV's aversion to them. The episode is also reported by Ponnelle and Bordet (1928), 74–75, 176–78. The prior was Angelo Cattani da Diacceto, Dominican at S. Marco in Florence and then in Rome, where he twice became prior of the Convent della Minerva, in 1550 and in 1557 (*Processo*, 1: 81, n. 264). He represents an important *trait d'union* between the Florentine years and the Roman period of Philip.
13 *Processo*, 3: 51; my translation.
14 The engravings, based on drawings by Guido Reni, illustrated the second edition of St. Philip's biography, written by the Oratorian Pietro Giacomo Bacci, published in 1625 (1st ed., 1622); see Melasecchi (1995), 45–47; Melasecchi and Pepper (1998), 596–603.
15 Ponnelle and Bordet (1928), 75, n. 2; cf. *Processo*, 1: 184.
16 Barbieri, Barchiesi, and Ferrara (1995), 111–13; Melasecchi (1995), 45.
17 Sight was not the only sense involved in Philip's religious culture. We must at least briefly mention the music that made the Oratory famous in the seventeenth century. In unifying sacred texts and melodious compositions, a delight to the ear, the Oratorians succeeded in attracting an incredible number of faithful who participated in their religious activities. See Morelli (1991).
18 See the milestone chapter on Suger in Panofsky (1955).
19 Scavizzi (1981), 236.
20 Lippomanno (1553), c. 200v, quoted in Scavizzi (1981), 240.
21 Barbieri (1995), 73, n. 55.
22 On the visual power of images as fundamental stimuli to spiritual elevation, from the Greek fathers to the Jesuits, see D. Freedberg (1989), 161–83.
23 *Giardino de Oratione* (Venice, 1563). The book, with St. Philip's inscription and originally in his library, is preserved at the Biblioteca Vallicelliana, Rome, with the signature "S Bor S III 8."
24 On these issues, classical references are Baxandall (1972), ch. 2; Ringbom (1984), 11–30; Gentili (1985), 118–28. See, more recently, Hamburger (2000); Nelson (2000).
25 Venturoli (1988), 46–47. Philip possessed several books by the Ferrarese, as indicated by the inventory of his properties after his death, still preserved in the Archive of the Oratory; see Barbieri (1995), 64.
26 R. Steinberg (1977), 7–9, 47; see also Tadlock (2005), 19.
27 See R. Steinberg (1977), 48 (for the translation of the *Trionfo della Croce*), and Tadlock (2005), 20.
28 In analyzing this belief, Tadlock (2005), 20–21, affirms that, as to emotions, Savonarola maintained that "heaven was a condition rather than a specific place, and this condition could be reached through contemplation." Cf. R. Steinberg (1977), 57.
29 See Barbieri (1995).

30 For Luther and Karlstadt on images see Scavizzi (1981), 43–83, 257.
31 Scavizzi (1992), 192.
32 For recent discussions see Frommel and Wolf (2006).
33 Scavizzi (1981), 278.
34 Scavizzi (1981), 282.
35 Scavizzi (1981), 286.
36 Scavizzi (1981), 56.
37 Scavizzi (1992), 93. See, more recently, Maniura and Sheperd (2006).
38 Scavizzi (1992), 99–100.
39 Cistellini (1989), 2: 292–93; Barbieri (1995), 75; see also Stenhouse (2005). Among the examples passed down by tradition was the so-called Madonna of Saint Luke, the most renowned version of which is the painting on wood kept at S. Maria Maggiore.
40 On Baronius see Jedin (1982); cf. *Dizionario biografico degli italiani* (1964), 470–78; on Baronio and the visual arts see Zuccari (1981), 77–92. See also the following note.
41 Toscano (1985), 409–23; Zuccari (1995b). See, more recently, Tosini (2009).
42 Scavizzi (1992), 135, 232, 279.
43 Scavizzi (1981), 160. At the same time, the well-known "Biblia pauperum" (formulated by St. Gregory the Great) afforded lay and illiterate individuals access to Scripture.
44 Scavizzi (1981), 192.
45 See the discussion on *honesta voluptas* among Erasmus, Luther, Pio, and Catarino in Scavizzi (1981), 159; see also Trinkaus (1970), 105.
46 For *gaudium* see Scavizzi (1981), 159–60.
47 *Processo*, 3: 309; from Oratorian Giovenale Ancina's deposition we learn that the Jesuit Antonio Possevino had frequented the Oratory and Philip since 1576.
48 Cardinal Paleotti had Philip as confessor; he regularly attended the Roman Oratory and dedicated to Philip his book *De bono senectute*, as testified in the *Processo*, 2: 68; 3: 296, 396; see also Ponnelle and Bordet (1928), 354.
49 Paleotti (1582), ch. 20, 212–13.
50 F. Borromeo (1932), 73, 104.
51 Valier (1975), 23.
52 Venturoli (1988), 114–15.
53 *Processo*, 1: 364.
54 Barbieri, Barchiesi, and Ferrara (1995), 52, 139–40, with bibliography.
55 *Processo*, 1: 95.
56 Barbieri (1995), 78.
57 Paleotti (1582), ch. 5, 144.
58 Paleotti (1582), ch. 7, 162: "Non avendo altra mira insomma tutte le sacre immagini ... che di unire gli uomini con Dio, che è il fine della carità; ne segue manifestamente che l'essercizio del formare immagini si ridurrà alla carità, et perciò diverrà virtù dignissima et nobilissima."
59 Zuccari (1984) 14, n. 18; see also Prodi (1962); Jedin and Prodi (1979).
60 Zuccari (1981), 83, analyzed the different approachs to the visual arts of Philip and Ignatius: "These images [from *the Spiritual Exercises*] are not visions but sight, as consecutive steps of a visual narrative" (my translation).
61 As Giuseppe Scavizzi has demonstrated in his fundamental works on this topic (1981, 1992).
62 R. Steinberg (1977), 40–50.
63 Bacci (1837), 87; Barchiesi (1995), 131.

64 R. Steinberg (1977), 47.
65 See Barbieri, Barchiesi, and Ferrara (1995), 22–24, for what the supervisor of the fabbrica said: "Si lascia ogni cosa rustica, che il padre messer Filippo non intende per conto alcuno stuccare, oltre che non ci è il modo, che il legato è già speso tutto." See also Zuccari (1981), 106.
66 C. Borromeo (1577), ch. 34, 112–13.
67 Graeve (1958), 234, and Kummer (1987), 119–21, referred mainly to the Rosary, but Barchiesi (1995), 131, reasonably considered the Rosary one of many sources of inspiration for Philip and his fellow Oratorians. On this topic see also the interesting relationship between the Oratorian sermons and the iconographic program of the Chiesa Nuova shown by Zuccari (1996).
68 Costamagna (1995), 150–73.
69 Barbieri, Barchiesi, and Ferrara (1995), 116–21.
70 Barbieri, Barchiesi, and Ferrara (1995), 122–26.
71 Barbieri, Barchiesi, and Ferrara (1995), 126–31.
72 Barbieri, Barchiesi, and Ferrara (1995), 131–35.
73 Barbieri, Barchiesi, and Ferrara (1995), 136–39.
74 Barbieri, Barchiesi, and Ferrara (1995), 139–42.
75 Barbieri, Barchiesi, and Ferrara (1995), 56–60.
76 Barbieri, Barchiesi, and Ferrara (1995), 60–65.
77 See the document in the Archive of the Congregation of the Oratory, C I 2, p. 10: "In the painting of the Ascension of Our Lord has to be painted the Madonna." See also Barbieri, Barchiesi, and Ferrara (1995), 67.
78 Later replaced by the painting with the same subject by Giovanni Maria Morandi: Barbieri, Barchiesi, and Ferrara (1995), 74.
79 Barbieri, Barchiesi, Ferrara (1995), 80.
80 For a discussion see Barchiesi (1995), 131–34, and Zuccari (1996), 173–93.
81 Zuccari (1981), 111–12; Barbieri, Barchiesi, and Ferrara (1995), 102–104.
82 Bacci (1837), 87.
83 As suggested by Carlo Borromeo (1577), 43.
84 Venturoli (1988), 116–18.
85 On Barocci and the Oratorians, see Emiliani (1985), 2: 217; Ferrari (1995), 111; and Verstegen (2003b), 56–87.
86 Cf. Verstegen (2003b), 64–65; Lingo (2001).
87 Verstegen (2003b), 64–65.
88 Paleotti (1582), 501–502: "Dipoi, che la pittura abbia seco quella maggior chiarezza si può, e dove accada sia distintamente compartita, talmente che chi la riguarda, subito con poca fatica riconosca quello che si vuol rappresentare.... Laonde è grandemente da deplorare l'abuso che corre cosi gagliardamente per l'opere della maggior parte dei pittori, che, intenti solo al magnificare sè stessi e al desiderio della propria eccellenza, pigliano nelle immagini sacre tutte le occasioni che possono di mostrare l'industria e l'artificio loro."
89 Paleotti (1582), 916.
90 R. Steinberg (1977), 45–47.
91 Barbieri, Barchiesi, and Ferrara (1995), 152; Melasecchi (1995), 535–36 (with bibliography); Melasecchi and Pepper (1998), 596–603.
92 Bacci (1837), 87.
93 Barbieri (1995), 74.
94 Venturoli (1988), 110–11.
95 Paleotti (1582), 496–97.

REBUILDING FAITH THROUGH ART

CHRISTOPH SCHWARZ'S *MARY ALTARPIECE* FOR THE JESUIT COLLEGE IN MUNICH

Jeffrey Chipps Smith

IN 1580 WILHELM V, duke of Bavaria (r. 1579–97, d. 1626), commissioned Christoph Schwarz (c. 1548–92) to paint an altarpiece for the aula, or great hall, of the Jesuit college in Munich. The resulting *Mary Altarpiece* (Illustrations 56–58), completed a year later, proved to be the opening artistic salvo in Wilhelm's campaign to transform his capital into a bulwark of the Catholic Reformation. The story of this altarpiece has been largely overlooked, since the duke soon afterward erected and decorated St. Michael's (1583–97; Illustration 59), the first great Jesuit, indeed late Renaissance, church in Germany.[1] On the basis of the success of the *Mary Altarpiece*, Schwarz, a Munich native, became Wilhelm's favorite painter of religious themes.[2] He completed two paintings, including *St. Michael Vanquishing Lucifer* (1587–89) as the high altar, for this Jesuit church, as well as many private devotional pictures for the duke and his wife, Renata of Lorraine. This essay examines the *Mary Altarpiece*, its original setting, its multiple audiences, including a newly established Marian confraternity, and how it and a closely related painting by Schwarz for the Jesuits in Augsburg functioned within the increasingly assertive confessional environment of late-sixteenth-century south Germany.

The Society of Jesus astutely recognized that to strengthen Catholic faith it needed to offer a dynamic religious alternative to Protestantism. The visual appeal of Schwarz's painting, with its rich Venetian-inspired coloration, would be matched by the aural delights of antiphons, notably those by the famed composer Orlando di Lasso, as well as the comforting familiarity of daily masses and recited litanies performed in the college hall. The Jesuits employed art, music, drama, and stirring oratory to appeal to the senses, minds, and hearts of the students, confraternity members, courtiers, and others who worshipped at the college. Unlike Protestants, who stripped most art from their churches, the Jesuits were beginning in the early 1580s to appreciate the affective power of the visual arts. Attracting the eye and ear was a strategy for engaging the individual.

Carefully cultivated personal spiritual formation was linked with communal acts of devotion through the Munich college and its sodalities.

The *Mary Altarpiece* is a triptych, the dominant pre-Reformation format.[3] It measures 1.98 by 1.53 meters when opened. Seated in the heavens on the crescent moon, Mary, Virgin of the Apocalypse (Rev. 12:1, 5), gently supports Jesus as she hands him a rose.[4] Countless angels joyfully serenade mother and son. Four play musical instruments while two others proudly bear the IHS monogram, adopted by the Society of Jesus, just above Mary's head. Careful scrutiny reveals two narrative episodes, the Flight into Egypt and the Massacre of the Innocents in Bethlehem, at the bottom of the painting. The inner wings display St. Catherine of Alexandria, holding the instruments of her martyrdom, and St. Jerome in penance. When closed, the wings depict the Annunciation. Given the theme of the central panel, painted or carved images of God the Father and the Holy Spirit adorned the upper reaches of the now lost original frame.

Before entering Wilhelm V's service as court painter, Schwarz enjoyed a flourishing career in Munich. As an assistant to Hans Mielich, he prepared decorations for Wilhelm and Renata's wedding in 1568 and contributed to the huge high altar, completed in 1572, for the Liebfrauenmünster in Ingolstadt, commissioned by Duke Albrecht V (r. 1550–79), Wilhelm's father.[5] After becoming a master in Munich in 1569, Schwarz traveled to Venice and Padua from 1570 to 1573.[6] Upon his return, he was appointed city painter, and in 1574 he succeeded Mielich as Albrecht's court painter.[7] During the last years of his short career, Schwarz also made paintings for the Fuggers in Augsburg and Emperor Rudolf II in Prague when his activities for Wilhelm permitted.

The Protestant Reformation had a profound impact on religious art in south Germany. Iconoclasm gained strength in many Bavarian and Swabian towns.[8] In 1531, the fifty-two altars in Ulm Münster were stripped of their "offending" decorations; only one altar, retrieved by the donating family, survives.[9] Six years later Protestants destroyed altars in the cathedral and St. Ulrich and Afra Basilica in Augsburg.[10] Towns controlled by the dukes of Bavaria, such as Munich and Ingolstadt, experienced little iconoclasm. Yet even in seemingly staunchly Catholic regions, the threat of iconoclasm as well as serious debates about the appropriateness and use of religious art limited orders for new altarpieces. Between the late 1520s and the decades after the Peace of Augsburg (1555), few noteworthy new painted and/or sculptured altarpieces appeared in south Germany. Albrecht V's high altar for Ingolstadt's Liebfrauenmünster, first contracted in 1560, plus several altars commissioned in Augsburg in the 1560s and 1570s specifically to replace those destroyed in 1537 are the only precedents for Schwarz's *Mary Altarpiece*.[11] The sheer rarity of new altarpieces underscores the significance of Wilhelm V's gift to the Jesuit college.

The Bavarian dukes labored to strengthen Catholicism in Munich.[12] The Peace of Augsburg recognized the existence of Lutheranism, though no

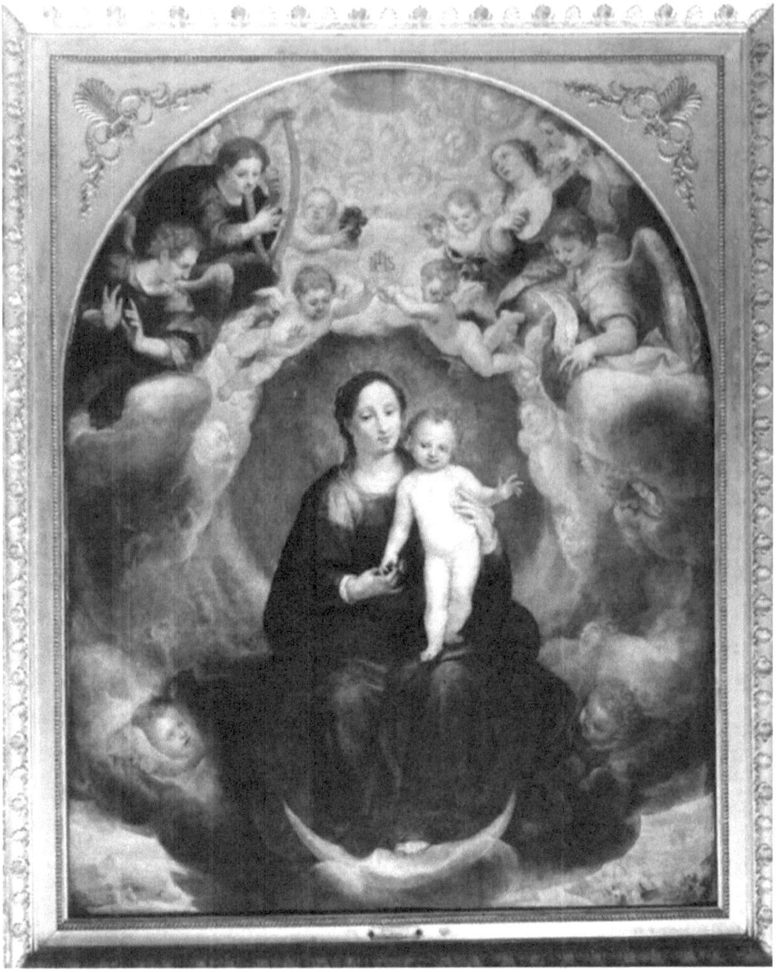

56. Christoph Schwarz, *Mary Altarpiece*, central panel: *Virgin and Child in Glory*, 1580–81. Nuremberg, Germanisches Nationalmuseum. Photo: Germanisches Nationalmuseum, Nuremberg.

other Protestant sects. The principle of "cujus regio, ejus religio" (he who rules a territory determines its religion) empowered authorities to determine local or regional confessional affiliations. Invited by Albrecht V, the first Jesuits arrived in Munich in November 1559 to establish a new school. Although Ignatius of Loyola initially resisted any ties that would restrict members' free movement, he soon made education one of the Society's core missions. Through their free schools, the Jesuits first gained local patronage and social access in many towns. Teaching proved highly effective for shaping the intellectual and spiritual formation of their students, whom they expected to be future lay and church leaders. Furthermore, they worked diligently to earn the support of their students' parents and families.

By December 1559 classes began in four provisional rooms in Munich.[13] The new Jesuit college, the second in Bavaria after Ingolstadt's, was consecrated on 3 March 1560. The enrollment that year reached about three hundred students. In August 1561, the Jesuits consecrated their own school building, erected on part of the garden of the Augustinerkloster adjoining Neuhauser Strasse. Duke Albrecht expanded the school buildings in 1575–76, and the enrollment soon swelled to about six hundred students. As Wilhelm V's plans for a glorious new church began to materialize, he addressed the college's needs. The foundation stone for a new school complex was laid on 10 January 1585. Construction was largely finished in 1590 when the church's tower collapsed on May 10 and damaged the choir. The church and college were not completed until 1597. By then, the enrollment had reached nine hundred students. The Jesuit complex, occupying a plot 140 by 140 meters, is recorded in Johann Smissek's etching (Illustration 59).

57. Christoph Schwarz, *Mary Altarpiece*, inner wings: *St. Catherine of Alexandria and St. Jerome*, 1580–81. Nuremberg, Germanisches Nationalmuseum. Photo: Germanisches Nationalmuseum, Nuremberg.

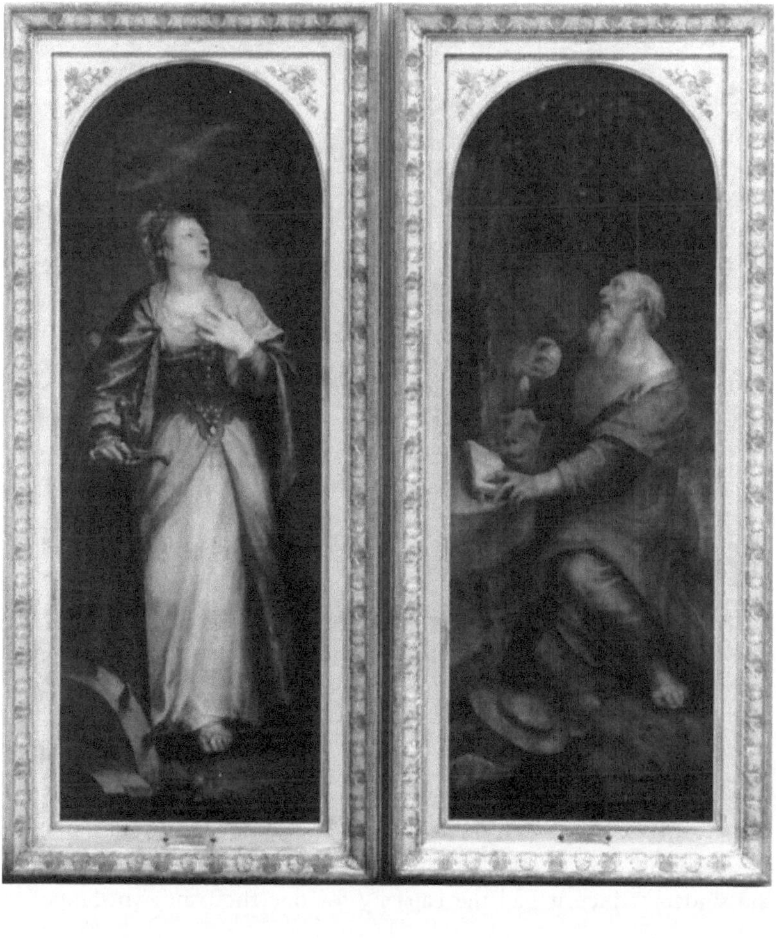

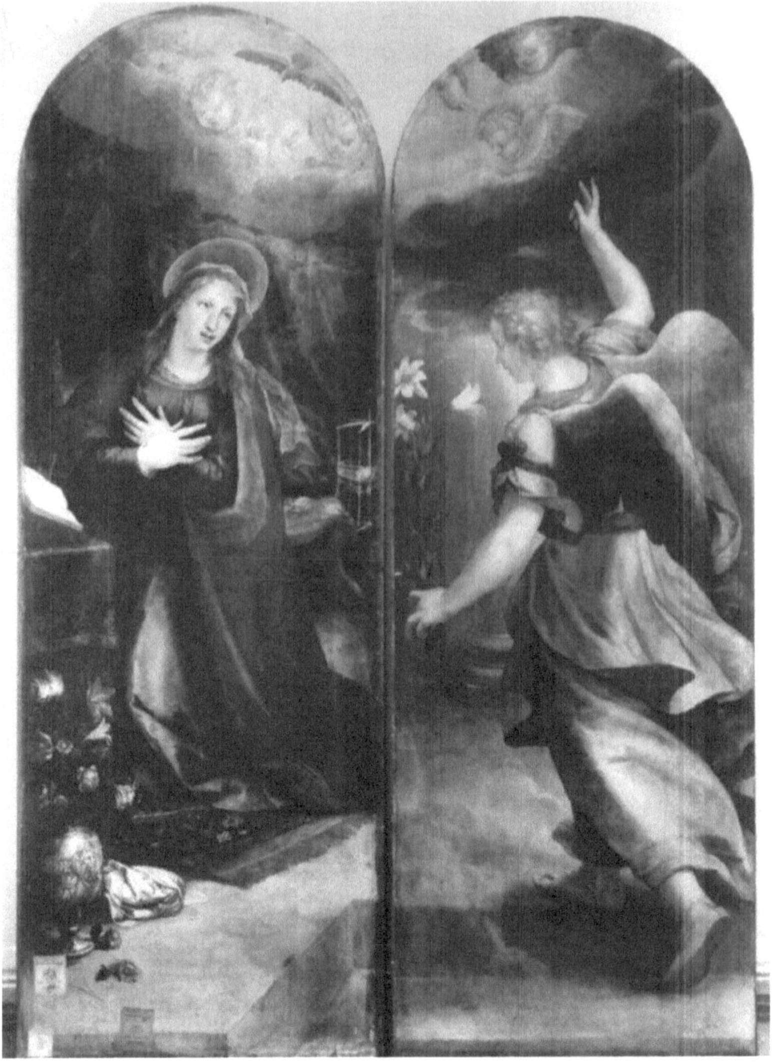

58. Christoph Schwarz, *Mary Altarpiece*, outer wings: *Annunciation*, 1580–81. Nuremberg, Germanisches Nationalmuseum. Photo: Germanisches Nationalmuseum, Nuremberg.

SCHWARZ'S MUNICH ALTARPIECE

Schwarz's *Mary Altarpiece* was designed for the original aula located on the second upper floor of Albrecht V's edifice. This structure was razed in 1592 when Wilhelm decided that St. Michael's needed a grander choir. The aula, measuring 44 by 21 meters, was the largest hall in the college. The room served multiple purposes. Prior to the completion of St. Michael's, the Jesuits and their students had use of a single chapel in the Augustinerkloster across the street. The aula, dedicated to the Assumption of the Virgin, was a better space for holding religious services involving the students, since it had the capacity for one thousand worshippers.[14]

Meetings and other school events, such as academic competitions and some theatrical productions, took place in this great hall. Schwarz's altarpiece also served the members of the Marian sodality, who met in this room until about 1592, when they transferred, along with the painting, to the new aula located in the wing along Neuhauser Strasse just to the left of the church facade in Smissek's print.[15]

The iconography and form of the altarpiece are ideally suited to the audiences and functions of this original hall. The ensemble glorifies the Virgin Mary. She was the subject of extraordinary Jesuit veneration and the patroness of their primary confraternities. Protestant critics decried what they perceived as the undue veneration accorded to Mary.[16] Luther and others honored her as Jesus's mother and as a paragon of humility; however, they rejected Catholic claims to her sanctity, notably her immaculacy and her powers of intercession. Mary's cause was championed by Peter Canisius, the brilliant Dutch Jesuit who more than anyone else was responsible for establishing the Society of Jesus in the German-speaking lands. While he was the provincial of the Order's Upper German Province

59. Johann Smissek, *St. Michael's and the Jesuit College in Munich*, c. 1644–50. Etching. Photo: author.

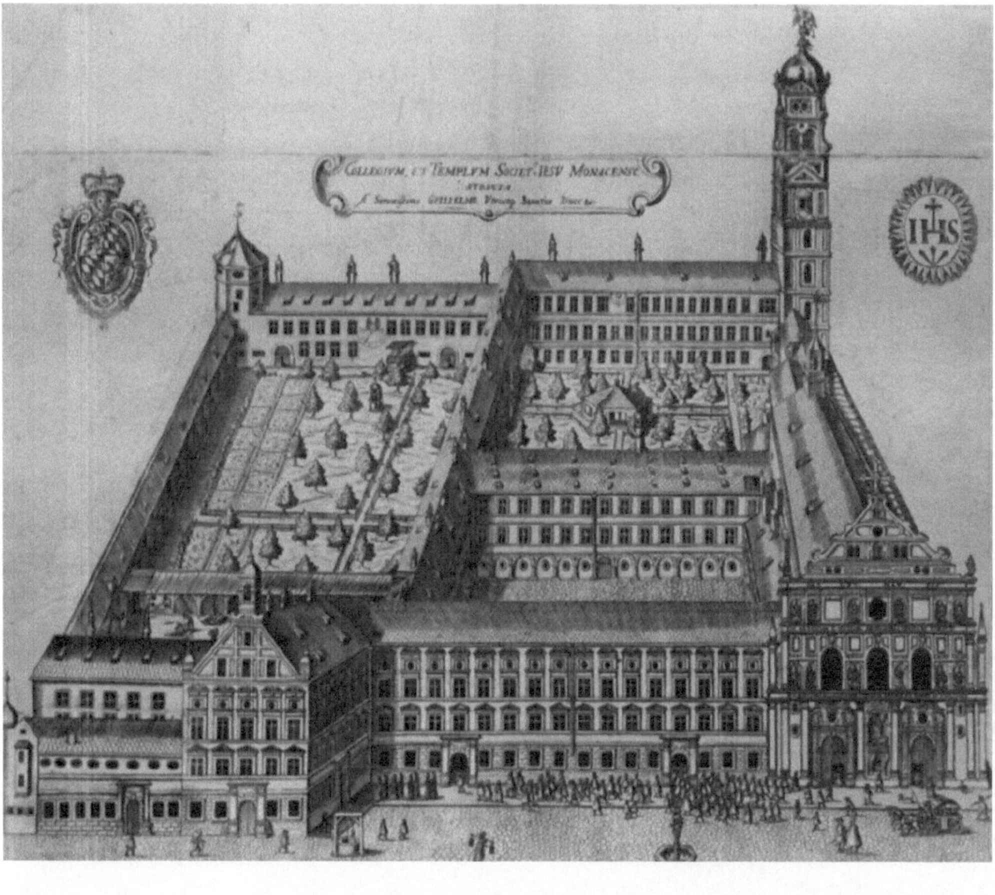

(1556–69), he founded new colleges in Ingolstadt (1556), Munich (1559), Innsbruck (1562), Dillingen (1564), and Würzburg (1567).[17]

Canisius's writing proved exceptionally influential for clerical and lay Catholics. In 1555 he published *Summa Doctrinae Christianae* in Vienna, the first of his catechisms.[18] Subsequent versions targeted young children or, in the case of the *Parvus Catechismus*, or *Small Catechism* (Dillingen, 1558), youths and adults. At the time of Canisius's death in 1597, more than two hundred editions of his catechisms had been printed. By 1615, these were available in twelve languages. In these texts, Canisius clearly explains basic Catholic beliefs and practices. These include how to greet Mary with the full grace of one's heart, how to ask her for help, how to pray the Hail Mary (Gabriel's greeting as recorded in Luke 1:28), which he considered second only to the Our Father in importance, and how to recite other Marian prayers, such as the *Salve Regina* (Hail Holy Queen). Canisius popularized the Litany of Loreto (*Letania Loretana*), which he published in 1558.[19] Using this prayer, the worshipper systematically meditates on Mary's symbolic associations and many roles, such as Queen of Angels. The Jesuits, their students, and their congregations placed this litany at the core of their devotions long before the Roman Church officially adopted it in 1587. At the request of Pope Pius V (r. 1566–72), Canisius wrote *De Maria Virgine Incomparabili* (Ingolstadt, 1577) as a response to Protestant criticisms about the Virgin Mary.[20] The book defending Mary includes thousands of citations of Scripture, patristic writers, and Scholastic authors. Canisius dedicated this volume to Albrecht V, who rewarded the Jesuit father with 50 guldens in 1578. Wilhelm V the Pious, as he was called, and his wife particularly venerated the Virgin Mary and sought her help when the future duke became gravely ill in 1575 and again in 1578. Wilhelm's copy of Canisius's Marian book is today in the Bayerische Staatsbibliothek in Munich.[21] Soon after becoming duke in 1579, he designated Our Lady of Altötting, named for Bavaria's foremost Marian pilgrimage shrine and the site of a famous exorcism performed by Canisius in 1570, as the protectress of Munich and the defender of Catholic faith.

Schwarz's central panel invites the worshipper's devotion. Even though ascendant and surrounded by angels, Mary is approachable and eminently human. The artist places her in the extreme foreground close to the viewer. Mary sits humbly on the clouds. Her attire is far simpler than that of St. Catherine in the adjoining panel. The Virgin's expression conveys tender maternal love and sad resignation. Fully aware of her son's sacrificial fate, Mary hands Christ a red rose, symbolizing his Passion.[22] The Litany of Loreto lauds Mary as the "mystical rose," while other texts refer to her as the "rose without thorns."[23] Mary is normally associated with white roses signifying her purity, though her co-passion and compassion link her with her son. Schwarz's Christ Child appears beguilingly innocent as he looks curiously past the worshipper. Mary and Jesus possess faint halos, though it is really the backdrop of the rich blue sky that frames the couple. Rather than the traditional heavenly crown, the two angels above Mary's head bear the flaming disk with the IHS monogram. This expresses the Society of Jesus's special veneration of the Virgin Mary as well as her reciprocal guardianship. In addition to playing various musical instruments, the large angel at the right holds a musical score on which is written "Regina coeli" in clear letters. This refers to the *Regina caeli [coeli] laetare*, or *Rejoice, Queen of Heaven*, that grew in popularity from the end of the twelfth century.[24] This is one of four Marian antiphons normally sung at the end of the office of Compline or sometimes Vespers if Compline was not celebrated. In Dante's *Paradiso* (canto 23:121–29), Gabriel and the saints chant this song as Mary ascends to the upper reaches of heaven, much as Schwarz's angels do in this picture.[25] The angels, just like the students and sodalitists worshipping in the Munich aula, joyously serenade the Virgin and Child.

Schwarz situates this apparition of the Virgin and Child above the Holy Land. Diminutive scenes of the Flight into Egypt and the Massacre of the Innocents are staged below. The Holy Family flees from Bethlehem, where Herod's soldiers slay all firstborn infant sons.[26] While these narrative episodes offer multiple possible devotional interpretations to the observant viewer, Schwarz uses them as geographic bridges to the side panels. Joseph, Mary, and their son head toward Egypt, the future home of St. Catherine of Alexandria, who in the early fourth century accepted martyrdom rather than renounce her Christian faith. On the opposite wing kneels St. Jerome, who from 386 until his death in 420, dwelled in Bethlehem.

Catherine and Jerome, venerated as the patron saints of scholars and learning, were well chosen for this Jesuit college context. Their body language expresses, respectively, rapture and intense religious fervor. Catherine offers a model of steadfast faith as she piously stares heavenward with her left hand placed on her heart. Almost casually she holds a sword, the final instrument of her martyrdom, while the broken death wheel rests by her feet. Jerome gazes intensely at the simple wooden crucifix. Although seated, his twisting body expresses his spiritual agitation. His left hand marks a biblical passage while he prepares to beat his chest in penance with the rock held firmly in his right hand. Jerome, wearing cardinal's attire, provides an exemplum of a life questing for spiritual betterment in the service of the Church. In Hans Mielich's Ingolstadt altarpiece, partially painted by Schwarz, the front side celebrates the life of the Virgin Mary. The elaborate reverse, fully visible from the ambulatory, honors St. Catherine. According to legend, the noble and highly educated Catherine rebuffed Emperor Maxentius's demand that she worship pagan idols.[27] As shown by Mielich, Maxentius assembled fifty learned men to dispute with her; however, her wise arguments converted most to Christianity, for which they suffered immediate martyrdom. The subject is especially relevant, since the Liebfrauenmünster served as the university church, and the altarpiece commemorates the centennial of the university's consecration in 1472. Mielich inserted faculty portraits among Catherine's questioners. The four Latin church fathers, including St. Jerome, adorn the predella. In the Munich and Ingolstadt pictures, Catherine embodies knowledge and rhetoric used in defense of one's faith, a message resonating in both academic communities.[28] The same points were conveyed in the St. Catherine play staged by the Jesuits and more than two hundred student actors in Innsbruck in 1577.[29]

Schwarz's St. Jerome (340/42–420) is an ascetic, a church leader who retreats in solitude to grapple with his faith and human weaknesses.[30] He is typically shown as a hermit in the wilderness or in a room writing. A prolific author, who translated the Bible into Latin, Jerome was the prototype for the Christian humanist in the early Renaissance. Prior to 1589, Ingolstadt's Jesuits and their students worshipped in the Hieronymuskapelle at their college. Duke Wilhelm commissioned Schwarz to paint a now lost *St. Jerome* (1581) for this chapel's main altar.[31]

When the wings are closed, Mary turns from her reading to attend to Gabriel's salutation. The Annunciation, signaling the inception of Christ and the Christian Church, was long popular on the outside of pre-Reformation altarpieces.[32] It represents the opening scene of a story whose later chapters are recounted within the altarpiece. The importance of Gabriel's message is presented brilliantly by Schwarz. As he sweeps in from the right, his forward motion suddenly halts in midstride. Gabriel, rather theatrically, offers the lilies held in his extended left hand. Gesturing toward the apparition of the Holy Spirit and angels, he reveals that he is God's messenger. Mary, in turn, humbly crosses her arms while inclining her body toward Gabriel. Schwarz's staging, with its actors and dramatic lighting, is visually alluring. One senses that a compelling story is commencing. In addition to its thematic aptness in Schwarz's painting, the choice of subject refers as well to the academic sodality of Mary of the Annunciation, which, since its founding in 1578, met in the Munich aula.

MUNICH'S MARIAN CONFRATERNITY

The original audience for the *Mary Altarpiece* consisted primarily of the Jesuits, their students, members of the Marian sodality, and important visitors. Let us briefly consider the creation and goals of the Jesuits' first confraternity in Munich, since these contextualize Schwarz's painting.[33] In 1563, Jean Leunis, a young Belgian Jesuit in Rome, fretted over the bad influences that his students encountered outside of class. He organized a group of students who prayed and read pious texts together after school and on weekends.[34] Gradually, the students participated in daily meditations and masses, weekly confessions, and monthly communions. They served the poor and sick, and during Holy Week performed penitential activities, such as carrying crosses. Leunis placed this informal sodality under the Virgin's protection. While religious congregations were hardly new – indeed, Ignatius of Loyola belonged to two and helped sponsor others – the Society of Jesus had been slow to establish its own for fear of limiting the mobility of its own membership.[35] Most Catholic brotherhoods were tied to a particular parish, economic group, or form of devotion, such as the Dominicans' rosary confraternities. Leunis, Franciscus (Frans) Coster, Canisius, and other Jesuits who shaped the emerging Marian congregations sought "to support and promote a more deeply interiorized ethical and religious life."[36] These men looked upon the Virgin Mary as the ideal patroness, the humble maiden chosen by God to bear Jesus; she experienced the joys and sorrows of motherhood, including her co-passion and compassion; and she reigns as the Queen of Heaven and humanity's foremost intercessor. Their veneration of Mary, while deeply rooted in pre-Reformation devotions, signaled one way the Jesuits and other Catholics distinguished their religious beliefs and practices from those of the Protestants.

One congregation soon became many. Leunis's initial protector was Cardinal Otto Truchsess von Waldburg, bishop of Augsburg. With the cardinal's encouragement, Jakob Rem established the first German Marian congregation in Dillingen in 1574. Franciscus Coster, like Rem an alumnus of the Roman sodality, founded other chapters, first in Douai in 1572 and, two years later, in Cologne. Oswald Redling initiated a new student sodality in Fulda around 1574.[37] Pope Gregory XIII formally approved of the sodality of the Blessed Virgin in 1577, the same year that Canisius started a fourth German brotherhood in Ingolstadt and others arose in Mainz and Würzburg. The year 1578 saw new congregations in Munich, Innsbruck, Hall in Tirol, Lucerne, Speyer, and Heiligenstadt. Dozens more soon followed.

As the number of congregations grew, so did the variations in their practices. Claudio Aquaviva, the Society's superior general from 1581 to 1615, moved to institutionalize the congregations. The Virgin Mary, patroness of the original Roman congregation (*congregatio primaria*), assumed an identical role for all of the other early Jesuit sodalities.[38] These were known as the congregations of Mary of the Annunciation, named for S. Maria Annunziata, the Society's first church in Rome, which was destroyed in 1626 to permit the building of S. Ignazio. As confirmed in Gregory XIII's bull (*Omnipotentis Dei*) of 5 December 1584, all existing and future Jesuit congregations were linked with the mother congregation in the Collegio Romano in Rome.

These brotherhoods were bound by common statutes based on Coster's *Libellus Sodalitatis*, first published in Cologne in 1576.[39] This text is a fascinating mix of practical rules (frequent confessions and how to listen to daily masses) and devotionals. It offers a method for stabilizing the heart, remedies against vices, preparations for death, explanations of Catholic ceremonies, and an elucidation of the Annunciation. The unillustrated book closes with more than one hundred pages of Marian hymns and meditations. To Coster, a congregation's main mission was the "restoration in all her glory of the Mother of God at the head of cities."[40] He voiced hope for a universal Marian sodality that would be an integral part of a universal Christian republic.[41] Later in the 1580s, Coster authored several other Marian devotional books for Jesuit sodalists and students.[42]

According to the *Libellus Sodalitatis*, new members recited the following vow to the Virgin Mary:

> Holy Mary Mother of God and Virgin, I ... choose you today for Lady and Mistress, Patron and Advocate, and I order and propose with all my heart, never to forsake you, and never so to say or do that by my deeds anything should be done against your honor; I beseech you therefore most lovingly that it should please you to receive me as your perpetual servant to assist me in all my actions, and not to abandon me at the hour of death. So be it.[43]

In 1582 Maximilian I (r. 1597–1651), Duke Wilhelm's son and heir, and two other nobles joined the Munich confraternity. According to one account, the young men physically expressed their piety by kneeling before the altar of the Virgin Mary, which by then was adorned with Schwarz's painting.[44] As Wilhelm, his courtiers, and the sodalists watched, they first recited their creed and then a series of pledges to Mary. The 1584 membership roster lists eighty students, thirty-two clergy led by the papal legate, and twenty-six laymen headed by Wilhelm V.[45]

Hieronymus Wierix's *Rosary of the Virgin* (Illustration 60), created for Marian congregation members (Sodalibus D.V. Mariae), though not specifically for the Munich brotherhood, reflects devotional practices common to these Jesuit groups.[46] The central image celebrates the Annunciation, which is framed by a giant rosary. Descending angels distribute rosaries to the members, who will use these when reciting the *Fifteen Mysteries of the Rosary* printed at the top of the engraving. The text includes the Litany of Loreto in the side panels and a prayer to Mary below. The Jesuits recognized that communal prayer, including the auditory sensation of reciting and hearing others recite popular devotions, bolstered individual and collective Catholic identity. The familiarity that comes with repetition can impart a sense of spiritual well-being and unity with the divine, goals central to Ignatius of Loyola's *Spiritual Exercises*.[47]

The Munich aula was the site of various devotional celebrations. Confraternity members attended daily mass and recited prayers every morning and evening.[48] Weekly meetings began with prayers and hymns. The members celebrated confession and communion at least once a month as well as on feast days. A partial description of how this hall was used during Holy Week in 1580 survives.[49] On Maundy Thursday the windows and walls of Munich's congregational hall were hung with black cloth that blocked out all daylight. Before the room's single altar stood a temporary sculpted (?) and painted scene showing Christ on the Mount of Olives just as the angel hands him the chalice. At about 5 P.M., Orlando di Lasso (Orlandus Lassus), Wilhelm's chapel master, and the court chapel performed the composer's *Penitential Psalms*. Then Ferdinand Alber, the Jesuit *praese* (or adviser) of the sodality, delivered a sermon to close the day's service. On Good Friday the aula was filled with burning candles, many set on the wall. Replacing Thursday's scene was an image of Jesus lying in the holy grave, above which were mounted statues of praying angels. Dolorous music was performed during the different liturgical hours. Paul Hoffaeus, Canisius's successor as the provincial of the Upper German Province (1567–81), and Alber expounded on Christ's bitter Passion and death. At these events, one's senses were fully engaged by the art, the music, the ritual, and even the texture and taste of the communion wafer. By these means, the Jesuits heightened the affective potential of the moment. The sodality members and other attendees, including Wilhelm and Renata, wore mourning clothes. That Friday, Munich's clocks were stopped, no wagons were permitted on the streets, and everything was still throughout the city. A procession, which included the duke, duchess, courtiers, and sodalitists, paraded somberly through the streets, stopping at the holy graves in local churches.

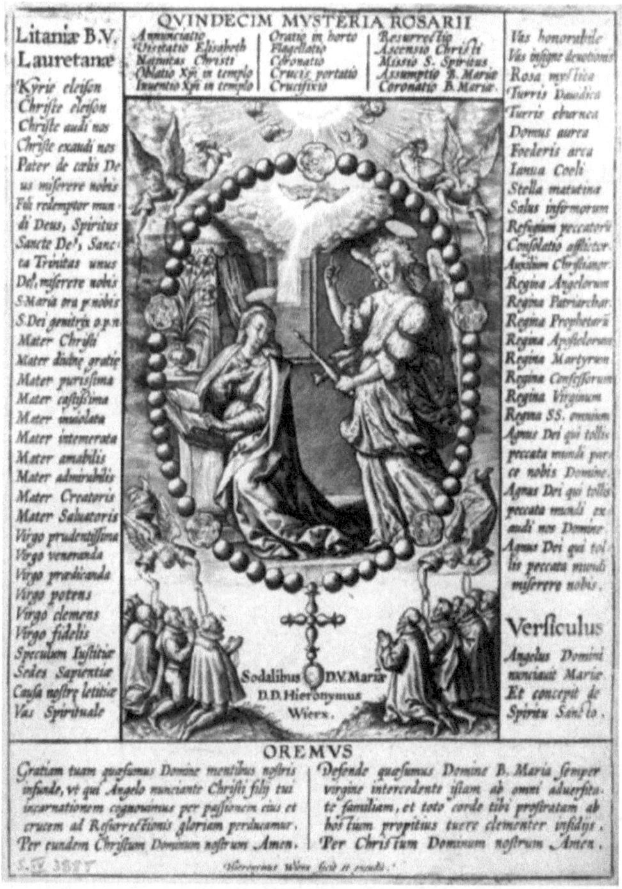

60. Hieronymus Wierix, *Rosary of the Virgin*, before 1595. Engraving. Photo: author.

Students and confraternity members sometimes staged plays in the aula. Best known are the elaborate productions such as *Constantinus* of 1574 and *Esther* of 1577. These involved hundreds of actors and were enacted in public settings, including the Marienplatz for the 1577 play. The college's aula was more suitable for simpler plays, rhetorical competitions, and other communal activities. The purpose of the plays was to instill virtue in the actors and audience alike. One contemporary Jesuit writes, "We shall continue to labor at it, even in the face of difficulties, as long as it will help to expel wickedness, increase piety, inflame a love of virtue, and afford becoming amusements."[50] Such plays, like Schwarz's altarpiece and the Marian sodalities, were tools deftly wielded by the Society of Jesus as it sought to build individual spiritual formation and communal Catholic identity.

ORLANDO DI LASSO AND MARIAN MUSIC IN MUNICH

The angels in the *Mary Altarpiece* laud the Virgin much as the students and sodalists would. The members of the congregation sang the Litany of Loreto, Marian hymns, and other songs during their daily gatherings and religious services in the aula.[51] The score of the *Regina caeli [coeli] laetare* held by the singing angel at right, can be linked with almost any Catholic group venerating the Virgin. Yet this is the only one of Schwarz's many Marian paintings to contain written music. Its inclusion suggests a more specific association with the Bavarian court and this Jesuit college. Does the score's insertion refer to the compositions of Orlando di Lasso, who served as court chapel master under both Albrecht V and Wilhelm from 1563 until his death in 1594?[52] In 1577, he composed his musical accompaniment for the antiphon. The text reads:

Regina caeli laetare, alleluia
Quia quem meruisti portare, alleluia
Resurrexit sicut dixit, alleluia.
Ora pro nobis Deum, alleluia.[53]

(Queen of Heaven, rejoice, alleluia,
for He whom you were worthy to bear, alleluia,
has risen as He said, alleluia.
Pray for us to God, alleluia.)

Lasso already enjoyed an especially close relationship with Wilhelm as early as 1567. He prepared the elaborate music for the young prince's wedding to Renata of Lorraine on 22 February 1568. Three years later the men reached an accord specifying that Lasso would work primarily for Wilhelm. In 1577, he dedicated two motets to the crown prince.

Lasso presented him with an elaborate choir book containing the magnificat *Quando lieta sperai* on 22 December 1580.[54] Although the edicts of the Council of Trent, which concluded in 1563, said little about liturgical music, a concerted effort was made to standardize the Divine Office throughout the Catholic Church.[55] Specifically, a reformed Roman Breviary (1568) and Missal (1570) were published. Their practices were obligatory; however, strict observance was still being called for when Pope Sixtus V established the Congregation of Rites in 1588. Early in his reign, Wilhelm embraced the new Roman Breviary, or Tridentine Rite, which in 1580–81 replaced the calendar, or Rite of Freising, that had been used in Munich's churches. This liturgical reform stressed the need to make musical texts clearly intelligible, which could be a challenge in polyphony; it meant considerable work for the composer. The duke commissioned Lasso's *Hymnarium*, which was completed in late September 1581. Between 1580 and 1583, Lasso wrote nine Marian antiphon settings, most of which presumably were performed in the Jesuit aula. The *Regina caeli [coeli] laetare* was performed from Holy Saturday, the day before Easter, until the feast of Holy Trinity, which occurred eight weeks after Easter and one week after Pentecost.[56] The Jesuits recognized the power of music to stimulate devotional memory. Tunes and lyrics, when repeated over and over, lodge firmly in one's mind and heart. These can be recalled as desired, whether to strengthen one's religious ardor or to console oneself in moments of difficulty.

Schwarz's Munich aula altarpiece, Lasso's compositions, the new college sodality, and Wilhelm's patronage in the early 1580s manifest the intense Marian devotions promoted by the Jesuits and the Bavarian court. Lasso accompanied the duke on pilgrimages to Mary's shrines at Altötting in 1581 and Loreto in 1585. The Jesuits actively encouraged pilgrimages to the Virgin's home, which legend holds had been physically transported by angels from Nazareth to Dalmatia and finally to Loreto, on the Adriatic coast of Italy, when threatened by Saracens and later Turks.[57] Lasso set the Litany of Loreto to music at least twelve times.[58] In 1619, Rudolph di Lasso writes about his father's devotion to the Virgin Mary: "The extent of the love that my father, Orlandus Lassus of blessed memory, bore toward the Virgin Mother of God may be gathered from the fact that he embellished with such great variety of voices and harmonies – more, in fact, than anyone else, that divine hymn commonly known as the Magnificat, in which the Most Holy Virgin sang the praises of god and gave thanks for all his blessings; so that it seemed that he wanted to pour out all his musical art (in which he was second to none) upon the praises of this one Lady."[59]

As the Jesuits' presence grew in Munich under the sponsorship of the duke, Lasso developed close ties with their college and church.[60] Writing in 1727, Ignatius Agricola claims that Lasso performed at the obsequy of Bartholo Portia, the first Jesuit to die in Munich, in 1578.[61] The service, attended by the sodalitists, was held in the aula. In 1580 Lasso and his wife,

Regina Wäckinger, donated 70 guldens, the equivalent of a quarter of his annual salary, to the college.[62] This grant signals their admiration for the Jesuits and their missions even if we cannot be certain about their precise intentions. Were they encouraging music at the college or promoting the activities of the sodality? At Wilhelm's request, Lasso composed music for the college on several occasions, most notably for the church's initial inauguration in 1591, as well as for some Jesuit dramas.[63] Thirty-four of his scores were transferred from the court to the fledgling music collection of St. Michael's. These include music for masses, prayers and devotions, penitential psalms, and the Marian Litany of Loreto. Although Lasso never seems to have taught at the college, eight members of his *Hofkapelle* did. At the very least, the score held by Schwarz's singing angel reminded contemporaries of the marvelous Marian music then being written for the Bavarian court and the college by one of Europe's foremost composers.[64]

SCHWARZ AND THE JESUITS

The *Mary Altarpiece* proved visually alluring and devotionally appealing. If this was a test to see whether Schwarz could create a compelling image in a land with few recent pictorial precedents, then the Munich painter succeeded. Within the next few years, Schwarz painted at least four other altarpieces for the Jesuits in south Germany. These include Duke Wilhelm's commissions for the Hieronymuskapelle (1581) in Ingolstadt and, for St. Michael's in Munich, the monumental *St. Michael Vanquishing Lucifer* for the high altar and, assisted by Alessandro Scalzi (Paduano), the *Martyrdom of St. Andrew*, executed between 1586 and 1589/90.[65]

In about 1584, the artist painted a larger (3.53 × 2.08 m) *Mary Altarpiece* (Illustration 61) for the new Jesuit church of St. Salvator in Augsburg.[66] The Fugger family and Duke Wilhelm funded the construction of the Augsburg church and college between 1581 and 1584.[67] Schwarz's picture adorned the side altar dedicated to the Virgin Mary. The patron is unknown, though he may have been Octavian Secundus Fugger, who was one of the church's primary supporters.[68] Also in 1585, he paid Schwarz for a design for a separate painting intended for his house chapel on the Weinmarkt.[69] As a young man, Fugger was greatly influenced by Peter Canisius, who served as Augsburg cathedral's preacher from 1559 to 1566. With Canisius's encouragement, he studied at the College Germanicum in Rome. Thus, it is not surprising to discover that Fugger acquired, presumably for the Augsburg college's use, three hundred copies of Canisius's *Catechism* in 1591 and that, eight years later, he commissioned an engraved portrait of the Jesuit father (and future saint), who died in 1597, by Dominicus Custos of Augsburg.[70]

Schwarz's Munich and Augsburg pictures treat the same basic theme; however, the latter's composition is more expansive. By pushing Mary and the Christ Child back into the near middle ground, he provides room for more angels, including the lively quartet dancing blissfully in midair just beneath Mary's feet, and additional instrumentalists. Schwarz arranges God the Father, the Holy Spirit, and four angels supporting the Jesuit's form of the IHS monogram on the central axis. We share this apparition of the Apocalyptic Woman with St. John the Evangelist, the diminutive figure seated below in the peaceful verdant field. Visionary scenes located above a deep ribbon of landscape can be found in pre-Reformation German art.[71] Schwarz encountered further examples by Titian, with whom he may have worked, Lorenzo Lotto, and Paolo Veronese in Venice. Rarely is the setting identifiable. Schwarz, however, portrays the skyline of Augsburg from the southwest. This presents Mary as the city's guardian patron, a role she also played in Wilhelm V's Munich. The artist most likely knew the Monogrammist A.C.'s engraving (Illustration 62) depicting the Virgin and Child in the sky above a very detailed prospect of Augsburg from the east.[72] They are accompanied by Ulrich, Afra, Simpertus, and other locally venerated saints and, higher up, God, the Holy Spirit, and angelic hosts. Since 1555, Augsburg had been officially a biconfessional city, a legal fact that did not necessarily defuse the remonstrations between Catholics and Lutherans. This print, perhaps more militantly than Schwarz's painting, proclaims Augsburg's long Catholic history, one that extends back to St. Afra, who was martyred there in about 304. Schwarz or his patron apparently liked this formula, since he and Peter Candid included an even more detailed view of Augsburg in their later *Enthroned Virgin and Child with Sts. Benedict and Francis* done for Octavian Secundus Fugger.[73]

Mary and Christ now look directly at the viewer/worshipper in the St. Salvator painting. The Virgin's attire is again simple, especially when contrasted with the jeweled diadems and sumptuous fabrics of the larger angels. Christ holds two red roses in his right hand while his raises his left in blessing. The four primary angels gaze more clearly on Christ than on Mary. This shift in emphasis, however slight, may reflect the Augsburg church's dedication to the Holy Savior as well as a conscious response to standard Protestant complaints about Christ's displacement by Mary in Catholic devotions. Canisius once sought to disarm this criticism by remarking, "When we venerate Mary as the Mother of God, we honor the whole Trinity."[74] Schwarz's picture reassures Augsburg's Catholics of their spiritual bond with the Holy Trinity and the Virgin Mary.

The success of Schwarz's paintings for the Jesuit communities in Munich and Augsburg can be judged in three ways. First, after several decades in which scarcely any major works of art were created for Catholics in south Germany, these altarpieces stand as important reaffirmations of the potent role of religious art. Between the 1580s and the 1630s, before Swedish and Protestant troops occupied the region, churches in Munich, Augsburg, Ingolstadt, and other Catholic strongholds were sumptuously adorned with new art. Second, Schwarz's altarpiece for the Munich aula long continued

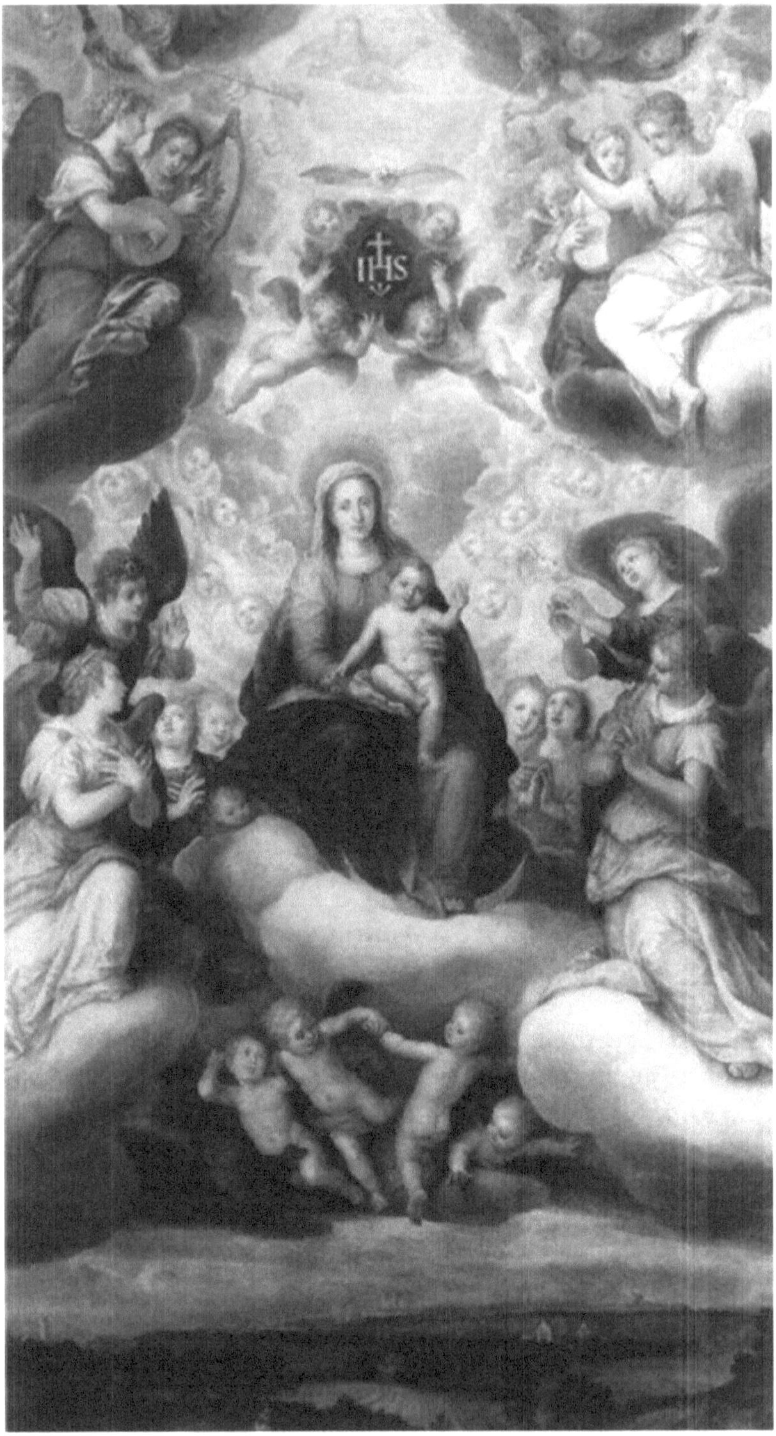

61. Christoph Schwarz, *Mary Altarpiece* (*Virgin and Child in Glory with a View of Augsburg*), c. 1584. Munich, Bayerische Staatsgemäldegalerie. Photo: Bayerische Staatsgemäldegalerie, Munich.

to address the devotional needs of the Jesuits, their students, and their Marian sodality members. Schwarz's *Mary Altarpiece* in St. Salvator functioned in much the same way. I have not located evidence about whether the original Augsburg student sodality, founded in 1589, prayed regularly at this altar; however, the Jesuits' Herren Bürger-Kongregation, or citizens' congregation, dedicated to the Assumption of the Virgin and established in 1613, worshipped there for many years.[75] This sodality grew quickly to 150 members. At its peak, it claimed 7,000 members and its own congregation hall down the street from the Jesuit church.

Finally, three later commentators extolled Schwarz's Marian paintings. Hippolytus Guarinonius, a former Jesuit pupil and medical doctor for the Damenstift in Hall in Tirol, touted the moral lessons to be gained from looking at Schwarz's altarpieces rather than at opulent and frivolous art.[76] In 1643, the famous Jesuit neo-Latin poet Jacob Balde composed a fourteen-strophe ode about the *Mary Altarpiece*, "the celebrated artifice by Schwarz's hand," which, as the *praese* of the college's main sodality from 1637, he often contemplated in the Munich aula. He lauds Mary's modest countenance, her humble attire, and her maternal love.[77] Writing in his *Teutsche Academie* (1675), Joachim von Sandrart praises this painting, which he saw in the great hall of the college, as exemplifying the very best of

62. Monogrammist A.C., *View of Augsburg from the East*, c. 1566. Engraving. After Schmidt (2000), fig. 32. Photo: author.

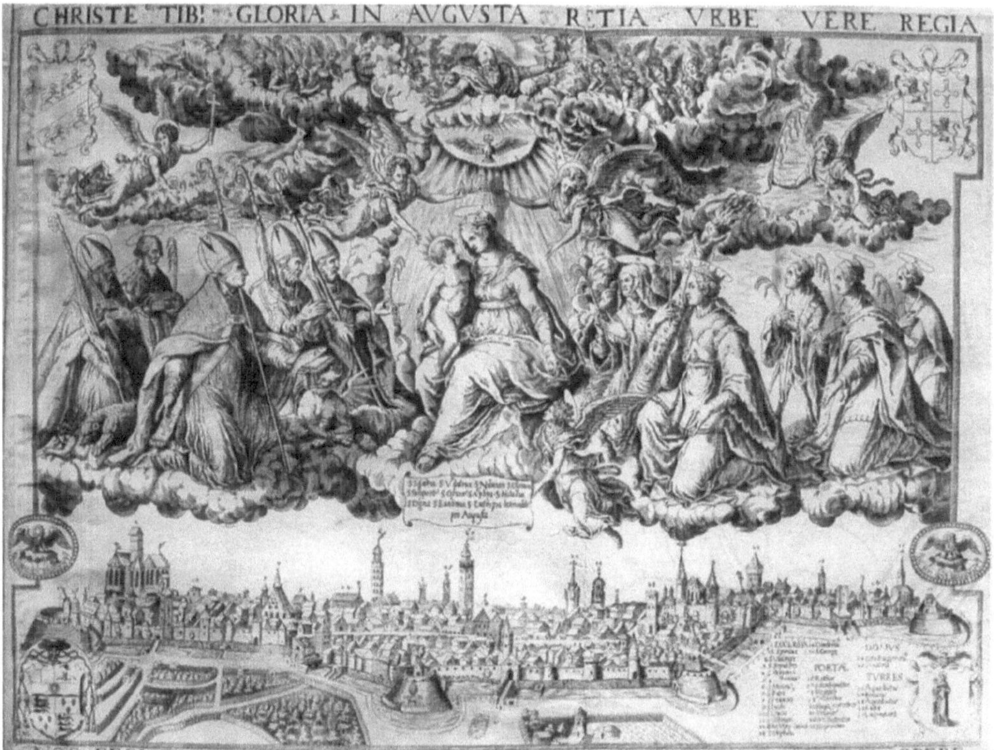

Schwarz's art. He stresses the painter's talent as a colorist and the beauty of his portrayal of Mary.[78]

Duke Wilhelm and the Jesuits discovered in Christoph Schwarz a highly skilled painter capable of devising exquisite, indeed poetry-inspiring, pictures promoting the veneration of the Virgin Mary and Catholic faith. Schwarz successfully combined a highly sophisticated modern style, one melding sensuous coloration and affective figures with a requisite clarity of design. He fully understood how the *Mary Altarpiece* would visually and thematically foster the diverse activities being performed in the great aula of the Munich college.

Notes

I wish to acknowledge the generous assistance of Alexander Fisher (University of British Columbia), Daniel Hess (Germanisches Nationalmuseum), and Susan Maxwell (University of Wisconsin, Oshkosh). The altarpiece remained in the college until 1804. It belongs to the Bayerische Staatsgemäldesammlungen, Munich, inv. nos. 88–90, and is on loan to the Germanisches Nationalmuseum in Nuremberg, inv. nos. 900–902. Heinrich Geissler, "Christoph Schwarz, ca. 1548–1592," unpubl. diss., Albert-Ludwig-Universität (Freiburg im Breisgau, 1960), 31, 58–59, 179, 322, cat. no. G I, 17, and doc. no. 17; Hubert Glaser, ed., *Wittelsbach und Bayern. Um Glauben und Reich: Kurfürst Maximilian I*, exh. cat., Munich, Residenz (Munich, 1980), II/2, no. 71 (text Peter Diemer); Kurt Löcher and Carola Gries, *Germanisches Nationalmuseum Nürnberg: Die Gemälde des 16. Jahrhunderts* (Stuttgart, 1997), 465–69; Freya Strecker, *Augsburger Altäre zwischen Reformation (1537) und 1635* (Münster, 1998), 299–301, 306; Katharina Krause, ed. *Geschichte der bildenden Kunst in Deutschland*, vol. 4: *Spätgotik und Renaissance* (Munich, 2007), no. 185 (text Esther Meier); Daniel Hess and Dagmar Hirschfelder, eds. *Renaissance, Barock, Aufklärung: Kunst und Kultur vom 16. bis zum 18. Jahrhundert* [Germanisches Nationalmuseum] (Nuremberg, 2010), 298–89, cat. no. 234.

1 On St. Michael's, see J. Smith (2002), 57–101 (with earlier literature); Nising (2004), 211–14; Sauter (2004), 124–30.

2 Geissler (1960), 28–37; Geissler (n.d.).

3 Rasmussen (1974); Laun (1982), 47–52; on winged altars, 1520–1600.

4 On this theme and its connection with the Immaculate Conception, see J. Smith (2006), 62–66.

5 J. Smith (1994), 123–25; Wimböck (1998).

6 Meijer (1999).

7 Vignau-Wilberg (2005), nos. A3, A12, D4–14, D25, E2, G2.

8 J. Smith (1994), 31–45.

9 Tüchle (1977), 126–82, esp. 127 ff.

10 Rasmussen (1980–81), 3: 95–114.

11 Strecker (1998), 363–66.

12 J. Smith (2008).

13 Schade (1960), 209–57; Nising (2004), 207–22, for a chronology of the Jesuit complex.

14 Strecker (1998), 300, cites Lipowsky (1819), 1: 166 on the room's dedication.

15 Daniel Papebroch provided a detailed description of his visit to the Jesuit church and college in Munich on 27 September 1660. By then, there were

several sodalities, not all of which met in the same hall. He remarks that the major Latin Marian sodality assembled in a room 50 by 25 feet (*Fuß*) on the third floor of the building along Neuhausser Strasse. The room was finely decorated with paintings, including pictures of the seven Marian feasts. Kindermann (2002), 229–30.

16 Heming (2003), 33, 66–74; Heal (2007), 64–115.

17 Duhr (1907–28), 1: 66–91; Brodrick (1935); Diez (1987); Oswald and Rummel (1996).

18 J. Smith (2002), 17–23.

19 Paulus (1902); Beissel (1910), 475–93; Bagley (1967), 7: 790–91; J. Smith (2002), 145–51.

20 Canisius (1933); Donnelly (1981), 149–50; Haub (1996), esp. 159–61; Baumstark (1997), esp. 41–54, 499–563.

21 Munich, Bayerische Staatsbibliothek, Rar. 167. The title page includes the Annunciation.

22 Jakob Sprenger, founder of the first rosary confraternity in Cologne in 1475, writes, "[A]fter ten white roses, insert a red rose, by which is meant a Paternoster. And at the same time meditate on the rose-red blood of Christ Jesus, that God, Our Father, wished to be shed on our behalf." Winston-Allen (1997), 68.

23 J. Smith (2002), 145.

24 Julian (1957), 2: 954.

25 Warner (1976), 169, 171; also 103–17 on the subject of Mary, Queen of Heaven.

26 The inscription on Johannes Sadeler I's engraving after Schwarz's *Rest on the Flight* urges Mary to protect "our salvation" by fleeing so that she can later return him to us. Hollstein (1949–), 21–22, no. 302.

27 Voragine (1969), 708–16; Wimböck (1998), 81–86.

28 Wilhelm V donated some of St. Catherine's relics to St. Michael's in Munich. In the *Trophaea Bavarica*, the commemorative book accompanying the church's 1597 consecration, St. Catherine is mentioned several times, including in an epigram in which she promises to be the patroness of poets. Hess, Schneider, and Wiener (1997), 78–81, 132–33, 194–95, 253.

29 McCabe (1983), 39–40.

30 E. Rice (1985), ch. 4. A drawing copying Schwarz's *St. Jerome* is in Stuttgart. Kaulbach with Messling and Geissler (2007), no. 633.

31 Geissler (1960), doc. no. 18, which he mistakenly associates with the Munich aula altarpiece; Ettelt (1991), 60; J. Smith (2002), 108–109, 111; Strecker (1998), 299.

32 Canisius (1933), 233–47, on the Annunciation and Ave Maria.

33 On Jesuit congregations, see Duhr (1907–28), 1: 357–71; Müller (1909); Villaret (1947); Châtellier (1989); O'Malley (1993), 192–99.

34 Rolle (1989), esp. 27–29; O'Malley (1993), 196–97, for what follows.

35 O'Malley (1993), 192–95.

36 O'Malley (1993), 196.

37 Duhr (1907–28), 1: 358–59.

38 Duhr (1907–28), 1: 365.

39 De Backer and Sommervogel (1960), 2: cols. 1510–14, list Coster's texts.

40 Châtellier (1989), 115.

41 Coster (1588), fol. ⋆1.

42 Coster's Latin texts, first published in Antwerp and then in German translations, include *Sieben Betrachtungen über das Andächtige alt und herzlich Lobgesang*

Salva Regina (Dillingen, 1588); *Fünffzig Betrachtungen von dem Leben und Lob der heiligen Jungfrauwen Gottes Gebärenin Mariae* (Dillingen, 1588); and *Sieben Betrachtungen über das uhralte Catholische Lobgesang Ave Marias Stella zu Teutsch* (Ingolstadt, 1590).

43 Coster (1588), fol. **6 (Oratio Sodalitatis in admissione à singularis recitanda); Villaret (1947), 64; Châtellier (1989), 6.

44 Schade (1960), 220–21, citing Agricola (1727–29), 1: 252, nn. 97–98.

45 Châtellier (1989), 15.

46 The undated engraving, made in Antwerp, circulated widely throughout Germany. Johann Bussemacher of Cologne published a crude copy in 1595. Mauquoy-Hendrickx (1979–83), no. 1342. The numerous variations of this print testify to its popularity. Hollstein (1947–), 63: 163–65, nos. 1069, and its pendant, 1070 (the *Circumcision with the Litany of Our Lord Jesus*). The copper plate is in the Dutch Jesuit Collection in Amsterdam. Begheyn (2001).

47 J. Smith (2002), 29–55.

48 Lazar (2005), 135.

49 Sattler (1864), 41–44.

50 Dimler (1974), 139.

51 B. Schneider (1991), 279–80.

52 Leuchtmann (1976); Hell and Leuchtmann (1982); Erb (1990); Leuchtmann and Schaefer (1994).

53 The translated text is given in the program notes to Lassus (1989), 8. Also see Lassus (1982), preface and score. Lasso's original manuscript score is Mus MS 15, fols. 94v–100, in the Bayerische Staatsbibliothek in Munich. A second version is Mus MS 48, fols. 189v–197. See Bente (1989), 81–83 and 173–75, respectively. Crook (1994), 75–76, lists the litanies.

54 Crook (1994), 38–39, 56, 79; also Zager (1995), esp. 219–21.

55 Dyer (n.d.); Monson (2002), esp. 18–28; Ditchfield (2007), 201–24.

56 Lassus (1982), preface (Clive Waring).

57 Richeôme (1604); J. Smith (2002), 50–51.

58 Crook (1994), 73–76.

59 Crook (1994), 3.

60 On the impact of Ignatian spirituality on Lasso, see A. Fisher (2007).

61 Agricola (1727–29), 1: 184, as cited by Leuchtmann (1976), 192–93.

62 Erb (1990), 18.

63 Herrmann-Schneider (1985), nos. MM 711–44, for what follows. The catalogue of the former music collection of St. Michael's lists six anonymous *Regina caeli laetare* motets of uncertain date.

64 On Jesuit sodalities and music, see A. Fisher (2004).

65 *St. Michael Vanquishing Lucifer* measures 5 by 3.5 meters, while the altarpiece's intricately carved frame, finished in 1591–93, fills the entire height of the choir. Geissler (1960), 180–81, nos. G I, 20–21; Wagner and Keller (1983), 90–92, 104, figs. 47, 59; Baumstark (1997), nos. 111, 146, plates IV–VI; J. Smith (2002), 86, 92–93.

66 Munich, Bayerische Staatsgemäldegalerie, inv. no. 5129; since 1950 on loan to St. Anna im Lehel in Munich. Schwarz's attractive preparatory drawing is in Stockholm's Nationalmuseum. Geissler (1960), 180, no. G I, 19; Baumstark (1997), nos. 152 (drawing) to 153 (painting), both texts by Claudia Denk; Strecker (1998), 297–315.

67 Nising (2004), 88–93; Sauter (2004), 78–79.

68 He is documented paying for the church's largest bell (the Salvator); the *Apostles Altarpiece* (now lost) located on the other side altar; the tabernacle

for the high altar; and, in 1585, the gilt silver chalice and paten for use on the Mary altar. Lieb (1980), 30, 201.

69 *The Enthroned Virgin and Child with Sts. Benedict and Francis* was completed after Schwarz's death in 1592 by Peter Candid, another of Duke Wilhelm's court artists. Sometime after Fugger's own death in 1600, the picture was transferred to his burial chapel in Augsburg's St. Ulrich and Afra Church. Geissler (1960), 33, 74, 141–43; Lieb (1980), 18, 26–27, 72 (for three other paintings by Schwarz), 189, 198, 209, 229, 274, figs. 25 and 28; *Welt im Umbruch* (1980–81), 2: no. 463; Strecker (1998), 366; Heal (2007), 171–76. Volk-Knüttel (1988), figs. 1–3, argues that this picture is by Candid, partially after a drawing by Schwarz, and that Fugger's house chapel painting, created by the two painters, is the *Virgin and Child with Sts. Ulrich and Afra*, today also in the Ulrich and Afra Church in Augsburg; Volk-Knüttel (2010), nos. G19–20, on these two pictures.

70 Lieb (1980), 174–75, 201; Baumstark (1997), 483 and no. 166.

71 For instance, see Albrecht Dürer's *Apocalyse* woodcuts (1498), his *Adoration of the Holy Trinity* (1511; Vienna, Kunsthistorisches Museum), and Albrecht Altdorfer, *Virgin and Child in Glory* (c. 1522–25; Munich, Alte Pinakothek). Hecht (2003), figs. 1, 2, 66–67, 78, 100, 105–106.

72 Schmidt (2000), 52–53, fig. 32. Lutherans developed their own scenes in which God appears above a city.

73 Lieb (1980), 174–75, 201; Baumstark (1997), 483 and no. 166.

74 Canisius (1933), 262; also cited by Claudia Denk in Baumstark (1997), 486.

75 Rolle (1989), 42–44.

76 Guarinonius (1610), 231, as cited by Claudia Denk in Baumstark (1997), 484, 486.

77 Balde (1990), 1: 212–13 (*Lyricorum* bk. IV, 13); Glaser (1980), II/2, no. 71; Woeckel (1992), 164; Baumstark (1997), 486.

78 Sandrart (1994), 1: 263–64.

"UNTIL SHADOWS DISPERSE"

AUGUSTINE'S TWILIGHT

Meredith J. Gill

When the voice of Jerome came to Augustine at the hour of Compline, according to an apocryphal medieval letter, his study became irradiated by a magical light. Carpaccio's depiction of this subject in 1502 (Illustration 63) contrasts with Georges de La Tour's Jerome of about 1622 (Illustration 64), who glimmers within the penumbra of his cell. Where Augustine looks out from his lighted space to a window, Jerome is absorbed in candlelit revelation, seen in partial luminescence that seems literally to battle with the shadows.

Augustine's complex philosophy of light bears not only on his portrait but also on Renaissance conceptions of sanctity, for philosophers and writers from Dante onward appropriated his rapturous first-person interrogations of God, fusing them with Platonic imagery relative to the senses. Marsilio Ficino (1433–99) brilliantly rephrased Augustine's theory of divine illumination wherein knowledge, as light, was a formation of the mind by God. "What is this light," Augustine had asked, with typical ardor, "that shines through the chinks of my mind, and pierces my heart? ... Wisdom it is, none other than Wisdom, that shines through my darkness, tearing apart the cloud that envelops me; yet I fall away from it."[1] For Augustine, as for Ficino, light was the "finest corporeal substance connected to the soul." Like the *spiritus*, light dwelled on the boundary between material and immaterial; it sparkled.[2]

What happened to the metaphysics of light in the sixteenth century, especially after the Council of Trent (1545–63), and can we discover in Christian controversy in these years a new voice of Augustine and, allied to it, a changed aesthetic sensibility? At the same time that discoveries in natural science and physics yielded new knowledge about optics and the behavior of light, can we speak of a metaphysics of light – or, rather, of a metaphysics of shadow – as bearing on the storied tenebrism of early modern painting?[3] Carlo Del Bravo, Maurizio Calvesi, and others have argued that light in late-sixteenth-century Venetian and Spanish painting, as well as that in Caravaggio and de La Tour, is an Augustinian metaphor – a severe Jansenist one in the case of de La Tour – for divine grace in an age of reform, modulated by what they term the new Scholasticism.[4] This essay began as a speculation: If Augustine's light, as his versatile metaphor for encapsulating the corporeal and incorporeal apprehension of God, is suggestive of his place in the Renaissance, could it be that his shadow – as his "almost nothing" before creation, as ambivalence, abyss, and falling away – aptly encapsulates a new convergence of Augustinian themes in the artistic culture of the Counter-Reformation?[5]

Shadows have always been a part of painting's history. In practical terms, Renaissance artists and theorists had always understood shadows and shadow projection as necessary indicators of the painter's mastery of three-dimensional representation – whether this was to give a sense of relief within an object, to establish the relation of one object to another, or to locate the positions of the observer before the work of art and a light source, either within or without the painting.[6] In the late sixteenth century, the painter and writer Giovanni Battista Armenini (c. 1525–1609) stated that, after the outline of a figure, *rilievo* is the most important aspect of a painting. The painter must here put the "larger lights" in accordance with the shadows they cause; he must know, then, the kind of light that comes from heavenly bodies as well as the light issuing from artificial sources, as required for *istorie* or *fantasie* of nocturnal scenes.[7] Giorgio Vasari and others had been equally preoccupied with the practical as well as dramatic possibilities of light effects, and they were aware, too, of the relative nature of the perception of contrast; we all look at shadows differently: at them, into them, or through them.

In painting, the representation of shadows has always relied on unstable conventions, and it turns, as well, on the problem of consistency with regard to the painting's context. To address this dilemma, Piero della Francesca – in his *Dream of Constantine* at Arezzo, for example – and others followed Cennino Cennini's (c. 1370 to c. 1440) advice, extending into their fictive spaces the physical conditions of light outside them. This still left, though, the question of recording the impression of a fleeting instant; for this, both Cennini and Paolo Pino (active 1534–65), who especially esteemed Giorgione, advised working in conditions of diffused light.[8] Leonardo recommended northern light, others the use of models, also set up in special conditions such as candlelight or lamplight.

It was Leonardo who adapted shadow projection, based on astronomy and optics, to the needs of the painter, and he also came very close to adapting Renaissance rules of perspective to the projection of shadows. Like Leon Battista Alberti, Leonardo mistrusted outline, which led him to probe a shadow's edges in relation to the shadow's geometrical delineation: "Shadows appear to me," he said, "to be of supreme importance in perspective, because without them opaque and solid bodies will be ill-defined; that which is contained within their outlines and their boundaries themselves will be ill-understood unless they are shown against a background of a different tone than themselves."[9] Leonardo's findings were further rationalized by the late sixteenth century, when Giovanni Paolo Lomazzo (1538–1600) linked shadows more precisely to perspectival theory. Other theorists became sensitive, further, not only to the implications of several lighting conditions, but also to the demands of multiple figural compositions, light's scatter, reflection, and, above all, *sfumato*.[10] In Caravaggio's day, Karel van Mander (1548–1606) identified point-source illumination as a property of candlelight, which he noted was then relatively rare but wherein "the shadows must fall all over the picture from the light as from a point."[11] The Jesuit scientist François Aguilon scrutinized the varying intensity of shadows in 1613, for he perceived that the air's luminosity factored among the different shadows within the shadow, and he made still more critical distinctions among lamps and the sun, windows, and the open air.[12]

By the early seventeenth century, just a decade before the appearance of such celebrated nocturnes as de La Tour's *Magdalene with the Smoking Flame* (c. 1638–40) (Illustration 65), theorists recognized what it was that Leonardo, the great maestro of "tonal unity," had anticipated: that the problem of shadows' *edges* could never find a fully objective – that is, geometric – solution.[13] Yet Leonardo's own shadow loomed large, so to speak, in this same century, when the imitation of nature became for artists

63. Vittore Carpaccio, *St. Augustine in His Study*, 1502. Oil on canvas. Venice, Scuola di San Giorgio degli Schiavoni. Photo: Alinari / Art Resource, NY.

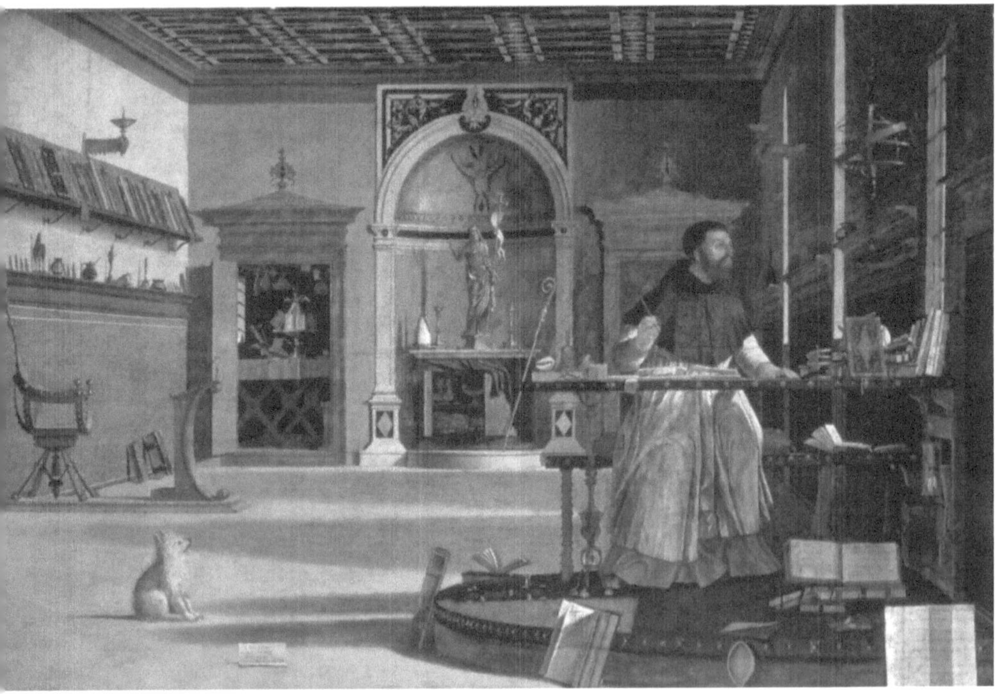

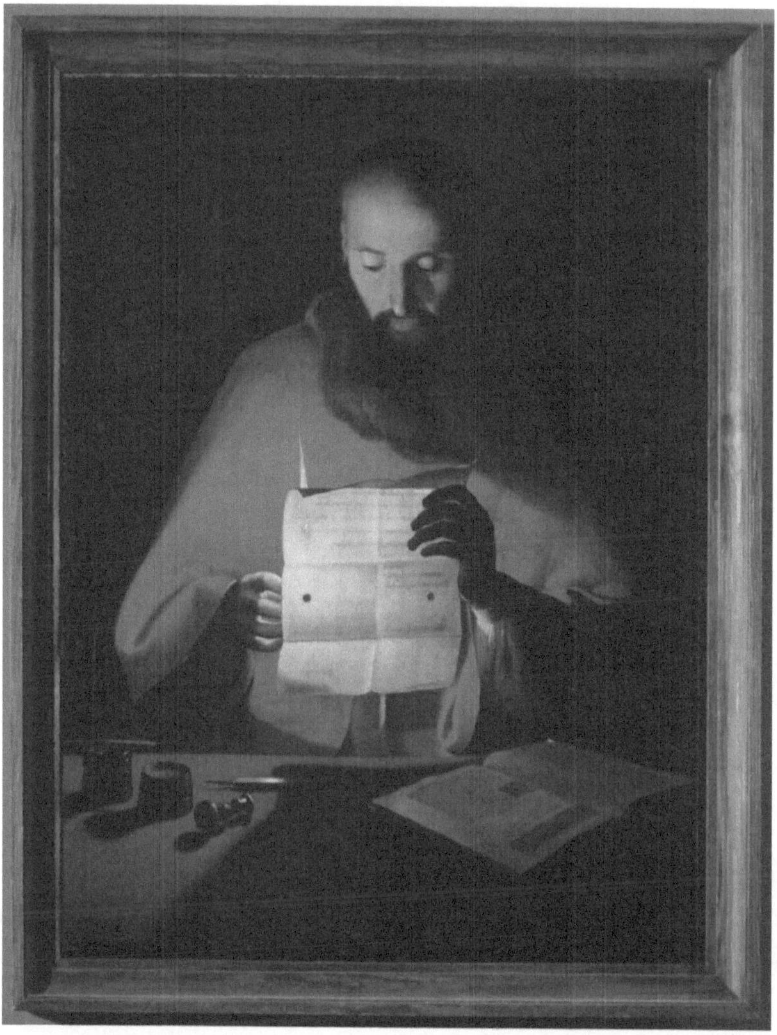

64. Georges de La Tour, *St. Jerome Reading*, c. 1621–23. Oil on canvas. Nancy, Musée Historique Lorrain. Photo: Réunion des Musées Nationaux / Art Resource, NY.

a conscious and well-publicized goal. Cast shadows became, in Janis C. Bell's words, "the 'hot' new topic in contemporary perspective treatises."[14] In the 1620s, a member of the Theatine Order and an almost obsessive admirer of Leonardo, Matteo Zaccolini, was at work on his massive study of perspective and optics, of which one volume, *Della descrittione dell'ombre prodotte da corpi opachi rettilinei*, was dedicated to the projection of cast shadows under various lighting conditions, including candlelight, sunlight, and broad illumination.

Zaccolini was not alone, for Pietro Accolti (1625), Jean Dubreuil (1642), Abraham Bosse (1648), and André Félibien (1666–1685), among others, also addressed the subject, if less expansively, in their own perspective treatises.[15] For all of these writers, as well as for the artists who both influenced and adapted their ideas, the supreme goal was to reproduce the effects of nature so that the observer entered into a persuasive fictive realm.[16] Among his audience, Zaccolini counted artists, including those without any training in either perspective or mathematics. His accessible *grisaille* demonstrations bear this out, for they provided a quick reference that circumvented mathematical calculations. When Domenichino came to paint his *Flagellation of St. Andrew* (1626–28) in the apse of S. Andrea della Valle in Rome, Zaccolini was likely close to finishing his treatises, having returned to that city from Naples. In the summer of 1623, just as Domenichino received a model of the conch of the apse, Zaccolini was lodging at S. Andrea's Theatine house. Domenichino approached his cast shadows at S. Andrea with new attention, and in a fashion that reflects the distinctive precision of Zaccolini's illustrations, such as those of the fall of shadows onto the planes of steps.[17] Bellori lauded the style of the evangelists in S. Andrea's pendentives (Illustration 66); they were, he commented, "represented as realistic apparitions detached from the surface of the wall, which forms the background for them in a whitish half-tint. The clouds underneath project forward from the surface, and cast shadows project over the gilded cornices."[18]

Such spilling shadows were not new to Rome, but they were a later component of Domenichino's design at S. Andrea, and they endowed the figures with a living presence. For the first time, plaster protrudes over the moldings, breaking through the architectural frame in a manner Zaccolini recommended; this technique also saved on the expense of gilding.[19] As in his earlier *Last Communion of St. Jerome* (1614; Pinacoteca, Vatican), which Bellori also admired, Domenichino had pushed his sovereignty in technique to new heights.[20] The plaster shadow resolved the dilemma of portraying shadows' edges in painting. It was, though, ultimately left to physics to wrest the study of shadows' edges from painting, leading eventually to modern-day propositions about light's behavior, including the finding that light does not travel in straight lines.[21]

What I have outlined here of the science of shadow projection describes discoveries that seem independent of metaphysics and theology, although I wonder whether we should ever fully separate these disciplines. Artists are always attentive to an exciting paradox of their craft: that religious mysteries can be affirmed by the material and the visible; painters can accomplish this by combining an apparent optical truth with reference to an ineffable one.[22] It is tempting to imagine the kinds of conversations that Zaccolini and Domenichino might have had about this very subject when the two were together in Rome. Zaccolini would have been mindful of his religious calling as a Theatine and likely held hopes, ultimately unrealized, to publish his volumes with the Order's publisher at S. Agostino, Naples.

The image that he uses in his noteworthy, because unusual, treatment of reflection and refraction of the broken appearance of the oar under

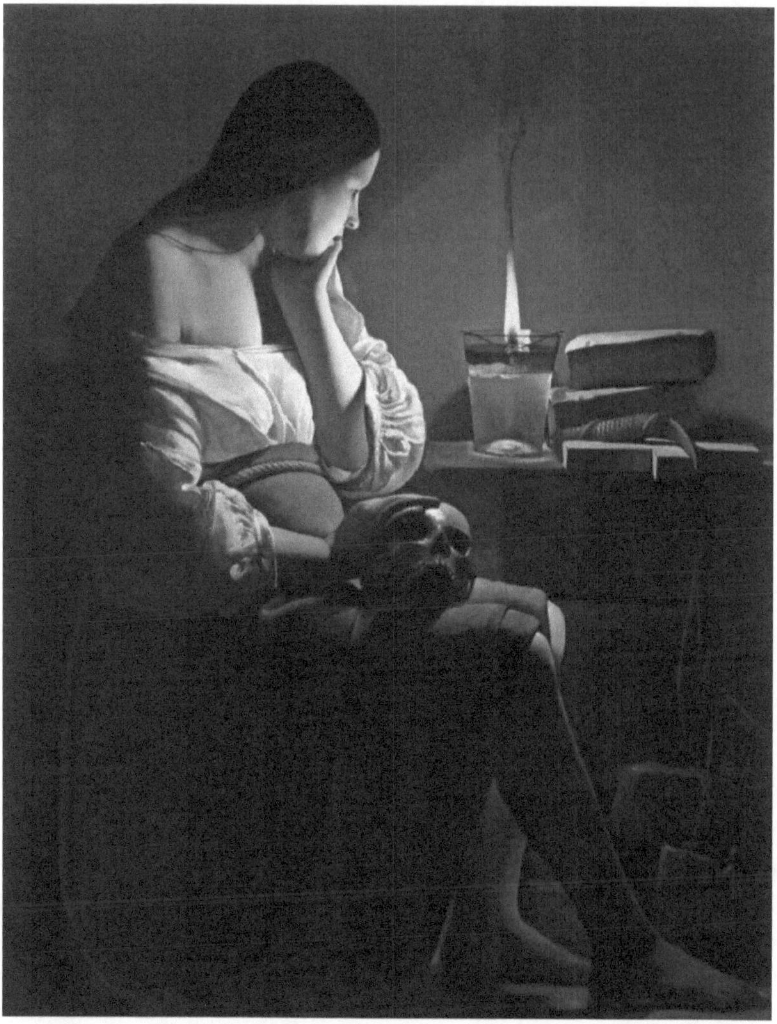

65. Georges de La Tour, *Magdalene with the Smoking Flame*, c. 1640. Oil on canvas. Los Angeles, Los Angeles County Museum of Art. Photo: Digital Image © 2009 Museum Associates / LACMA / Art Resource, NY.

water strikes a chord with any reader of Cicero and Augustine. In the context of Augustine's analysis of corporeal and noncorporeal sight in the *Soliloquies*, the figure of Reason points out that, among other illusions, the "false break in the oar in the water" is false only because it "resembles the true."[23] The highest kind of sight, for Augustine, "intellectual" sight, encapsulated the discriminating and self-aware mechanics of the mind in being able to judge things for what they really are.[24] Zaccolini's reasonableness about the artist's need to look for himself, to judge his work and nature alongside one another, and not simply by means of rules, seems very much in the spirit of Augustine's Reason. At the same time, and somewhat like Augustine himself, Zaccolini maintained – as his magisterial volumes testify – that the sense of sight answered to a higher calling, not just to the truths of nature but, with them, to the superior operations of the intellect. In this, the seventeenth-century theorist upheld a long-standing belief in the artist's capacity to outwit nature in the process of imitating nature's forms.

As early as the 1420s, St. Peter's shadow, moving miraculously over the infirm and the disabled in Masaccio's *St. Peter Healing with His Shadow* (Illustration 67), only loosely conformed to the real light issuing from the chapel's window, as well as the symbolic light emanating from the altar onto the form of Peter himself.[25] In a subtle way, too, Filippo Lippi, in his *Annunciation*, used the shadow of objects at the boundary of his picture space to announce the Incarnation. In Victor Stoichita's incisive reading, not only do certain of Lippi's objects, such as a pilaster, column, or a transparent vase, indicate the border between "fiction and reality," but in the case of the vase, which is itself a symbol of the Incarnation, the cast shadow resting on the space where the Incarnation happens also becomes an attribute of that same dogma.[26]

Both Masaccio and Lippi denote, then, the ambivalence or, to put it more precisely perhaps, the multivalence of the shadow as a sign of transcendence, for the shadow has a mixed symbolic history. In diverse cultures, it represents the soul or "essence of the person who casts it"; this also harks back to customs in which shadows can be metaphors for the misery of the human state, as they are, for example, in Job 14:2.[27] For Cicero, however, a shadow suggested protection.[28] In the Greek New Testament, shadow (*skia*) appears as "a shade caused by the interception of the light; [or] an image cast by an object and representing the form of that object; [or] a sketch, outline."[29] In his Vulgate, Jerome translated shadow as *umbra*, meaning "shade" or "shadow"; but this could imply both the "shadow" of death in the book of Job and Peter's healing "shadow" of Acts.[30] Masaccio's renderings of shadow seem to bear out a feature of the text of Acts 5:15, namely its Near Eastern character in combining a Greek inflection, in which a shadow can be a double for a man, and a Roman one, evoking the idea of shadow as protective. In early exegetical writings, as well as in vernacular sources, it was only Peter's healing – not his shadow – that became symbolic of the continuity of Christ's miracles, such that Peter embodied the Church.[31] Peter's ministry heralded the Church's sacramental mission. This typology is borne out by the humble figures in Masaccio's painting who assume the ritualized postures of persons present at mass.[32] It would not be until 1588 that an interpretation of Peter's *shadow*, as opposed to his healing, would appear wherein the shadow itself is an image with healing power. This would be in the *Annales Ecclesiastici* (1588–1607) of the cardinal, librarian, and papal confessor Cesare Baronius.[33] The fifteenth-century artists hint at what I argue becomes even more evident from the later sixteenth century onward: the shadow assumes a tactility, a physical presence, and, at the same time, an uncertainty that sharply distinguishes it from the metaphor of light.[34]

Shadow in Scripture and in scriptural commentary can be even more profoundly ambiguous, for its meaning devolves, further, to clouds and even to light itself. In the New Testament, a verb form of the Greek *skia* (shadow) is rendered as *episkiazo*, "to throw a shadow upon, to envelop in shadow, to overshadow."[35] This form, "to throw a shadow upon," is used in the New Testament to record three miraculous events: the Transfiguration of Christ, when a "bright cloud overshadowed them; and behold a voice out of the cloud [spoke]";[36] the Annunciation, when "the power of the Highest shall overshadow" the Virgin;[37] and, for Peter, the laying out of the sick so that "at least the shadow [*umbra*] of him [Peter] passing by might overshadow some of them."[38] The overshadowing cloud is, in all cases, paradoxically a source of brightness. In the three textual accounts

66. Domenichino, *St. Mark the Evangelist*, 1620s. Fresco. Rome, S. Andrea della Valle. Photo: Scala / Art Resource, NY.

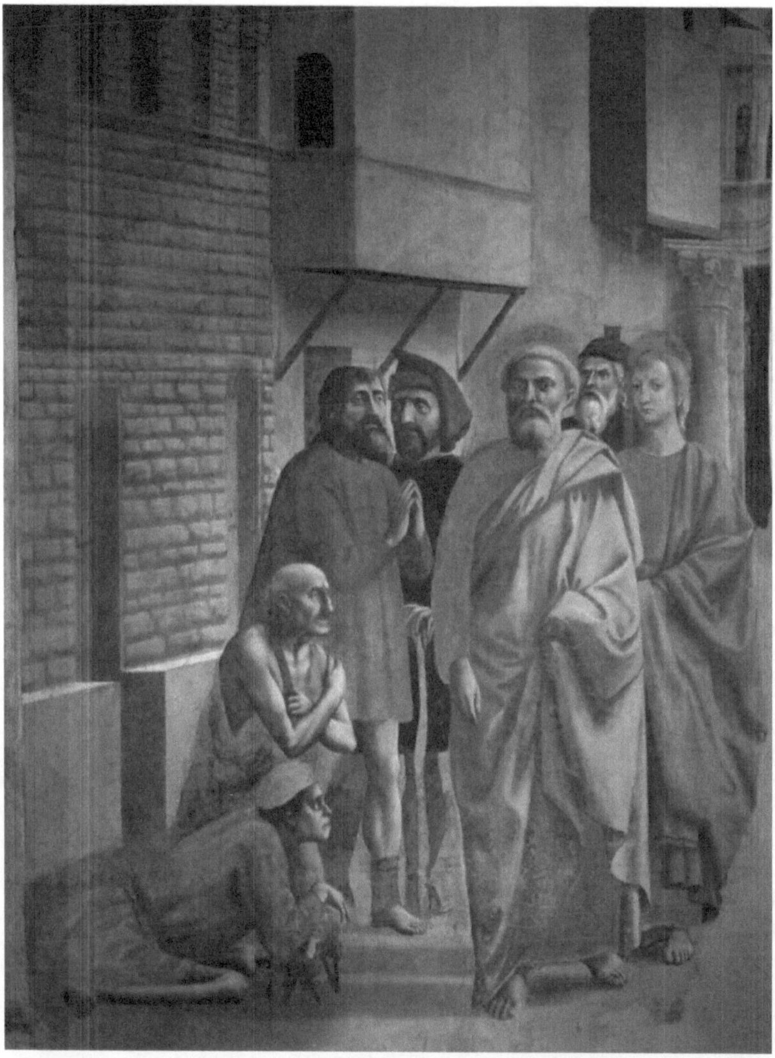

of the Transfiguration, to which we must add Raphael's famous altarpiece of c. 1518, "shadow" transfers meaning "from a vaporous cloud that casts a shadow" to "a shining cloud surrounding and enveloping persons with brightness."[39] Light and shadow are thus here fused in the term *episkiazo* (to throw a shadow upon); when translated in the Bible into Latin, as *obumbro*, it becomes "overshadowing" with an attendant richness of meaning.[40]

Art theorists did not explicitly associate light with expressive, as opposed to symbolic, values until the late seventeenth century, but artists themselves may always have perceived their conjunction.[41] This seems to be the case, to cite only one extraordinary Venetian example, in Tintoretto's *Last Supper* for S. Giorgio Maggiore (1592–94; Illustration 68), where the drama of light and shadow, magnified in and through the actions of Christ and the apostles, seems to offer the observer the perfect vehicle for the expressive force of the miracle of the Transubstantiation.[42] In the spirit of the Counter-Reformation, Tintoretto also squarely faced the ticklish problem of representing the unrepresentable by painting his angels as diaphanous beings, part light and part shadow, both and yet neither, on the boundaries between the visible and invisible worlds.[43] Such subtleties in visualizing shadows do not disappear. We could say, in fact, that the ambivalence of the shadow, in its otherness from light and yet its sameness, becomes more manifest through the years of Trent and beyond. And it is here, too, perhaps, that Augustine, who often paraphrased or rephrased Scripture and who frequently deferred to Paul, might be heard in a different way.

It is received wisdom that justification by faith alone, as a constituent of the Reformation understanding of personal salvation, depended on Augustine and Paul as part of the doctrinal discourses of Catholic renewal.[44] But as many recent scholars have demonstrated, the language of reform and its very definition are not easily arrived at. Luther, of course, was not alone in his critique of the Church. Another Augustinian, the Order's prior general and a prominent figure at Trent, Girolamo Seripando (1492–1563), also preached the doctrine of justification by faith: "And everybody thronged there [Rome] because they liked this doctrine."[45] Long before Trent, too, though critical to its legacy, writers anticipating change in Catholic practices turned to the Augustinian themes of conversion, will, and grace. They broached, as well, a long-standing notion in the history of spirituality, that of faith as an affective phenomenon.

Since the Middle Ages and into the period of Trent, mystics and spiritual authors had appealed to anticlerical and individualistic religious sensibilities. In the 1540s, for example, the Spanish dissenter Juan de Valdés, who had fled to Rome to escape the Inquisition, encouraged the reception of *alumbradismo* in Italy – that is, simply expressed, a practice of listening to the urgings of one's spirit and conscience as a means to apprehend God, rather than paying unthinking obeisance to the teachings of the

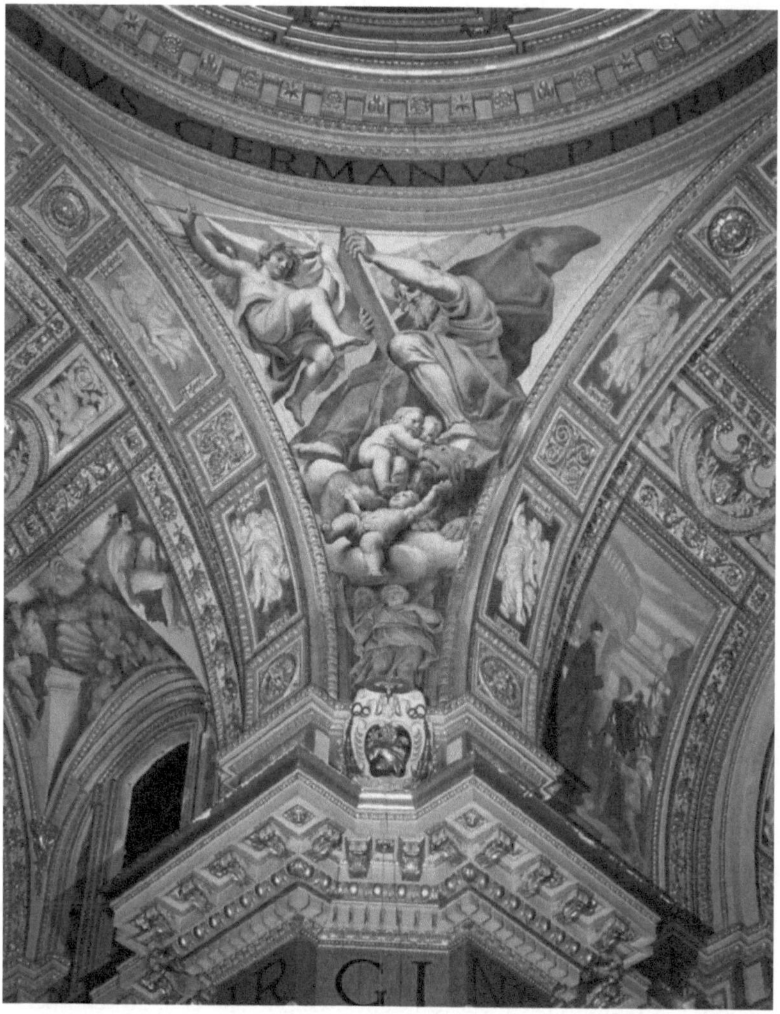

67. Masaccio, *St. Peter Healing with His Shadow*, 1420s. Fresco. Florence, S. Maria del Carmine, Brancacci Chapel. Photo: Erich Lessing / Art Resource, NY.

Church and Scripture.[46] The same Augustinian culture that had nurtured Seripando, Valdés, and others who were ardently hoping for a transformation of Catholic practices had also fostered Protestant theologies. As the Tridentine Church emerged – if we might speak of such a monolithic enterprise – that same, shared Augustinian inheritance came more sharply into focus.[47]

Pius IV reconvened Trent in part for fear of John Calvin's growing authority, even if this was only one element of the story.[48] Calvin's influence embraced an affectional, very Augustine-like apprehension of the Bible: "[T]he assent which we give to the divine word," Calvin wrote, "is more of the heart than the brain, and more of the affections than the understanding.... [F]aith is absolutely inseparable from a devout affection."[49]

Can we speak, then, of much in later-sixteenth-century painting – and sculpture, too – as attempting a greater, somehow unmediated fidelity to scriptural meaning, a concern of Catholics and Protestants alike, but also in a very Augustine-like awareness of the passions, and of the passionate struggle for faith shared by each side of an increasingly divided Christendom? In this context, the sensual communion intrinsic to the work of art had the potential to effect a reconciliation of divergent religious values. In their solitary devotions, many shadowy subjects of works of art – the hermit reading, the saint visited by a mystical vision – invited active sympathy on the part of their late-sixteenth- and early-seventeenth-century viewers.[50] That art could be transformative and that it activated the senses were assumed by the Jesuits, for example, and their patrons after Trent, especially in Italy. Since the edict on art tabled toward the end of the Council had nothing specifically to do with painting, it left open the role of art within newly renovated interiors, at least until the publications of figures such as Gabriele Paleotti in the late sixteenth century.[51]

Among the heirs to the medieval, spiritual tradition were Teresa of Ávila (1515–82), John of the Cross (1542–91), and Ignatius himself (1491–1556). They each described darkness as a palpable, meditative locus, postulating what has been called "a theology of darkness." This theology seems to have its correlative, after the Counter-Reformation, in the slow, meditative inspection engaged by new kinds of religious subjects, including the single saintly figure, and by their visual language, namely the glimmering dimness of a tenebrism.[52] The Carmelite John of the Cross identified the soul's progress as an affirmative passage across three nights, including active nights of the spirit and the senses.[53] "It is called Night," he said, "because of the way or the means which the soul must use in order to achieve the union. That means is faith, which is such a darkness for the mind as the shadows of night.... [I]t is called Night owing to the end, this end being God. In life on earth He is also a dark night for the soul." When John turns to the active night of the spirit, he says:

> Deeper is the obscurity in the spiritual part, similarly as pitch darkness is deeper than the shadows of night. Even in the depth of night it is still possible to see something, whereas in total darkness one cannot see anything. Also in the night of the senses some light still remains; there remain the mind and reason, as they are not dimmed then. However, the spiritual night, i.e. faith, is deprived of any light from either the reason or the senses.

He differentiates between faith and God, both being akin to the pitch black of night, and the penumbral gloom that is the habitat of the "mind and reason." "According to theologians," he wrote in his *Way to Mount Carmel*, echoing the linguistic polarities of shadow and overshadow in Scripture,

> faith is the soul's faculty, sure and dark. It is a dark faculty because it makes one believe in the truths revealed by God Himself, which are above all

> natural lights.... This mighty light flowing from faith is deep obscurity for the soul, as it deprives the reason of light just as sunlight eclipses all other lights.... Faith is a night for the soul but it also gives it light. And the more it obscures it the more light it imparts to it.[54]

Each of these saints was receptive in their personal spiritual formation to Augustine: not least to his inward-dwelling consciousness, his yearning, and unquiet self-examination. Inspired by the *Confessions*, in particular, each would write in the subjective mode, responding, as well, to the tenor of his interrogation of time, the character of memory, belief, and the question of predestination. Their reflections seem all too naturally to implicate the art of Caravaggio.

Although we cannot classify the artist as a straightforward paradigm of the Counter-Reformation, his work has often been viewed as emblematic of Counter-Reformation ideals. He was certainly a magician of light and an original colorist who achieved astonishing effects of "forced chiaroscuro." His tenebrism relies on deep, "obscuring shadows with no reflected light at the edges of forms, and small delimited areas of illumination."[55] His colors range from very light to very dark tones in the lit areas of his portrayal of the Supper at Emmaus; in the apostle on the right, for example, and in the innkeeper at left.[56] Rather than the gradations of modeling recommended by Leonardo, Caravaggio's forms shift sharply from dark shadow to bright light without halftones, and yet – this is the

68. Tintoretto, *Last Supper*, 1592–94. Oil on canvas. Venice, S. Giorgio Maggiore. Photo: Cameraphoto Arte, Venice / Art Resource, NY.

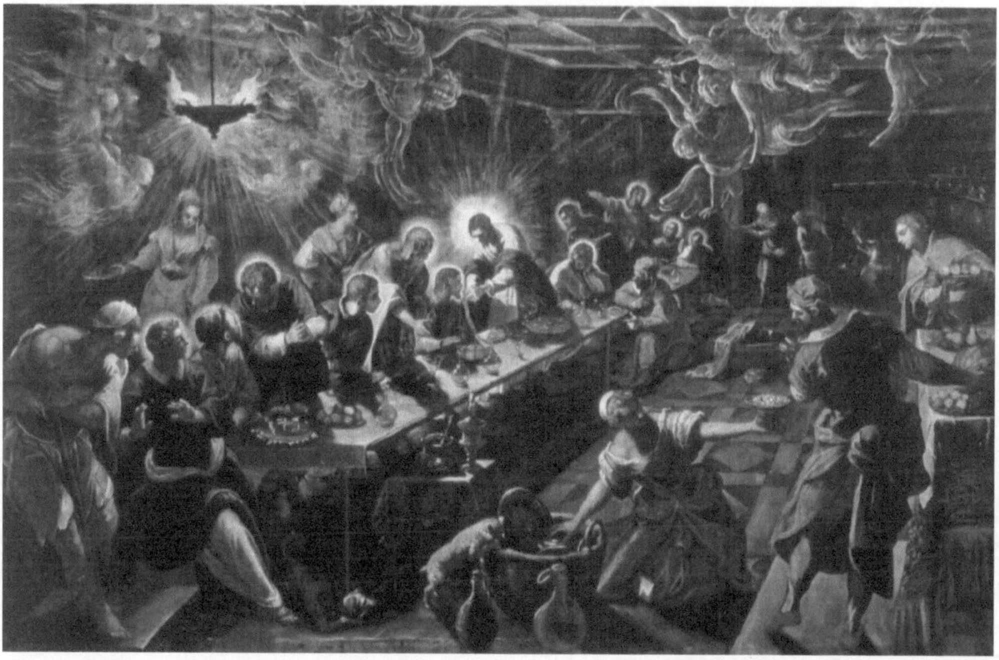

mystery – we still perceive a system of lighting that seems consistent. It was not, however, for his tenebrism or violent contrasts that Caravaggio's coloring was admired in his day, as Janis Bell and others have shown, for his lighting was oftentimes criticized as "unnatural."[57] It was rather more for his "somiglianza del vero," as Malvasia expressed it – his "appearance of truth" – that he was praised: "His textures, relief, and light looked real," so that, in fact, his achievement combined the semblance of color constancy and a masterful *imitation* of light.[58] Yet with all of this, the *effect* of the artist's light in no way seems to me to be identified with a simplistic Augustinian metaphor of grace – and for Augustine, there never really *was* such a simplistic metaphor. If there is an Augustinian relation to be drawn out here, it is to an analogy – one that was implicit in Scripture itself – of the shadow. Such a relation accommodates itself to the cultural and doctrinal climate of Trent and to the perceptual reasoning of late-sixteenth-century and early-seventeenth-century observers.

Caravaggio was an iconoclast who was recognized in his day both as his age's "greatest exponent of naturalism and the man almost singlehandedly responsible for destroying the art of painting."[59] For some commentators, his chiaroscuro gave the body a powerful relief that heightened its realism and produced deep emotional resonance. For the viewer in the Cerasi Chapel, the anamorphic effect of his *Conversion of St. Paul* (Illustration 69) reenacts that very conversion by requiring in the viewer "physical displacement parallel to the spiritual turn it represents.... And what makes for the dramatic necessity of this turn is our 'place' in the broadest sense: not just our relative position before the altar, but our home in the fallen world of carnal darkness that both image and beholder share."[60]

The painting's primal contrast between light and enveloping dark, to which we are directed by Paul's blind and "unenlightened" companion, "inscribes," in Christopher Braider's words, "the severe Pauline and Augustinian theology of original sin soon to take shape as the unyielding Jansenist rejection of man and world."[61] In keeping with contemporary reformatory themes, Caravaggio suggests that it is an "unmerited" grace, and grace alone, that redeems us. For this reason, as if to portray grace's unexpected and ineffable nature, the source of his light is invisible; it is absent to us and to Paul's attendant, though it was once present to Paul before his eyes closed.[62] This refusal on the artist's part to give in to an ideal of light as ubiquitous and dominant is itself a Pauline construct, for in Paul, as in Augustine, divine light and worldly darkness, incorporeal and corporeal, are in mortal contest.[63]

Shadows and darkness were ubiquitous for Augustine, as they were for his great model, Paul: from his extended meditations on the creation of light in Genesis, before which a "darkness of ignorance" prevailed, to his allegory of darkness as that of the unbaptised soul

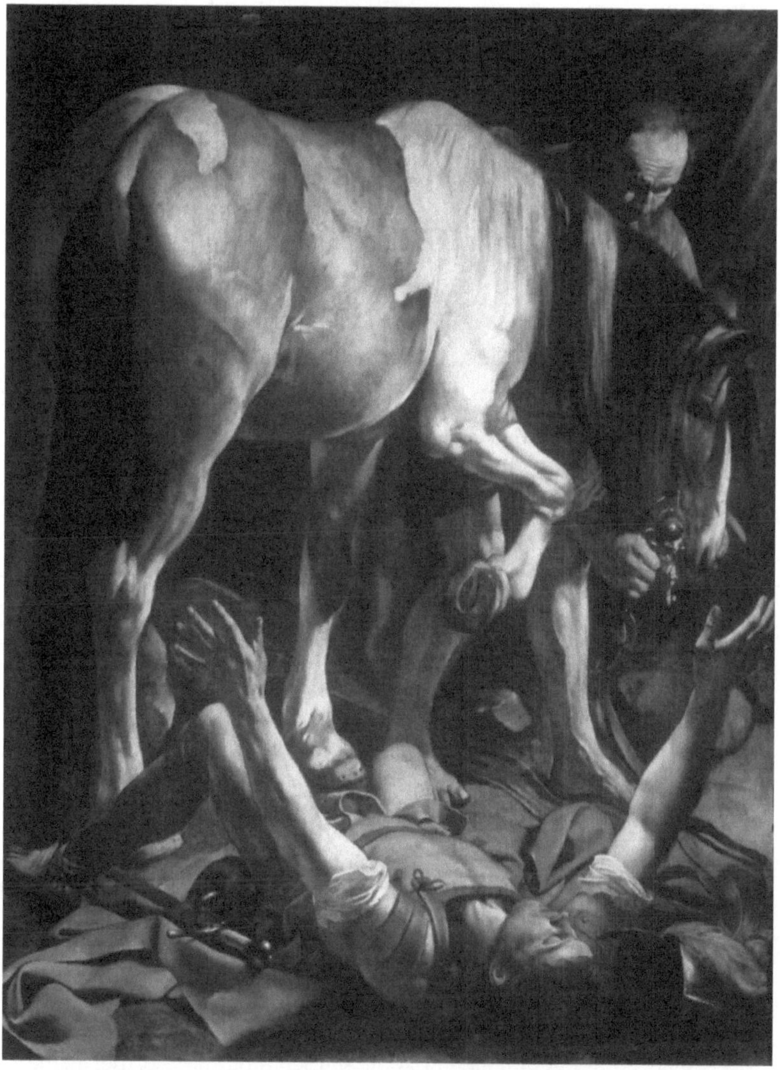

69. Michelangelo Merisi da Caravaggio, *The Conversion of St. Paul*, 1600. Oil on canvas. Rome, S. Maria del Popolo. Photo: Scala /Art Resource, NY.

longing for God.[64] In book 13 of his *Confessions*, he expressed this in emotive terms:

> Yet my soul is sad, because it slips back and becomes an abyss once more, or rather, it feels itself to be still in the depths. But my faith takes it to task, that faith that you have kindled, lamp-like, on my nocturnal path. We too were once children of his wrath; once darkness, we carry that residual gloom in bodies marked for death because of sin, but hope on until day dawns and shadows disperse.[65]

In his work *The Literal Meaning of Genesis*, Augustine also considered the "proper" and "metaphorical" senses of "body," approaching the exact scriptural sense of shadows – the dualistic sense – as "embodiments" (his word) of God himself. And here we have an Augustine of the Counter-Reformation perhaps: creatively linking light and shadow to the past and the present, and linking them both, as well, as crucial indications of divine purpose:

> Now the Godhead is not a body, but because St. Paul calls the religious observances of the Old Testament shadows of what is to come (using the analogy of shadows in the physical world), he says that the fullness of the Godhead dwells in Christ corporeally; for in Him was fulfilled all that was prefigured by those shadows, and thus in a certain sense He is the embodiment of the shadows; that is, He is the truth of those figures and symbols.[66]

Augustine reprises here the dualistic sense of the overshadowing cloud of the New Testament that is both dark and light, apprehended by mortals yet an emanation of the divine.

The shadow is, after all, a remarkable sensory phenomenon, dynamically oscillating as it does between presence and absence, inviting slow, empathetic vision and invoking, too, the sense of touch. A shadow courts our imagination and our emotions. Paul's and Augustine's perceptions of the two sides of darkness had a part to play in reifying the shadow as analogy and metaphor, as a positive sign of the inadequacy of the human person and of a necessarily emotive approach to God. As artists from the mid-sixteenth century onward incorporated the tenets of Catholic renewal and the findings of science into the lights and shades of their pictures, they had no choice but to be mindful of the dark.

Notes

1 Augustine (1997), 11, 9, 11, p. 292.

2 For Augustine, as for Ficino, light also issued from the eye; the eyes of lovers sent out beams of light. Just as the sun sends out rays, so, too, the heart emits *spiriti*. These "liminal substances," for both Augustine and Ficino, were at once corporeal and incorporeal. See Fehrenbach (2005a), 10–11; also my chapter, "Augustine's Light," in Gill (2005), 125–47. Fehrenbach points out how Augustine "found common ground with ... the Aristotelian tradition. In his biological writings, Aristotle characterizes *pneuma*, the bearer of the *thermon*, as glimmering, placing it in the category of shining substances, such as oil, which contain a great deal of *calor nativus*."

3 In its day, the "soverchia oscurità" of seventeenth-century painting was viewed negatively. Rzepińska (1986), 91.

4 See, e.g., Del Bravo (1983). The teachings of the Catholic theologian Cornelius Jansen (1585–1638), which were inspired by Augustine, articulated clear concepts of predestination and the action of grace relative to human will. His posthumously published *Augustinus* (1640) was condemned by the Inquisition.

5 I am persuaded by John W. O'Malley and Robert Bireley that, instead of "Counter-Reformation," the term "Early Modern Catholicism" might be preferable. See Bireley (1999), 1–8.

6 Kaufmann (1975), 258; Bauer (1987); Gombrich (1995).

7 Armenini, *De'veri precetti della pittura* (Rome, 1587), in Kaufmann (1975), 258.

8 Kaufmann (1975), 259–60.

9 In Kaufmann (1975), 269. "Shadow," Leonardo wrote in the Codex Atlanticus, "is the obstruction of light." For his changing definitions, see Nagel (1993); Fehrenbach (2005b). See also Thro (1966), 42–50, app. 1; Baxandall (1995), "Three Notes on Leonardo and Early Renaissance Shadow," 146–55. Albrecht Dürer was more successful in his attempts to resolve the challenge of projecting shadows in painting according to perspective; yet his (and others') idea that any light source could be treated as a point was misleading for artists after him. More recently (since my paper at the Renaissance Society of America's meeting in March 2007), see Francesca Fiorani's excellent essay, including a discussion of Leonardo's painting technique, as well as his ambitions to produce a book on theories of light and shadow: Fiorani (2008), 271–78 (and her forthcoming book on Leonardo and shadows).

10 Kaufmann (1975), 260–61, 262–63. Lomazzo divided perspective into optics (medieval *perspective naturalis*), sciagraphy (Renaissance *perspectiva artificialis*), and the study of reflections. Outside painting, shadow theory had belonged to classical tropes, such as those of Quintilian and Pliny – the lover's shadow in the wall – or to astronomy, which in turn linked the cast shadow to geometry. See, further, D. Summers (2007), esp. ch. 1, "Shadow-Painting and Scene-Painting: The Beginnings of Optics and Classical Art," 16–42. Summers makes the important distinction between *skiagraphia* and *skenographia*, the former as engaged with shadow painting itself, the latter attaching to more general optical themes.

11 In Kaufmann (1975), 279.

12 The geometer Girard Desargues (1591–1661) subsequently correctly demonstrated the projection of shadows from the sun. Kaufmann (1975), 283.

13 See Shearman (1962), 30; Nagel (1993), 9–10. Tonal unity, Shearman argued, "is the essential and inevitable pre-requisite for the classical plasticity of the High Renaissance, by which painting achieved the corporeal homogeneity and *rilievo* which would rival sculpture." See, further, Farago (1992), 63–88; Bell (1995), 141: "Tonal unity is the organization of colors in a painting according to their lightness and darkness, such that the lightness of colors in the illuminated parts is approximately equal, and the darkness of colors in the shadowed parts are approximately equal, as they would be in an achromatic chalk or wash drawing."

14 Bell (2003), " 'hot' new topic," 81.

15 Bell (2003), 81, 84–85.

16 Bell (2003), 87. In the preface to his companion volume, *Prospettiva del colore*, Zaccolini wrote, "The learned painter, who in practice has been noticing the whimsy of nature and observing its variety with the acumen of scientific knowledge, can imitate its superficial appearance, as is required by this superhuman profession." Unlike Agucchi or Bellori, for whom the exemplars of classical sculpture and Raphael supplied the theoretical counterpoint to nature, Zaccolini "continued the tradition of Leonardo: knowledge of the laws of nature would guide the painter to choose the most typical and universal examples. Both sides, however, shared the idea that vision is not a passive sensory experience but an intellectual activity affected by education and experience." Bell (2003), 87.

17 This is an argument eloquently made by Bell (2003), 88–99.

18 Giovan Pietro Bellori, *Le vite de'pittori, scultori e architetti moderni* (1672), in Bell (2003), 92.

19 Bell (2003), 92–93.

20 Bell (2003), 93–95.

21 In a provocative study, Roberto Casati (2004) sees in the depiction of cast shadows a means by which to investigate the connections among art, cognition, and cognitive science. He addresses the history of the science of shadow perception and lists types of shadows in a sample of early Renaissance paintings.

22 See the argument (and other early examples) in Eisenberg (2002).

23 Bell (2003), 98, notes Zaccolini's "admonition" about the oar under water (but not Augustine's or Cicero's image from his *Academics*) and the deft way in which seventeenth-century artists avoided representing it, if they could. In the *Soliloquies*, Reason points out: "We also speak of a false tree which we see in a picture, a false face which is reflected in a mirror, the false motion of towers as seen by those sailing by, a false break in the oar in the water: these are false for no other reason than that they resemble the true." Rotelle (2000), 66; Gill (2005), 129–32.

24 See Augustine's *De Trinitate* 16, 6, 8. In Summers's apt summation: "Intellectual vision looks upward, so to speak, to the ideas to which it is nearest, and spiritual vision looks downward, and is a kind of reflection upon corporeal sense. But just as the spirit is a mean between body and intellect, spiritual vision is a mean between corporeal and intellectual vision. It is only through cogitation that the mind can be brought under its own gaze." D. Summers (1987), 200. Ignatius, a great reader of Augustine, would make a similar distinction, based on Aquinas, except that he referred to the senses rather than types of vision, distinguishing "between the external, or affective, senses, such as sight, and the internal, or cognitive, senses." J. Smith (2002), 38–39.

25 Eisenberg (2002), 236; Freedman (1990).

26 Stoichita (1997), 81–82: "The painter's intentions would have been obvious not only to anyone possessing great theological knowledge.... Experts have pointed out that Italian hymns had for a long time conveyed the idea illustrated by Lippi and that contemporary theological opinion had also written extensively on the theme of light penetrating the vase without destroying it. The small shadow cast by the decanter in the S. Lorenzo *Annunciation*, on the 'spot' where the incarnation takes place, is the metaphor of the latter.... Lippi's intention was that it [the shadow] should depict – not the fathomable, but its absolute opposite: the mystery. Although, in response to the demands of hermeneutics, we could say that to Lippi the shadow as a symbol, is *an interminably interpretable symbol* [emphasis added]."

27 Freedman (1990), 17–18, citing, among others, Frazer (1951), ch. 4, "The Soul as a Shadow and a Reflection." She notes that for writers such as Aeschylus and Sophocles the shadow was always a negative construct.

28 Freedman (1990), 18.

29 See, e.g., *Blue Letter Bible* (1996–2012); s.v. "*skia*," www.blueletterbible.org/lang/lexicon/Lexicon.cfm?strongs=G4639; Thayer (1996), s.v. "*skia*." It occurs seven times in the New Testament and is translated by Jerome as *umbra*, or a version of it, in all instances (Matthew, Mark, Luke, Acts, Colossians, Hebrews). I am indebted in this analysis and in the following discussion of the text in Scripture to an excellent study of shadow in

relation to Carpaccio's *St. Augustine in His Study* by Hannah Wong, seminar paper in "Studies in Italian Renaissance Art: The Science of Sight in the Renaissance" (University of Maryland, Fall 2005). See also Freedman (1990), 17–19.

30 As Wong (see n. 29) notes, in the Latin Vulgate, Jerome does not translate Hebrew words connected to shadow (e.g., *tsêl* and *tsalmôwn*) with the same Latin word. In the passage from Job, Jerome translates these as *umbra*, which also appears in a positive sense in the New Testament. *Blue Letter Bible* (1996–2012), s.v. *umbra*, www.blueletterbible.org/search/translationResults.cfm?Criteria=umbra&t=VUL&sf=5.

31 "The Church, like St. Peter, by invisible power performs the actions that help visible, corporeal beings." Freedman (1990) (on Bede), 21, 19–21. She isolates three instances of commentary on Acts 5:15 between the fourth and thirteenth centuries, in Oecumenius, Arator, and Bede. For Rabanus Maurus, "shadow" had contradictory implications: present human life; Christ's protection; impiety; and the shades of damnation. In c. 1309, Nicholas of Lyra, whose *Postillae Perpetuae, sive Breva Commentaria in Universa Biblica* was in the library of S. Maria del Carmine in the fifteenth century, summed up the three authors, adding that St. Peter's facility for curing with his shadow testified to his virtue, which was of divine essence.

32 Freedman (1990), 26–30.

33 Baronius (1588–1607); Freedman (1990), nn. 22, 20.

34 As Freedman notes in discussing the paucity of examples of the curative powers of a shadow, "the followers of St. Peter in the role of healer appeared only in the Age of the Baroque." Freedman (1990), nn. 9, 18.

35 *Blue Letter Bible* (1996–2012), s.v. *episkiazo*, www.blueletterbible.org/lang/lexicon/Lexicon.cfm?strongs=G1982; Thayer (1996), s.v. *episkiazo*. In the Vulgate, it is consistently translated into *obumbro* and its forms. As in Wong (see n. 29). Luke, who is the generally accepted author of Acts, invariably used the verb "overshadow." Freedman (1990), 18.

36 Matthew 17:5; Mark 9:7; Luke 9:34. In all of these, "a voice from the cloud" spoke almost the same words. Luke notes, however, that the disciples became afraid "as they entered the cloud," while Matthew mentions the cloud's brightness.

37 Luke 9:34.

38 Acts 5:15. As in Wong's (see n. 29) treatment of these three subjects. *Blue Letter Bible* (1996–2012), s.v. *umbra*, www.blueletterbible.org/search/translationResults.cfm?Criteria=umbra&t=VUL&sf=5.

39 *Blue Letter Bible* (1996–2012), s.v. *episkiazo*, www.blueletterbible.org/lang/lexicon/Lexicon.cfm?strongs=G1982; Thayer (1996), s.v. *episkiazo*. This is not contradicted by the argument of Van Eikema Hommes (2000), that the lower portion of Raphael's composition has darkened over time and, perhaps more significantly, that it was only in the seventeenth century that the treatment of light in paintings was accorded an expressive, as opposed to symbolic, function relative to a figure's mental state or the meaning of a subject.

40 The paradox of the shadow can be read into the paradox of light, too, in these subjects. When Renaissance artists portrayed the Transfiguration and the Annunciation, they typically depicted the presence of God as light, even though the Bible refers to "shadows" and "clouds." The cloud of the Transfiguration, from which a voice "broke forth" – much like Jerome's

voice from the supernatural glow in Augustine's study – comprises a mandorla of light. Similarly, the Holy Spirit of the Annunciation that "overshadows" the Virgin is accompanied by slivers of light that convey her impregnation.

41 By the later decades of the seventeenth century, theorists writing about the modes, as much in relation to music as to art, articulated the notion that light expressed mood in painting. Van Eikema Hommes (2000), 38, refers to Félibien's *Conférences de l'Académie Royale de Peinture et de Sculpture pendant l'année 1667* (Paris, 1669) as an example, since he noted that Poussin accommodated his color and light to his subject's mood. See, as she notes, Montagu (1992). See also Bätschmann (1992). Poussin's striking shadows in his *Eucharist* (c. 1635; Belvoir Castle), not to mention his own understanding of the classical tradition in which shadows gave rise to painting itself, seem very much to the point.

42 See Bohlmann et al. (2002).

43 "Tintoretto behandelt dieses Problem als Maler und benutzt dabei seine raffiniertesten künstlerischen Mittel. Seine Engel befinden sich an der Grenze zwischen sichtbar und unsichtbar, was eigentlich ein Problem der gegenreformatorischen Malerei schlechthin ist, die die 'höheren Regionen' mit Farbe und Pinsel darzustellen hatte." Stoichita, in Bohlmann et al. (2002), 20. As he goes on to note, "this is not so far from a medieval understanding of *umbra* as pertaining to an ungraspable manifestation. We might note that it was Venice, as a major European publishing center, that was the "real 'door' to the Lutheran and Calvinist doctrines in Italy." Firpo (2004), 172.

44 Hsia (2005), 13. Luther's famous positions on "justification by faith" and the "priesthood of all believers" must be set within the history, pluralism, and internationalism of religious cultures in the Reformation. See Hsia (2004), esp. Cameron (2004), 3–21; Firpo (2004), 169–84; O'Malley (2004b), 223–36.

45 Quoted by Firpo (2004), 170, 172.

46 Firpo (2004), 177: "the inner revelation of the spirit, on the light that it instilled in everyone's conscience allowing genuine understanding of God's word."

47 Ozment (1980), 403–405.

48 For recent reassessments of Trent, see Bireley (1999); Luebke (1999); O'Malley (1999a, 2000).

49 In Bouwsma (1990), 47; Ozment (1980), "Catholic Reform and Counter Reformation," 397–418.

50 To mention only several examples: Guercino's *St. Paul the Hermit* (Luigi Koelliker Collection, Milan); Jusepe de Ribera's two versions of *St. Paul the Hermit* (Prado, Madrid; Luigi Koelliker Collection, Milan); and Giuseppe Vermiglio's *St. Jerome* (Luigi Koelliker Collection, Milan), in Sgarbi (2006), nos. 30; 38; 39. See also the brilliant analysis of de La Tour's nocturnes, with a consideration of the sense of hearing in relation to the divine Word, in Judovitz (2006), 143–63.

51 See the helpful summary in J. Smith (2002), esp. ch. 2, 29–55 (and bibliography).

52 See the suggestive essay by P. Fisher (2002): "We could think of darkness as one important precondition of searching. Its presence signals the pace of prolonged attention. Little or nothing is delivered to our first glance.... The

generosity of darkness, and of locally staged, partially lit places within darkness, is one guarantee of how time can be demanded by the work of art" (98–99); see also Stafford and Terpak (2001), esp. 66–79.

53 See the observations of Rzepińska (1986), 100–101; De Courcelles (2004).

54 In Rzepińska (1986), 100. "An image of this night was the cloud which separated the Israelites from the Egyptians as they went into the Red Sea.... From what we have said it can be concluded that faith as a dark night lends some light to the soul plunged in darkness." Quoting the second Epistle of St. Peter, he reflects: "The statement that we should regard the faith preached by the prophets as a candle in a dark place indicates that we should remain in darkness, shutting our eyes to all other lights.... Reliance on other lights, on clear comprehension, leads us to abandon that dark light of faith, shining for us, according to St. Peter, in a dark place." As the author notes (101), he was influenced by Pseudo-Dionysius.

The astronomer Johannes Kepler praised darkness, as well as "active" shadow and eclipses, noting that these gave rise to astronomy itself: "It is on these eclipses of the heavenly bodies that the whole of astronomy is based, so much so that this very darkness is the eyes of astronomers, these flaws illuminate human minds with the most precious images. How magnificent and recommendable to all nations are the considerations of the eulogy of the shadow!" *Ad Vitellonum Paralipomena. Astronomia Pars Optica* (1604), in Rzepińska (1986), 102. The author (103ff.) notes, too, the importance in the sixteenth century of the philosophical side of alchemy, in which *nigredo* assumes a positive value and gives rise to new life; she refers to Athanasius Kircher's *Ars magna lucis et umbrae*. On Kircher, Galileo, and others, see Brusatin (1987), 26–33.

55 Bell (1995), 141.

56 *The Supper at Emmaus* (1601–1602) (National Gallery of Art, London); see Bell (1995), 141, whom I follow closely.

57 Bell (1995), 141–42.

58 Bell (1995), 142.

59 Braider (1998), 291.

60 Braider (1998), 295: "Just as Paul, knocked flat by the sudden outbreak of celestial light, is driven from the road of his persecutory intent – both stopped in his tracks and turned in the entirely new direction of devoted apostleship – so the beholder is turned, abandoning the normal frontal posture relative to the image in favor of one dictated by the painting's placement."

61 Braider (1998), 295.

62 Braider (1998), 295.

63 "The Cerasi *Conversion* thus tells its story in such a way as to comment on, and condemn, at once the art that tells it and the hellish carnal nature that requires such a telling to image the light that escapes nature." Braider (1998), 296. More recently, in her paper at the Annual Graduate Student Symposium on the History of Art (Philadelphia Museum of Art, April 2010), "Darkness in a Positive Light: Negative Theology in Caravaggio's *Conversion of St. Paul*," Tiffany Racco explicitly connected Caravaggio's patronage to the Augustinian Order.

64 "Disgusted with our darkness, we were converted to you, and light dawned. See now, we who once were darkness are now light in the Lord. But as yet we know this only by faith, not by anything we see; for we have been saved

indeed, but in hope, and hope that is seen is hope no longer.... Paul himself, even Paul, who says, Not as spiritual persons could I speak to you, but only as carnal, even he does not consider himself to have laid hold on his salvation already, but, forgetting what lies behind him, he stretches out to what lies ahead, groaning and oppressed because his soul is athirst for the living God." Augustine (1997), 13, 12, 13; 13, 14, pp. 350–51.

65 Augustine (1997), 13, 14, 15, p. 352. See also his writings on creation in *On the Literal Interpretation of Genesis, an Unfinished Book* [*De Genesi ad litteram liber imperfectus*, c. 393] and in *On the Literal Interpretation of Genesis* [*De Genesi ad litteram liber*, c. 400–15]; he also wrote on many of the same themes in his first work on Genesis, an allegorical reading, *De Genesi adversos Manicheos*, as well as in *The City of God*, 11, and several minor works, such as *De fide et symbolo*, 2, 2.

66 "The figures, therefore, are called shadows in a metaphorical rather than proper sense of the word; and similarly, in saying that the fullness of the Godhead dwells corporeally, Paul is using metaphor." Taylor (1982), 187.

A MACHINE FOR SOULS

ALLEGORY BEFORE AND AFTER TRENT

Amy Powell

GODS DON'T BURY easily – which is why the Good Friday celebrations of the Latin Church were so peculiarly fraught with ambiguities and outright contradictions, both before and after Trent. During the Middle Ages, the Good Friday ritual commemorating Christ's burial emphasized his human death, chastening vision by ceremonially removing an effigy of the dead Christ from view. In the wake of the Protestant Reformation and the Council of Trent, the Catholic ceremonies surrounding the sepulcher came to focus on the Eucharistic Host – the "true and living body of Christ" (*uerum et uiuum corpus Christi*). This shift in emphasis brought with it a new focus on the divinity of Christ and a new degree of sensuous gratification. Greater attention to the Host, along with an intensified appeal to the senses, during the sepulcher ceremonies was in keeping with the Catholic campaign to reaffirm the truth of Transubstantiation, which had been called into question by Protestant Reformers, but it was not, according to some, consistent with the mourning appropriate to Good Friday. The incongruity of the joyful display of the Host during the darkest days of the liturgical year was symptomatic of the conceptual complexity of the sepulcher ceremonies, which were charged with representing a death that was understood to be synonymous with life.

When the ninth-century Irish philosopher Johannes Scottus Eriugena apostrophizes this peculiar death, he acknowledges the impossibility of speaking its proper name: "O death, death of life, if it is to be called death and not life / I would not dare to call that which supplies life death."[1] As different as they were – the one chastening the senses, the other gratifying them – the medieval and baroque commemorations of Christ's burial attempted a doublespeak comparable to Eriugena's, relying on the rhetorical mode of allegory (literally, "other speaking" or saying one thing and meaning another) to do so. "Allegory works like a machine for souls that are far removed from God so that through it they will be raised toward God," writes Gregory the Great in his commentary on the Song of Songs. It is because humankind is fallen, according to Gregory, that the soul needs a machine to elevate it again: "Since the human race was cast out from the joys of paradise, entering into this exile of the present life, it has had a heart blind to spiritual understanding." Such a heart, Gregory believes, requires allegories to move it: "[B]y a certain kind of enigma [i.e., allegory] the divine discourse addresses itself to the numbed and cold soul, and, by means of things that the soul knows, it secretly inspires in it a love that the soul does not know."[2] On Good Friday, one such enigma was the death of Christ – a seemingly ordinary death that could lead the soul to know an entirely unfamiliar life.

In his 1928 book on baroque tragedy, Walter Benjamin argues that the machine of allegory runs on all ordinary matter but most efficiently on the dry bones of the dead: "[T]he allegorization of the physis can only be carried through in all its vigour in respect of the corpse. And the characters of the *Trauerspiel* die, because it is only thus, as corpses, that they can enter into the homeland of allegory."[3] The irony of this operation is that the allegorical machine runs on the same terrestrial matter from which it seeks to separate the soul: "By the grace of a terrestrial language," Gregory explains, "[the soul] is separated from the earth."[4] Because allegory works best where the contrast between its terrestrial language and its unearthly aim is clearest, the corpse is its most powerful image. Only by mortifying, dismembering, and finally giving up its own fallen images and words can allegory fulfill its intention: "Ultimately in the death-signs of the baroque the direction of allegorical reflection is reversed," Benjamin writes, "on the second part of its wide arc it returns, to redeem."[5] In this redemptive movement, the stuff of allegory – the sensuous image – is finally relinquished, for according to Benjamin, allegory does not redeem its own means; on the contrary, it renounces them.

Both before and after Trent, I will argue here, Good Friday celebrations in northern Europe entailed a renunciation of the sensuous image, as if in recognition of the irremediable deadness of ritual and its objects. For all their differences, the medieval and baroque commemorations of Christ's burial shared the same difficulty: yoking a dead effigy to the concept of a god who is nothing if not life-giving but only for as long as it takes to move what Gregory calls the blind heart and cold soul.[6] Where the medieval commemoration found a solution in death, darkness, and the chastening of the sense of sight, the baroque celebrations turned to life, light, and sensuous gratification. But subtending these differences was a shared renunciation of the effigy. Attention to this renunciation reveals Good Friday to have been, both before and after Trent, not only a day for reckoning with the deadness of a god – that much is explicitly avowed – but also a day for confronting the deadness of his *image*.

THE MEDIEVAL DEPOSITION RITE

In the Middle Ages, Christ's burial was commemorated each year by lowering his image from the cross, wrapping it in linens, and placing it in a structure built to resemble a sepulcher. The Deposition Rite belongs to a group of quasi-dramatic embellishments of the Roman liturgy that date to about the tenth century and that continued to be popular until the Council of Trent. Although the Deposition Rite, like the other paraliturgical rites, was never included in the Roman liturgy, from which the liturgy of most of Western Christianity derived, textual and material artifacts attest to its regular performance throughout Europe and especially in the north. The earliest extant record of such a rite belongs to the *Regularis concordia*, a compilation of Continental and English monastic practices assembled in the tenth century in conjunction with the reform of the Benedictine monasteries of England:

> On that part of the altar where there is space for it there shall be a representation as it were of a sepulcher, hung about with a curtain, in which the holy Cross, when it has been venerated, shall be placed in the following manner: the deacons who carried the Cross before shall come forward and, having wrapped the Cross in a napkin there where it was venerated, they shall bear it thence, singing the antiphons *In peace, in the selfsame; He shall dwell;* and *My flesh shall rest in hope*, to the place of the sepulcher. When they have laid the cross therein, in imitation as it were of the burial of the Body of our Lord Jesus Christ, they shall sing the antiphon *After the Lord was buried.*[7]

The Deposition Rite was staged as a funeral, with some combination of candles, mourning robes, aspersion, censing, and a shroud.[8] The receptacle into which the crucifix was deposited took different forms, the simplest of which was an altar outfitted with curtains, like the one described in the *Regularis.*[9] Other accounts refer to temporary constructions of wood and cloth set up separately from the altar. Independent coffer-shaped sepulchers with and without shrine structures built around them are extant, some still containing an effigy of the dead Christ (Illustration 70). More elaborate sepulchers took the form of freestanding chapels – either temporary wooden structures or permanent stone buildings, like the one from around 1260 in the Cloister Church of Our Lady in Constance, which is modeled on the Holy Sepulcher in Jerusalem (Illustration 71).

After being deposited in the sepulcher, the crucifix remained hidden there for the time known as the "grave rest." Candles were burned, psalms sung, and prayers said continuously during the vigil: "In that same place the holy Cross shall be guarded," the *Regularis* mandates, "with all reverence until the night of the Lord's Resurrection. And during the night let brethren be chosen by twos and threes, if the community be large enough, who shall keep faithful watch, chanting psalms."[10] The guarding of the sepulcher had the practical purpose of preventing theft.[11] It also served the symbolic function of representing the mourning of the community. In addition to the guards paid to hold the forty-hour vigil, laypeople were sometimes welcome, providing them a rare opportunity to participate in the church's ceremonies.[12]

Darkness played an important role during the last days of Holy Week, when Matins and Lauds took the name *Tenebrae* (darkness) from the responsory *Tenebrae factae sunt* (There was darkness). During Matins, candles were lit and then extinguished one by one as the antiphons and responsories were sung. This continued through Lauds until, at the end of the last psalm, darkness enveloped the church.[13] The darkness that fell over the church during the *Tenebrae* service marked the withdrawal of the Savior from visibility. In some cases, the church remained darkened for all of Good Friday. Rabanus Maurus (d. 856) explains that on this day "the candles are not lit in the churches, because when the Redeemer himself was crucified the stars were hidden."[14] The darkening of the church on Good Friday reinforced the withdrawal of the *imago Dei* pictured in the Deposition Rite, which traced Christ's movement from the visibility of the cross to the

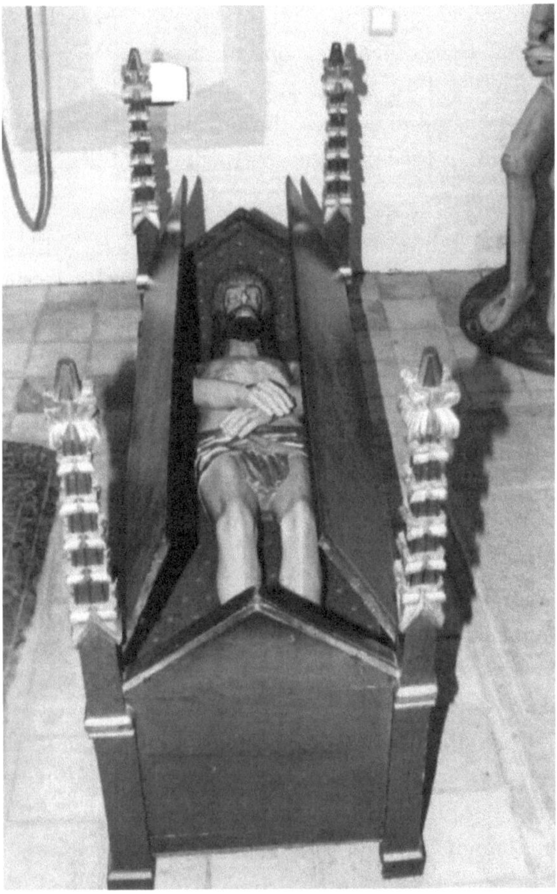

70. *Holy Sepulcher with Effigy*, c. 1500. Mariager, North Jutland, Denmark, Bridgettine convent church. Photo: Justin Kroesen and Regnerus Steensma.

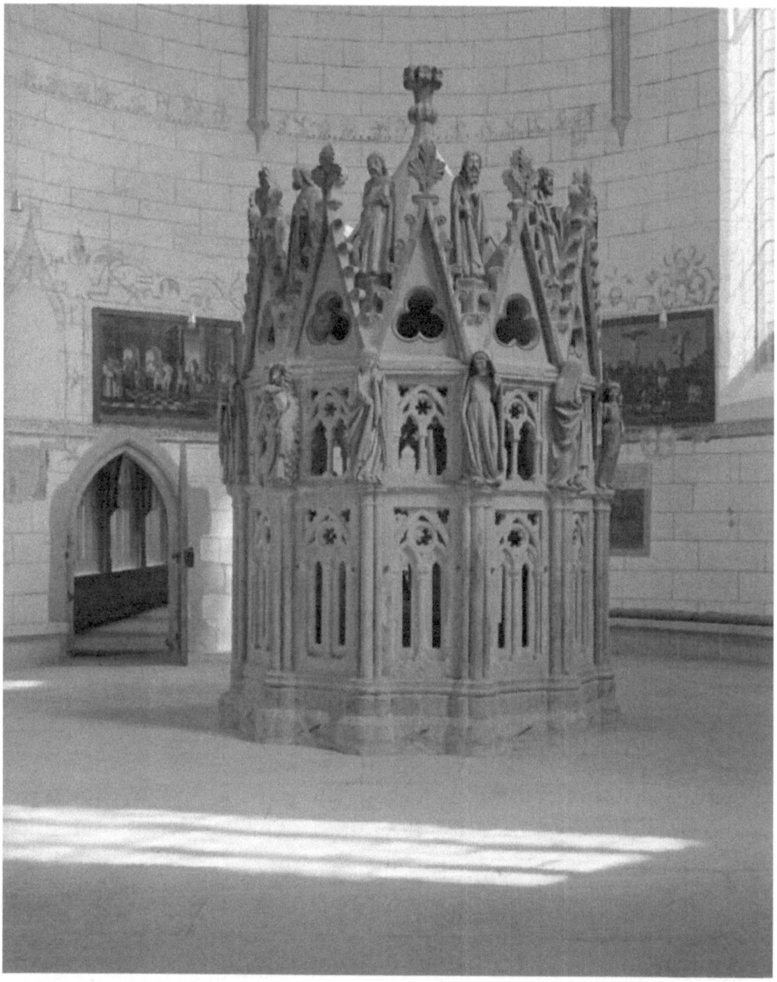

71. *Holy Sepulcher*, c. 1260. Konstanz, Constance cathedral, Mauritius Chapel. Photo: Wikimedia Commons.

invisibility of the tomb, moving the viewer from an ocular experience of the *imago Dei* to an inward understanding of the invisible God.

On Easter morning, an image of Christ was brought forth from the sepulcher in celebration of the Resurrection. While the *Regularis* describes an unceremonious Elevation, the rite performed in the church of Durham before the "suppression" of the monasteries was a splendid and public affair:

> Then they both risinge came to the Sepulchre, out of the which, with great reverence, they tooke a maruelous beautifull Image of our Sauiour, representinge the Resurrection, with a crosse in his hand, in the breast whereof was enclosed in bright christall the Holy Sacrament of the altar, throughe the which christall the Blessed Host was conspicuous to the behoulders. Then, after the eleuation of the said picture, carryed by the said 2 monkes

> uppon a faire ueluett cushion, all embrodered, singinge the anthem of *Christ is risen*, they brought [it] to the high altar, settinge that on the midst therof, whereon it stood, the two monkes kneelinge on theire knees before the altar, and senceing it all the time that the rest of the whole quire was in singinge the foresaid anthem of *Christ is risen.*[15]

Because the image of the crucified Christ was not well suited for the Easter celebrations, the crucifix deposited in the sepulcher on Good Friday was sometimes replaced during the grave rest with an image more appropriate to the Resurrection, like the one described in the Durham Rite. The ceremonial display of an image of the living Christ thus brought to an end the forty-hour period of the crucifix's occultation and the mourning that accompanied it.

CRUCIFIXES WITH MOVABLE ARMS

With their minimal dialogue and costumes, paraliturgical rites like the Deposition Rite were mimetically restrained. They were a far cry from the full-fledged religious plays that began to be performed in the thirteenth century. Religious plays were written in the vernacular instead of the Latin of the liturgy, performed by actors rather than clergy, and elaborately staged outside the church with sets and costumes. Where the religious plays tended toward a literal, historical re-creation of biblical events – affording what Rainer Warning has described as a magical return to mythical origins – the paraliturgical rites evoked the past only insofar as was necessary to remember the act of salvation effected in it, perpetuated by the liturgy in the present, and fulfilled in a future still to come.[16]

The development of the paraliturgical rites coincided with the flourishing of the allegorical mode of liturgical exegesis. Although he did not invent it, Amalarius of Metz codified the allegorical mode that would dominate liturgical exposition in the West from the ninth century up until the Council of Trent.[17] Pope Innocent III (c. 1160–1216), William of Durandus (c. 1237–96), and Thomas Aquinas (1225–74) are only some of the better-known exponents of Amalarius's method. To each gesture, action, object, and word of the liturgy, the allegorist attributed a meaning corresponding to an event in Christ's life, an Old Testament event prefiguring that life, an allusion to the end of time, an abstract spiritual truth, an ethical admonition, or some combination of these. The narrative of the life of Christ is the backbone of most allegorical expositions of the liturgy. In fact, these expositions sometimes make it seem as if the liturgy did little more than tell Christ's story in a manner much like that of the vernacular religious plays.[18]

But allegory is based – in theory, if not always in practice – on a distinction between what is said and what it represents. "Allegory is present when what is said literally has another meaning spiritually," writes Durandus, "for example, when one word or deed brings to mind another."[19] While they may have brought to mind the historical events of the life of Christ (and other things), the words and deeds of the liturgy also had to function – if they were to function allegorically – as a celebration *in the present* of the salvation those events had brought about. Insofar as the words and gestures of the late medieval liturgy were an "outward representation of that which is spiritual," as the *Regularis* calls them, they were distinct from the spiritual truths they called to mind.[20] Without this distinction, liturgical allegory would have collapsed into something like storytelling. Florus of Lyon objected to Amalarius's liturgical allegoresis for precisely this reason, among others.[21]

Although relatively restrained, the paraliturgical rites of the later Middle Ages sometimes tested the limits of allegory – just as the allegorical interpretations of liturgy did – pushing so far into the territory of mimetic narrative as to obscure the liturgy's kerygmatic function, its "announcement of a fulfillment still to come."[22] When, for example, the Deposition Rite delayed the celebration of the final, triumphant outcome of Christ's sacrifice in order to linger over his human death, conducting a funeral for a man who had long since ascended to the right hand of God the Father in heaven, it became easy to forget on Good Friday that Christ's death was not to be understood as a death in any simple sense but rather as the death that undoes all death, including itself. In other words, while tarrying over Christ's death on Good Friday made a good deal of narrative sense, isolating the moment of death and dramatizing it as if it were magically recurring in the present obscured the relation between that death and salvation. The inclusion of a Eucharistic Host in the Good Friday rite was one means of clarifying this relation.[23]

Hosts were sometimes buried alone, for example, at the Benedictine monastery of St. Blaise in the Black Forest; and they were sometimes buried along with the crucifix, as in the *Use of Sarum*, the variation of the Roman Rite used in most of England, Wales, and Ireland.[24] The use of the Host in the burial rite softened the emphasis on Christ's human death because the Host was considered to be the true and *living* body of Christ. Some people objected to the burial of the Host for precisely this reason. A Zurich ordinal of 1260 complains: "It is against all reason, that in certain churches the Eucharist is customarily deposited and closed up in a chest of such a kind that represents a sepulcher. There the Eucharist, which is the true and living body of Christ, actually represents the dead body of Christ, which is indecent, sinful, and absurd."[25] As far as narrative is concerned, it may have been absurd to bury an object that represented the living body, but the Host's inclusion in the Good Friday rite made it possible to celebrate the death of Christ without forgetting entirely the everlasting life that his death, it was believed, would bring about.

A special type of crucifix with hinged shoulder joints invented specifically for the Deposition Rite toward the end of the thirteenth century

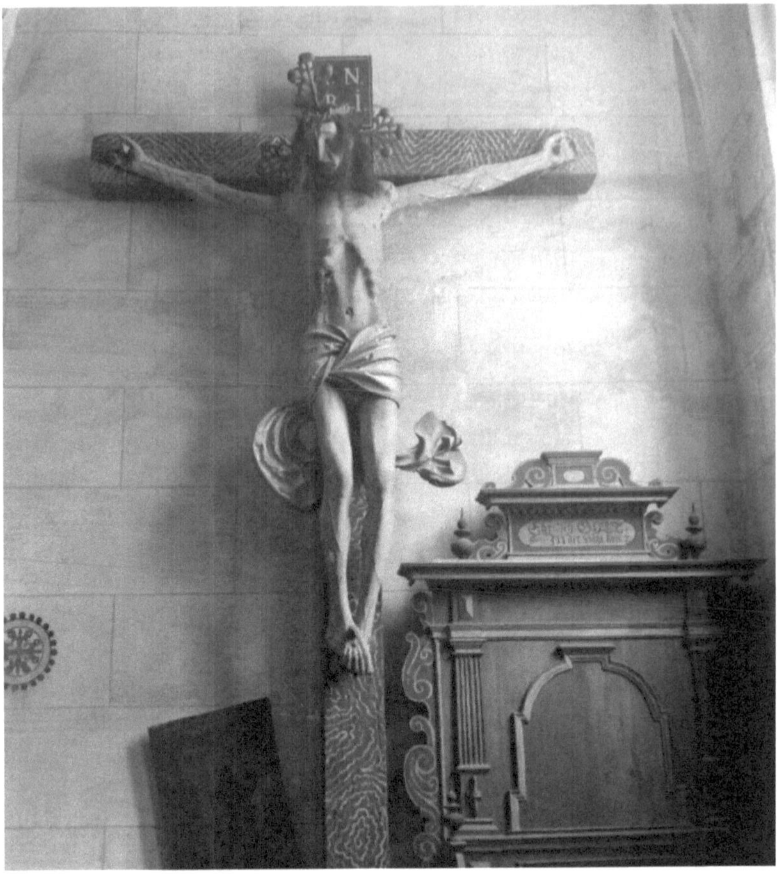

72. Oswald Bockstorfer aus Memmingen, *Crucifix with Movable Arms*, 1481. Polychromed wood. Bad Wimpfen am Berg, Evangelical church. Photo: Bildarchiv Foto Marburg.

offered another means of countering the rite's emphasis on Christ's human death – and one that did not contradict the Rite's narrative structure as did the burial of the Host.[26] The crucifix with movable arms stands as the culmination of the medieval development of an increasingly realistic image of the crucified body. The hinged shoulders of these sculptures allowed the same figure seen hanging on the cross to be lifted off the cross and to be placed in a narrow coffer. This strengthened the illusion of the deadness of the figure, which might have been taken for a representation of the still-living Christ before it was lifted off the cross and its arms were laid by its sides. To heighten this realism still further, a 1481 crucifix from Bad Wimpfen was adorned with human hair and beard (Illustration 72). And along with the shoulders, the elbows of an early, nearly life size crucifix from Kempten were articulated so that when the body was deposed its hands could be folded over its chest (Illustration 73). How might objects like these have countered the Deposition Rite's emphasis on the death of Christ, as I claim? The answer to this question lies in the specific way in which these movable sculptures were moved and in the impression that that movement was intended to make.

Modern scholars have naturally tended to associate crucifixes with movable arms with the other movable sculptures used in and around Holy Week. On Palm Sunday, for example, a statue of Christ seated on an ass was wheeled in procession through the streets as viewers scattered palm leaves before it in celebration of Christ's entry into Jerusalem.[27] And On Easter Sunday, Christ's Resurrection was performed by raising a sculpture of the triumphant Christ from the sepulcher, as I described earlier. This

73. Swabian, *Crucifix with Movable Arms*, c. 1350. Polychromed wood. Kempton, Basilica of St. Lorenz. Photo: Kunstverlag Peda.

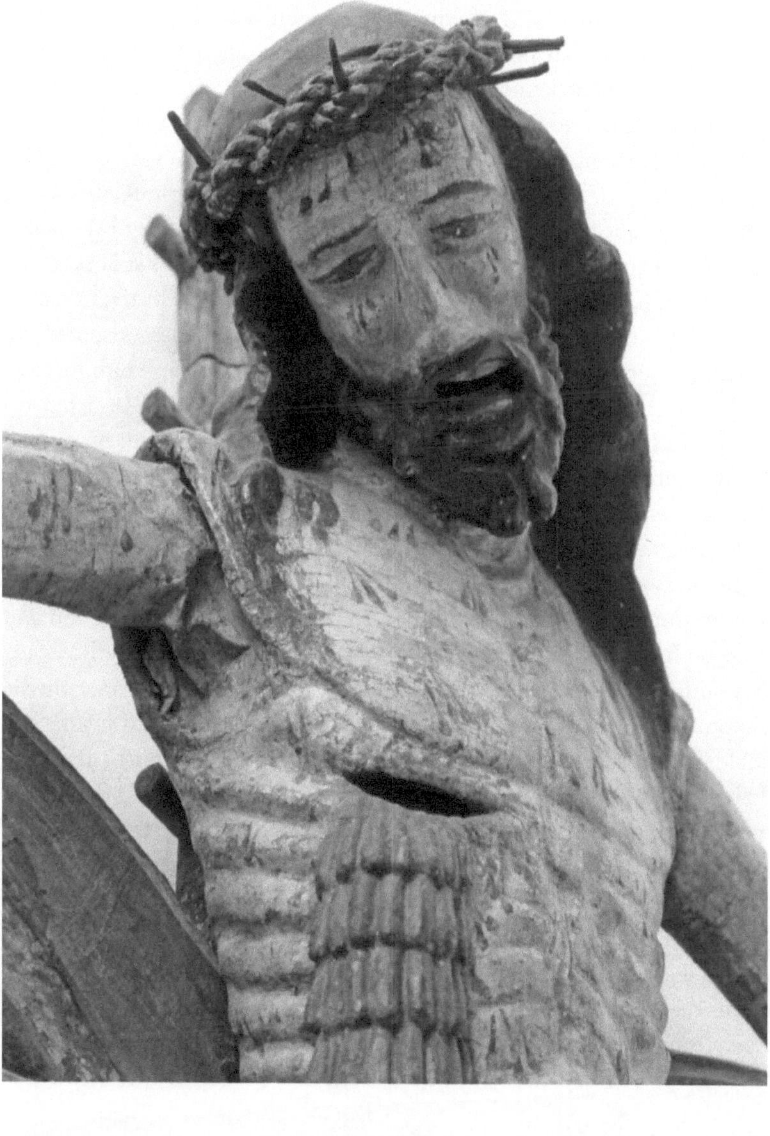

same figure was used to dramatize Christ's ascension to heaven forty days later, when a rope was attached to a metal ring in the head of the sculpture, by means of which it was pulled up through a hole in the vaulting of the church. Once the sculpture had disappeared through the hole, roses, lilies, Eucharistic Hosts, and sometimes – much to the chagrin of the less theatrically minded – a burning devil rained down from the hole onto the congregation.

The crucifix with movable arms, the Palm Sunday ass, and the Resurrection figure are all mobile in the sense that they can be made to move; they cannot move independently. This the three sculptures have in common. But insofar as the crucifix represents the dead Christ, its movements differ from those of the other two. When the Palm Sunday ass was rolled through the streets of town and when the Resurrection figure was hoisted up through a hole in the vaulting of the church, the fiction was that they were moving of their own accord or, at least, not by virtue of any human intervention. By contrast, when the crucifix with movable arms was taken down from the cross and its arms were laid by its sides, the fiction (and the fact) was that it had no volition whatsoever. This difference determined how the various movable sculptures were handled. With the help of ropes, wheels, and pulleys, the ass and the Resurrection figure were put into motion from a distance great enough to dissociate the mover from the moved. Because the fact of the crucifix's stillness coincided with its fiction, it could, by contrast, be handled directly; in fact, it had to be handled directly since it was its handler who demonstrated the crucifix's motionless passivity. Instead of setting the sculpture into motion, as did the manipulations of the Palm Sunday ass and the Resurrection figure, the handling of the crucifix heightened the impression of its dead passivity; and it was from this passivity that the object's allegorical function derived.

Calling the image dead or simply pointing to its inability to do what the living do was perhaps the central trope of late medieval and early modern iconoclasm. In the period leading up to the Protestant Reformation and then with renewed vigor during it, iconoclasts paired the words "dead" and "image" to impress upon their readers just how utterly not alive a sculpture or painting could be. To call the image dead was to invoke the Bible, where the trope appears in Jeremiah's condemnation of Babylon: "Their gods of wood, overlaid with gold and silver, are like a thornbush in a garden on which every bird perches; or like a corpse thrown out in the darkness" (Jer. 6:71). The idea also recurs throughout the Wisdom of Solomon: "[M]iserable, with their hopes set on dead things, are those who give the name 'gods' to the works of human hands" (Wisd. of Sol. 13:10). As old as the Bible, if not much older, the phrase "dead image" and the taunts that reveal the image's corpselike immobility had considerable currency toward the end of the Middle Ages. Whether a person employed them or not, everyone would have been conversant in them, and few would have been able to see the image buried on Good Friday without hearing an echo of this iconoclastic trope.

For Benjamin, the idol is second only to the corpse in its allegorical function: "It is ... no accident that the Middle Ages and the baroque took pleasure in the meaningful juxtaposition of statues of idols and the bones of the dead."[28] The Good Friday effigy is just such a juxtaposition, idol and corpse all in one. Doubly dead, it represents the dead Christ, while it also makes a point of revealing itself to be what iconoclasts liked to call a "dead image." Not suprisingly, it was the iconoclasts who recognized this double deadness most clearly. In the Deposition Rite's insistence on the deadness of its historical character, iconoclasts saw a humiliating spectacle of the deadness of the *image*. Writing critically about Catholic ritual in 1534, Sebastian Franck mocks the Deposition Rite: "[O]n Good Friday before Easter one carries a crucifix around in a procession and lays a great dead man-image [*eyen gross gestorben Menschen-Bild*] in a grave."[29] Franck positions himself outside the belief system that gives meaning to the liturgy's gestures and words: "As if I were a heathen, I was greatly astonished by the Christian folly."[30] Describing the ritual at face value, he reveals how inadequate its clunky maneuvers are to the task of representing the mystery of Christ's death and sacrifice, how ugly and silly its objects and gestures are in comparison with what they are meant to represent. Franck's rhetorical strategy capitalizes on the self-evidence of this disparity; he need only describe the proceedings, or so he makes it seem; their inadequacy speaks for itself.

But the ease with which Franck reveals the Deposition Rite to be theater – and bad theater at that – is not to be credited to his rhetorical skill alone. Before Franck recorded it, the Rite had already declared the paltriness of its means so as to open a gap beween what it says and what it signifies – the gap on which allegory depends. This gap permitted the burial of the image to represent the historical event of Christ's human death, while still calling to mind the ongoing presence of the *imago Dei* at the right hand of God the Father in heaven, beyond the reach of the human senses, incapable of being seen, much less pictured in wood and stone. No one who performed or watched the late medieval Deposition Rite is likely to have described it as a comment on the status of the sacred image, but few would have disagreed that it was an *image* of Christ rather than the man himself that reposed in the grave for forty hours each year. By invoking the trope of the "dead image," the Deposition Rite put the "deadness" of the image on display – renouncing the image under the guise of burial in order to better point the way to the real thing.

The renunciation of the image on Good Friday permitted Christ to go on living as the immortal and incorruptible God, while some*thing* held his place for forty hours in the grave, and it protected the invisible God from prying eyes seeking an image where there is none. But to invoke the trope of the "dead image" was to join ranks with the iconoclasts; or, perhaps, it was just to agree with those exegetes, including Durandus, who held ritual and its objects to be lifeless stony matter: "Whatever belongs to the liturgical offices, objects, and furnishings of the Church is full of signs of the divine and the sacred mysteries, and each of them overflows with a celestial sweetness when it is encountered by a diligent observer who can extract *honey from rock and oil from the stoniest ground* [Deut. 32:13]."[31] The allegorical function of the crucifix with movable arms was not exactly iconoclastic, then, but it was close – its purpose being to remind the viewer, as Durandus does, of the difference between rock and honey.

THE BAROQUE EXPOSITION GRAVE

The desire to remember the immortal body even in the depths of the darkness of Good Friday led to a new use for the Host in the last decades of the fifteenth century. It was around this time that Hosts began to be *displayed* on or near the Good Friday sepulcher. Some sepulchers were constructed with a built-in tabernacle, in which the Host could be made visible while the image was hidden in the grave.[32] Where sepulchers lacked built-in tabernacles, a monstrance could be used instead. This trend became even more pronounced in the wake of the Protestant Reformation and the Catholic response to it.[33] It was then that the Host moved to the center of the Good Friday celebrations and became the focus of the new exposition grave, much to the detriment of attention to the effigy itself. This turn to the Host on Good Friday reflected a preference for the real presence of the sacrament over the image and was in keeping with the Council of Trent's assertion that the Host was literally the body of Christ and not the mere symbol that some Protestants held it to be.

An elaborate theatrical ensemble devoted to glorifying the Eucharistic Host, the new exposition grave replaced the more modest sepulcher used in the medieval Deposition and Elevation Rites. This shift in form reflected a change in function. During the Reformation, the paraliturgical rites performed on Good Friday through Easter Sunday, including the Deposition Rite, fell out of favor – although they would never completely disappear. Protestants tended to reject them along with other quasi-dramatic aspects of the Catholic liturgy, and the Counter-Reformation looked unfavorably on them as well. The Council of Trent banned the singing of "tropes," those musical and textual additions to the liturgy that were integral to the paraliturgical rites. And the *Missale Romanum* of 1570 pointedly ignored the paraliturgical rites.[34] At the same time, a new sacred theater began to emerge, quickly becoming an organ for Catholic propaganda. After initial skepticism, the Jesuits took the lead in developing this theater and in promoting the exposition grave as part of it.[35] (On the Jesuits, theater, and an appeal to the senses, see the introduction to this volume by Hall.)

The Jesuits probably began commissioning exposition graves in the 1550s.[36] By 1580, the Jesuits of Munich had incorporated the exposition of the Host into their Holy Sepulcher celebrations. And by the turn of the century, exposition graves had spread to most areas where the Jesuits were active.[37] In 1628, Philipp Hainhofer reported on visiting nine exposition graves in Innsbruck alone.[38] Vienna had more than thirty in the seventeenth century.[39] By 1728, Munich had somewhere on the order of twenty-seven.[40] Exposition graves were built through most of the eighteenth century, before Enlightenment disdain for theatrical church displays brought the period of their widespread use to an end.[41]

With the Host at its center, the exposition grave was essentially an oversized tabernacle. Alessandro Galli-Bibiena's austere design is one of the clearest expressions of this (Illustration 74). But baroque exposition graves took many forms, including banners, stage sets made of painted canvas flats, and full-scale temporary architectural structures adorned with lights and mechanized figures that transformed the high altar into a vision of lofty spaces extending up as far as heaven. Many exposition graves had moving parts; one such grave, built in Prague in 1570, was equipped with angels that circled the monstrance, bowing as they moved in front of it.[42] In an account of his pilgrimage to Rome in 1575, Johann Jakob Rabus marvels over the movement of one of the several exposition graves he saw there:

> The whole church of the Order of the Jesuits in the Collegio Romano, named S. Maria della Strada, was covered with beautiful tapestries. High above swayed large angels made out of paper and paints in such a way that one might have thought they were alive. They leaned as if subservient spirits toward the most Holy Sacrament, which stood above in the heights. At the very top was a machine of the celestial spheres filled all around on the inside with little lights. These shone very prettily through several silver stars and also the sun and moon; the larger and smaller stars were different from one another. Also, the planets and the corpus [Christi] moved by means of a hidden weight; all of this moved the pilgrims to a great, inexpressible joy and grace.[43]

Not only does Rabus fail to mention the dead effigy – assuming there was one – he places all his descriptive emphasis on liveliness and movement: the movement of the angels, the mechanized celestial orbs, and the "corpus" itself, all of which "moved" the pilgrims in turn. The stillness and sadness of death play no role whatsoever in the spectacle Rabus describes.

Although effigies of the dead Christ had a place in baroque sepulchers, they were less prominently displayed than the Hosts that swayed high above them. Nor was the sepulcher any longer simply the setting for the ceremonies directly associated with the effigy, including the Deposition and Elevation Rites. It had become the stage for a whole series of dramatic and musical events stretching from Palm Sunday to Ascension Day. On

Maundy Thursday, for example, the exposition grave might serve as the setting for a performance of the Last Supper and Christ in the Garden of Gethsemane.[44] Although the Deposition Rite continued to be performed in some places, it rarely seems to have involved placing the effigy in a closed structure. Instead, the effigy was laid out on an open bier below the monstrance as part of the exposition grave. Gone was the central gesture of the medieval rite: the removal of the abject and immobile image from view.

Largely gone as well was the darkness associated with Good Friday. Although the church itself might be darkened, exposition graves and particularly the Hosts at their center were spectacularly lit. Hundreds of glass vessels filled with colored water were placed in front of candles and oil lamps surrounding the effigy. Lights illuminating the Host were strategically hidden behind and between canvas flats, so that the Host appeared to glow like a celestial body.[45] In comparison with these baroque ensembles, the late medieval sepulchers, even with their candles, cloths, and painted chests, were relatively modest affairs, and they certainly made none of the baroque claims to lead the gaze to celestial heights. On the contrary, their primary function was to chasten the sense of sight by demonstratively removing a "dead image" from view. It was through this chastening effect that the medieval sepulcher performed its allegorical function of elevating the soul – rather than the gaze – above the earth.

Darkness, mourning, and the hiddenness of the motionless image of a dead body gave way in the late sixteenth century to light, celebration, and a vision of the magically animated living body of Christ, leaving hardly a trace on Good Friday of the death that precedes the Resurrection. The baroque conversion of the sepulcher into a spectacular sensuous display was not without its detractors. In a 1679 treatise on the Host, Jean Baptiste Thiers writes disapprovingly of the display of the Host during the *Triduum sacrum*: "Of all the expositions of the uncovered Holy Sacrament in use in our century, there is none that is more universally condemned than that one performed in certain churches on Holy Thursday, Friday, and Saturday."[46] Thiers goes on to list dozens of examples of churches in which the Host is properly hidden during the *Triduum*, preferably under lock and key. He then poses a rhetorical question: "For finally what relation is there between the sadness of these three days and the joy that should be inseparable from the divine Eucharist displayed on our altars? Between darkness and the splendor of our Father?"[47]

Despite objections like this one, exposition graves continued to display and celebrate the Hosts at their center well into the eighteenth century. Johann Anton Gumpp's 1691 design for the exposition grave in the Theatine Church in Munich – here reproduced in an engraving by Michael Hartwanger – shows a sculpture of Abraham's sacrifice of his son, an Old Testament prefiguration of Christ's sacrifice on the cross

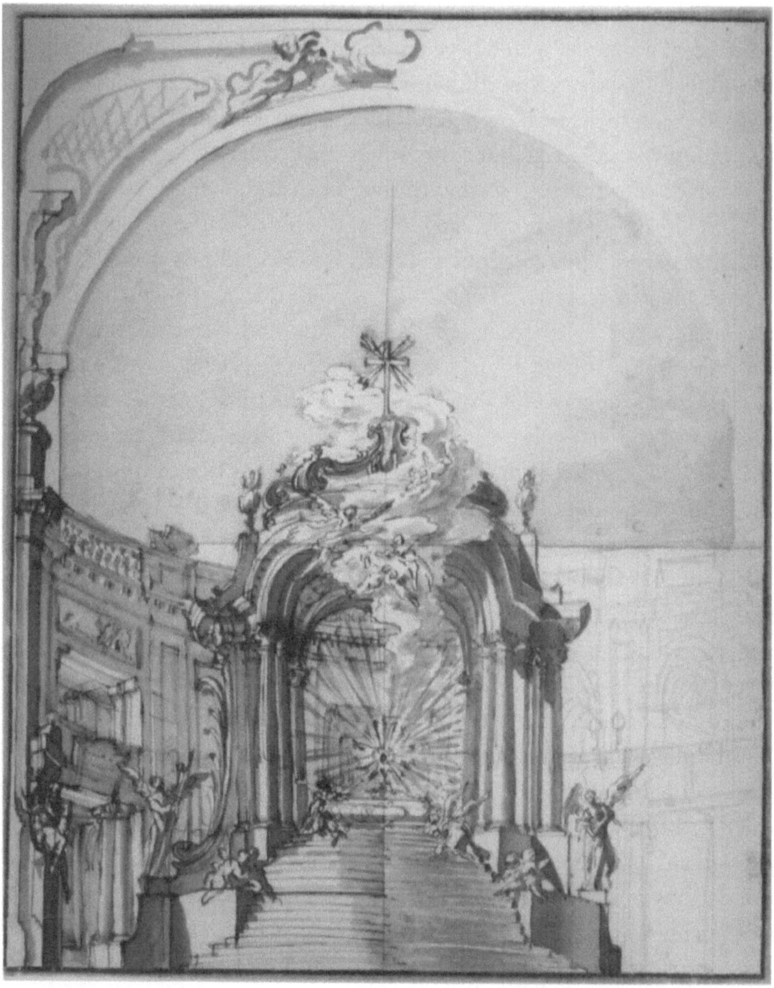

74. Alessandro Galli-Bibiena, *Design for an Exposition Grave.* Pen and wash on paper. Munich, Staatliche Graphische Sammlung München. Photo: Staatliche Graphische Sammlung München.

(Illustration 75). An extant record of payment for an exposition grave following Gumpp's design informs us that while the foremost columns of the arch and the platform supporting the sculpture were built in three dimensions, the rest of the architectural and sculptural decorations were painted on canvas flats placed one in front of another to create the illusion of deep space, including a vista opening onto Golgotha, where three crosses are faintly visible. On Good Friday, the Abraham and Isaac sculpture was replaced with the effigy of Christ on a bier, which was removed in turn on Easter to signal the Resurrection. (The sculptures were made by Andreas Faistenberger in wood with Venetian glass for the eyes and real cloth for the drapery.)[48]

The changing of sculptures according to the days of Holy Week was a common feature of exposition graves. But the central element of Gumpp's ensemble – the Host in a monstrance surrounded by a corona of light and worshipping angels – would have remained unchanged. Perfectly framed by the coffered vault, which springs from an elaborate entablature supported by twisted columns, a real Host in a real monstrance would have hung in front of Gumpp's stage-set architecture.[49] Sebastian Sailer, writing in the mid–eighteenth century, suggests that this rather than the effigy was the object of adoration: "Do we not see in most of the temples of our Christendom the most glorious presentations, in which art and costliness sparkle? ... They are illuminated with lamps and candles. The Holy Sacrament, as the true and living body of Christ, is displayed in the most beautiful monstrances for public adoration."[50] Equally unaffected by the changing of sculptures at the base of the ensemble was the image at the top: God the Father with one arm raised in a gesture of banishment, the other resting on the orb of the world. To his left is the expulsion of Adam and Eve from paradise, to his right the casting out of the rebel angels – the very events, according to Gregory, that set the allegorical machine into motion.

Gumpp's exposition grave pictures an apotheosis that connects the real architecture of the church, which it resembles, to the heavenly realm above.[51] The glowing sun that crowns the arch of stars above God's head resembles the light-emanating Host below it. The heavenly light above the architectural frame, thereby, finds its double beneath the vault, within the illusionistic space that merges with the real space occupied by the viewer. This doubling allows the Host to do its work of reversing the consequences of human and angelic disobedience. The Fall – here represented by humans and angels driven to the edge of an impossibly tall arch from which they are bound to plummet – is reversed by the gentle ascension of the angel-borne monstrance. This reversal includes the sublimation of death, that frightened and frightening skeleton shadowing Adam and Eve. But in what sense is death undone here?

The sacrificed body of Christ *in the form of the Host* is being taken up again to its heavenly abode, and along with it must eventually disappear the death that afflicts humankind. The fabulous animation of this sacramental machine, with its writhing figures, flickering lights, and twisting columns, guarantees that the imminent downward motion of the panicked figures – traced in the lance used to cast out Lucifer's rebel angels – will be recuperated by an upward movement along the central axis that connects the sacrificial victim (whether Isaac or Christ) to the Host, God the Father, and the sun. But the gap, the great, white, empty opening onto the sky above Golgotha, interrupts this otherwise unimpeded sublimation of death, marking the ineradicable difference between below and above, rock and honey, signifier and signified, enigma and truth, what one knows through the senses and what one can only imagine. Although the Host – that incorporeal corporeal thing – may pass through the invisible barrier between heaven and earth, according to the laws of allegory, the effigy cannot.

Andreas Wolff's 1689 design for the exposition grave in the Frauenkirche in Munich makes this distinction between below and above still clearer (Illustration 76). Wolff consigns the allegorical figures of Death, Sin (in the guise of Cupid), and the Devil to the decorative surface of the sarcophagus at the bottom of the scene. Here they appear defeated and bound – bound to one another and hopelessly entangled in the drapery and swags of

75. Johann Anton Gumpp, *Holy Sepulcher in the Theatine Church, Munich*. From engraving by Michael Hartwanger (1691). Photo: Bayerische Staatsbibliothek, Munich.

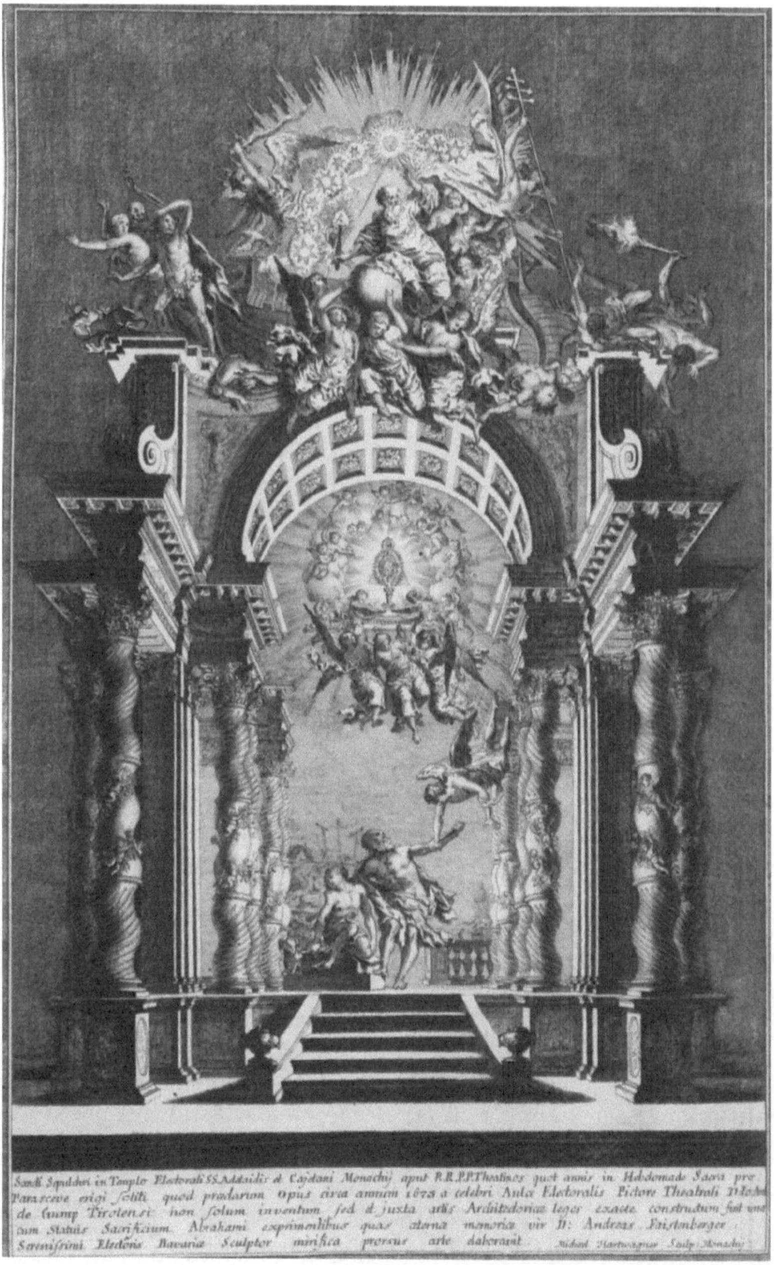

greenery together with which they form a decorative whole. As if to show that death is built into the very architecture of this allegorical machine, each column capital is decorated with a death's-head framed by volutes. Above the body, the monstrance, and the two angels carrying the cross, God the Father holds the orb of the world and indicates the scene of original sin pictured on it. This is how the death that now cowers beneath Christ's sacrificial body – a body fit to fuel the machine of allegory but not to be elevated by it – entered the world.

CONCLUSION

If the late medieval Deposition Rite reminded viewers of the invisibility of God, chastening the sense of sight by ceremonially removing a "dead image" from view, the baroque exposition grave offered an unmitigated spectacle of apotheosis, turning the vigil at the sepulcher into a period of Eucharistic devotion marked by the uninterrupted display of the Host and all the pomp befitting it. But the baroque exposition grave demanded, in the end, an act of renunciation no less rigorous than the medieval burial of the image. In its massive overgrowth of historical and allegorical figures, its bombastic architectural setting, and its subordination of the effigy to a wafer too small to be seen, the baroque Good Friday scenography elaborates the stuff of allegory for the sake of turning against it. When allegory returns to redeem, it turns away from its idols and its corpses, and the Host, whose appearance says nothing of its essence, leaves all this sensuous pomp and circumstance behind.

To mark the difference between the Real Presence of Christ in the sacrament and his merely symbolic representation in the image, Wolff places the effigy in the earthbound space of the proscenium at the bottom of the scene. Too freighted with original sin to ascend, the image is nonetheless the very foundation of the exposition grave – without it the machine of allegory could not get the viewer, fallen as he or she is, off the ground. Benjamin describes the crucial moment of the dialectic of allegory as a violent about-face in the depths of melancholic meditation, the moment when all the sensuous words and images to which the melancholic has attached himself or herself are given up as so much allegory, as so much self-delusion, for the sake of redemption.[52]

This renunciation at the bottom of allegory entails the loss of everything material but most tellingly the loss of those abject things that seemed in their baseness the least likely to deceive: "And this is the essence of melancholy immersion: that its ultimate objects, in which it believes it can most fully secure for itself that which is vile, turn into allegories, and that these allegories fill out and deny the void in which they are represented, just as ultimately, the [allegorical] intention does not faithfully rest in the contemplation of bones, but faithlessly leaps forward to the idea of

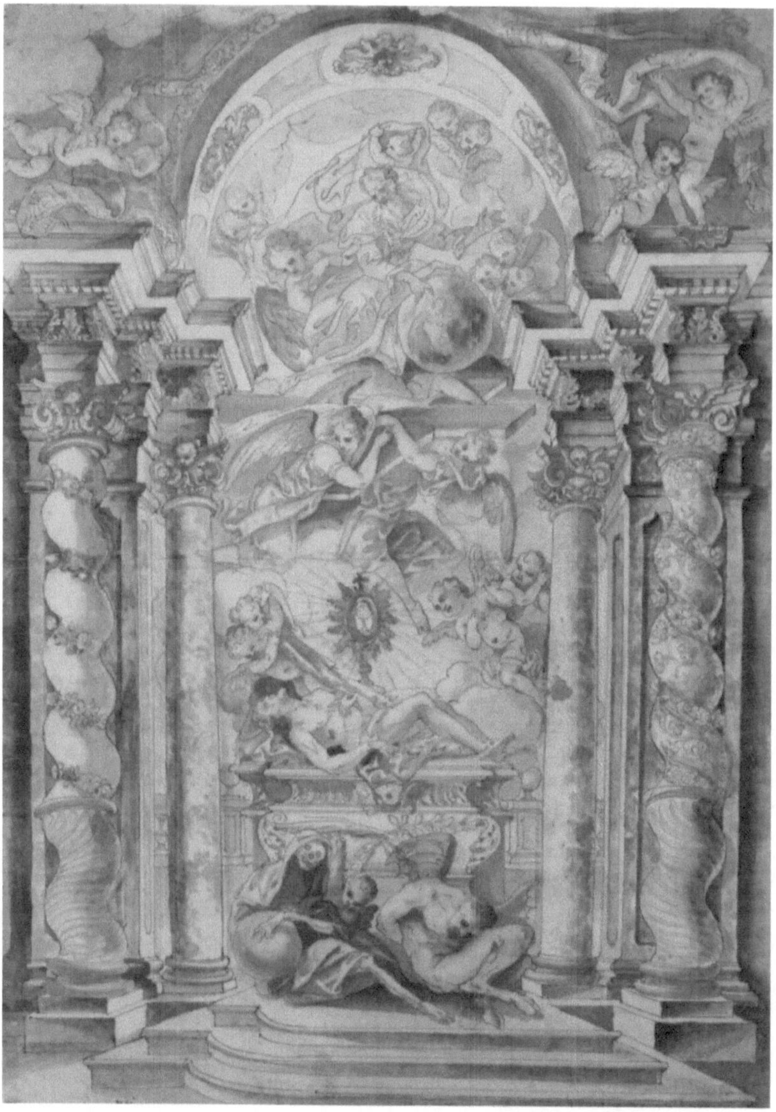

76. Johann Andreas Wolff, *Design for an Exposition Grave*. Ink and watercolor on paper. Munich, Staatliche Graphische Sammlung München. Photo: Staatliche Graphische Sammlung München.

resurrection."[53] By already diverting attention from the corpse to the Host on Good Friday, the baroque exposition grave made precisely this leap from bones to Resurrection.

The *imago Dei* would ascend to heaven and the soul might manage to ride its coattails, but the effigy – the image made by human hands – had to be left behind as so much unredeemed matter. "In allegory the observer is confronted with the *facies hippocratica* of history as a petrified, primordial landscape. Everything about history that, from the very beginning, has been untimely, sorrowful, unsuccessful, is expressed in a face – or rather in a death's head."[54] In the medieval burial of the "dead image" *and* in the baroque subordination of the effigy to the Eucharistic Host, the petrified landscape of ritual and ritual objects was confronted *in order to be renounced.* According to the thoroughly theological logic of allegory, to turn away from the effigy in this manner was – strange as it may seem – to stare death in the face, neither the death of a god nor one's own personal death, but rather the still stranger death's-head of the sensuous material present.

Notes

1 "O mors, mors vitae, si mors, non vita vocanda / (Quod praestat vitam, non ausim dicere mortem." Traube (1881), 3: 543.
2 "Postquam a paradisi gaudiis expulsum est genus humanum, in istam peregrinationem uitae praesentis ueniens caecum cor ab spiritali intellectu habet.... Idcirco per quaedam enigmata sermo diuinus animae torpenti et frigidae loquitur et de rebus, quas nouit, latenter insinuat ei amorem, quem non nouit." Gregory I (1984), 68.
3 Benjamin (1998), 217–18. Benjamin's theory of baroque allegory is based on readings of Protestant mourning plays. But baroque allegory cuts across denominational lines, and Benjamin's theory of it reveals a good deal about Catholic baroque aesthetics.
4 "Interpositis quippe enigmatibus, dum quiddam in uerbis cognoscit, quod suum est, in sensu uerborum intellegit, quod non est suum, et per terrena uerba serparatur a terra." Gregory I (1984), 70.
5 Benjamin (1998), 232.
6 On the differences between the medieval and baroque Good Friday celebrations, see Jezler (1983), 236–49.
7 Symons (1953), 44–45.
8 Manuals from Brixen dating to 1494 and c. 1553 describe both aspersion and censing. Taubert and Taubert (1969), 106, 108; Gschwend (1965), 95.
9 For an overview of sepulcher types, see N. Brooks (1921), 59–66; Sheingorn (1978); Ogden (2002), 25–68; Kroesen and Steensma (2004), 290–303.
10 Symons (1953), 45.
11 Young (1962), 1: 173.
12 For an example of lay participation, see Sacristy Manual of the Cathedral of Brixen in Lipphardt (1975), 6: 122. For a discussion of such participation, see Maisel (2002), 81–82.
13 On the *Tenebrae* service, see Young (1962), 1: 101; Scribner (1987), 26–27; Harper (1991), 141–42; Dupeux, Jezler, and Wirth (2000), 230–31.
14 "Hac die in Ecclesia luminaria non accenduntur, quia in ipso Redemptore crucifixo sidera obscurabantur." Rabanus Maurus, "De clericorum Institutione libri tres," in *Patrologia Latina* (1996), 107: 349A.
15 From *Rites of Durham, being a Description or Brief Declaration of all the Ancient Monuments, Rites and Customs belonging or being within the Monastical Church of Durham before the Suppression. Written 1593*, as transcribed in Young (1962), 1: 138.
16 Warning (2001), 14–22, 36.
17 On Amalarius's major work, the *Liber officialis*, see Cabaniss (1954), 52–65; Schnusenberg (1988), 193–220.
18 Hardison (1965), 44.
19 Durand (2007), 4.

20 Symons (1953), 36.
21 On the debate between Florus and Amalarius, see, e.g., Warning (2001), 31–39.
22 Warning (2001), 14.
23 The earliest known account of the burial of the Host occurs in the life of St. Udalricus, bishop of Augsburg (d. 973), written within about twenty years of his death. This is close in date to the *Regularis concordia* (c. 970), which contains the earliest instance of the burial of the cross. Young (1920), 17. On the infrequency of Host burial without a crucifix before the sixteenth century, see N. Brooks (1921), 40; Young (1962), 1: 132; Taubert and Taubert (1969), 95, 111–12.
24 For the ceremony at St. Blaise, see Young (1962), 1: 112–13. For the ceremony dictated by the *Use of Sarum*, see Frere (1898), 2: 165–66. For other examples of the Host and crucifix buried together, see Chambers (1903), 2: 21; N. Brooks (1921), 38.
25 "Nam contra omnem rationem est, quod in quibusdam ecclesiis Eucharistia in huiusmodi archa Sepulchrum representante poni consuevit et claudi. Ibi enim Eucharistia, que est verum et vivum Corpus Christi, ipsum Christi Corpus mortuum representat, quod est indecens penitus et absurdum." Leuppi (1995), 254.
26 Taubert and Taubert (1969), 79–121.
27 See, e.g., Haastrup (1987); Jezler (1989); Tripps (1998); Jung (2006).
28 Benjamin (1998), 222.
29 "Am Karfreitag vor Ostern tregt man aber eyn Creütz herumb in eyner Procession, leget eyen gross gestorben Menschen-Bild inn eyn Grab." Franck, fol. 137r.
30 "Ich hab mich als ein heyd der Christen torheit nit gnugsam verwundert." Franck (1534), fol. 137r.
31 Durand (2007), 1; emphasis added.
32 On built-in tabernacles, see Schwarzweber (1940), 63, 71; Kroesen (2000), 68–76, 182.
33 In the *Decreta authentica Congregationis Sacrorum Rituum* (1898–1900), 4: 433, the Catholic Church explains the turn to the Host on Good Friday as a reaction to Protestant attacks on the doctrine of Transubstantiation. Discussed in N. Brooks (1921), 45.
34 On the banning of tropes and their absence from the *Missale Romanum* of 1570, see H. De Boor (1967), 17; Jezler (1983), 240.
35 On the Jesuits' role in promoting the exposition grave, see N. Brooks (1928), 155–58; Grass (1957), 223–26; Jezler (1983), 240; Brossette (2002), 44, 184.
36 Berliner (1955), 32, 181 n. 222; Vetter (1994), 219.
37 Lipowsky (1816), 1: 200; Berliner (1955), 181–83, n. 222.
38 Grass (1957), 226.
39 Brossette (2002), 184.
40 Besch (1983), 196–97, n. 170.
41 On Enlightenment attitudes toward exposition graves, see Grass (1957), 253–57; Gschwend (1965), 135–36; Brossette (2002), 53, 598.
42 Berliner (1955), 182, n. 222.
43 "Die ganz Kirch der Herrn Jesuiter in Collegio Romano, zu S. Maria auf der Strassen genannt, war mit schöner Tapezerei überzogen, oben in der Höh schwebten große Engel, von Papier und Farben dermassen zugerichtet, daß einer hätte meinen mögen, sie lebeten, die neigten sich als dienstbare Geister gegen dem hochheiligen Sacrament; das stund oben in der Höh,

zu oberst droben war ein machina globi coelestis, inwendig mit kleinen Lichtlin umb und umb besteckt, die schienen durch etliche silberin Sternen gar fein samt Sonn und Mon mit Unterschied der größen und kleinern Sternen, item der Planeten und das Corpus moviert sich durch ein heimlich Gewicht, das alles bewegt die Pilgram zu großer unaussprechlicher Freud und Anmut." Rabus (1925), 113.

44 On the use of the exposition grave for many different performances, see Feuchtmayr (1989), 16–18; Brossette (2002), 182–83, 190–92, 204.

45 Besch (1983), 84; Imorde (1999), 108; Brossette (2002), 196.

46 "De toutes les expositions du saint Sacrement à découvert qui sont en usage dans notre siécle, il n'y a en a point qui soit plus universellement condamnée que celle qui se fait en certaines Eglises le jeudi, le Vendredi & le Samedi saint." Thiers (1777), 175.

47 "Car enfin quel rapport y a-t-il entre la tristesse de ces trois jours, & la joie qui doit être inseparable de la divine Eucharistie exposée en evidence sur nos Autels? Entre les tenébres & la splendeur du Pere?" Thiers (1777), 191.

48 For a discussion of Gumpp's exposition graves, see Rittershausen (1788), 133–34; Strieder (1951), 281–87; Besch (1983), 78–80; Wegmann (1985), 251–55.

49 Brossette (2002), 190, n. 86.

50 "Sehen wir nicht in den meisten Tempeln unsers Christenthumes die herrlichsten Vorstellungen, an welchen Kunst und Kostbarkeit glänzen? ... Sie werden mit Lampen und Lichtern beleuchtet. Das hochwürdigste Gut, als der wahre und lebendige Leichnam Christi, ist in den schönsten Schaugefässen zur öffentlichen Anbethung darinn ausgesetzet." Sailer (1997), 215–16.

51 On the relationship between real and fictive architecture in exposition graves, see Feuchtmayr (1989), 50; Vetter (1994), 219; Brossette (2002), 186–87, 190, 194.

52 Benjamin (1998), 166.

53 Benjamin (1998), 232–33.

54 Benjamin (1998), 166.

BIBLIOGRAPHY

Archival Sources

Archivio Segreto Vaticano (ASV)

ASV Cod. Borghese s. II, vols. 51a–52. *Ragionamenti fatti dal Papa in occasione della visita, di mano di sua Santità.*

ASV Cod. Borghese 764, s. II, vol. 3. *Diarorum Jo. Pauli Mucantii Magistri Caerimoniarum ab anno 1594 ad annum 1598.*

ASV Cod. *Borghese 869, s. I, ff. 1–50. Commentarius Visitationis Clementis VIII Anno 1592.*

ASV Misc. Arm. VII, 111. *Acta Sacrae Visitationis Apostolicae S.D.N Urbanus VIII Pars Prima Continet Ecclesias Patriarchales Collegiatas & Parochiales tam Seculares quam Regulares.*

ASV Misc. Arm. VII, vol. 3, ff. 1–98. *Decreta Sant.mi D.ni Clementis Papae Octavi facta in visitatione Ecclesiarum Urbis.*

ASV Misc. Arm. VII, vol. 4, ff. 1–50. *Commentarius Visitationis Clementis VIII Anno 1592.*

Archivio Storico del Vicariato di Roma (ASVR)

ASVR scaff. 64, tom. 38. *Liber Edictorum Tribunalis E.mi at R.mi Cardinalis Vicarii ab anno 1566 usque ad 1607.*

Biblioteca Apostolica Vaticana (BAV)

BAV Urb. Lat. 1060. *Avvisi di Roma 1592.*

BAV Urb. Lat. 1061. *Avvisi di Roma 1593.*

BAV Urb. Lat. 1062. *Avvisi di Roma 1594.*

BAV Urb. Lat. 1063. *Avvisi di Roma 1595.*

BAV Urb. Lat. 1064. *Avvisi di Roma 1596.*

BAV Vat. Lat. 5479. *Commentarius Visitationis Clementis VIII Anno 1592* [Agostino Valier].

BAV Ferraioli 374. Theodoro Ameyden. *Summorum Pontificum, et S.R.E Cardinalium Suo Aevo defunctorum Ad Phillipum Nepotem.*

Printed Sources

Abromson, Morton Colp. 1978. "Clement VIII's Patronage of the Brothers Alberti." *Art Bulletin* 60.3: 531–47.

1981. *Painting in Rome During the Papacy of Clement VIII (1592–1605): A Documented Study*. New York: Garland.

Acta ecclesiae mediolanensis. 1890–96. Vols. 2–4. Ed. Achille Ratti. Milan.

Affò, Ireneo. 1784. *Vita del graziossimo pittore Francesco Mazzola, ditto il Parmigianino*. Parma: Filippo Carmignani.

Agoston, Laura. 2006. "Michelangelo as Voice versus Michelangelo as Text." *Journal of Medieval and Early Modern Studies* 36: 135–67.

Agricola, Ignatius. 1727–29. *Historia Provinciae Societatis Jesu Germaniae Superioris*, 2 vols. Munich: Typis Mariae Magdalenae Riedlin.

Aikema, Bernard. 1994. "Titian's *Mary Magdalene* in the Palazzo Pitti: An Ambiguous Painting and Its Critics." *Journal of the Warburg and Courtauld Institutes* 57: 48–59.

Albèri, Eugenio, ed. 1857. *Relazioni degli ambasciatori veneti al Senato*, vol. 4.2. Florence: Società editrice fiorentina.

Alberigo, Giuseppe. 1981. "De concile de Trente au tridentisme." *Irenikon* 54: 192–210.

1984. "Carlo Borromeo Between Two Models of Bishop." In *San Carlo Borromeo: Catholic Reform and Ecclesiastical Politics in the Second Half of the Sixteenth Century*. Ed. John M. Headley and John B. Tomaro, 250–63. Washington, DC: Folger Shakespeare Library / London: Associated University Presses.

1988. "The Council of Trent." In *Catholicism in Early Modern History: A Guide to Research*. Ed. John W. O'Malley, 211–26. Saint Louis: Center for Reformation Research, 1988.

Alberti, Leon Battista. 1966. *On Painting* [*De pictura*]. Trans., with intro. and notes, John R. Spencer. New Haven, CT: Yale University Press.

1991. *On Painting*. Trans. Cecil Grayson. London: Penguin Books.

Alberti, Romano. 1585. *Trattato della nobiltà della pittura*. Rome: Zannetti.

1604. *Origine e progresso dell'Academia del Dissegno de' Pittori, Scultori, & Architetti di Roma*. Pavia: Bartoli.

Aldrovandi, Ulisse. 1962. *Avvertimenti del Dottore Aldrovandi all' Ill. mo e R.mo Cardinal Paleotti sopra alcuni capitoli della pittura*. In Barocchi (1960–62), vol. 2.

Alexander, John. 2007. *From Renaissance to Counter-Reformation: The Architectural Patronage of Carlo Borromeo During the Reign of Pius IV*. Milan: Biblioteca Ambrosiana; Rome: Bulzoni.

Ames-Lewis, Francis, and Anka Bednarek, eds. 1992. *Decorum in Renaissance Narrative Art*. Department of History of Art, Birkbeck College, University of London.

Ammannati, Bartolomeo. 1962. "Lettera agli Accademici del Disegno" [1582]. In Barocchi (1960–62), 3: 117–23.

Andersson, Christiane. 2008. "The Nude in German Art, ca. 1490–1830." In *The Language of the Nude*. Ed. William Breazeale, 128–59. Aldershot: Lund Humphries.

Angelis, Paolo De. 1621. *Basilica S. Mariae Maioris de Urbe a Liberio Papa I usque ad Paulum V Pont. Max Descriptio et Delineato*. Rome: Bartholomaei Zanetti.

Annali della Fabbrica del Duomo di Milano. 1877–1885. 9 vols. Milan: Libreria editrice G. Brigola.

Antinori, Aloisi. 1997. "La cantoria con organo di Alessandro VI e la 'Capella del S. Pietro di Bronzo.' " In *L'architetture della Basilica di San Pietro. Storia e costruzione*. Ed. G. Spagnesi, 129–36. Rome: Boncompagni.

Antoniano, Silvio. 1926. *Dell'educazione cristiana e politica dei figlioli libri tre*. Ed. L. Pogliani. Turin: Paravia.

Arditi, Jorge. 1998. *A Genealogy of Manners: Transformations of Social Relations in France and England from the Fourteenth to the Eighteenth Century*. Chicago: University of Chicago Press.

Aston, Margaret. 1990. "Segregation in Church." In *Women in the Church*. Ed. W. J. Sheils and D. Wood, 242–81. Oxford: Oxford University Press.

Attridge, Derek. 1986. "Puttenham's Perplexity: Nature, Art, and the Supplement in Renaissance Poetic Theory." In *Literary Theory / Renaissance Texts*. Ed. Patricia Parker and David Quint, 257–79. Baltimore: Johns Hopkins University Press.

Augustine of Hippo. 1997. *Confessions*. Trans. Maria Boulding, O.S.B., ed. John E. Rotelle, O.S.A. Hyde Park, NY: New City Press.

Bacci, Francesca, and David Melcher, eds. 2011. *Art and the Senses*. Oxford: Oxford University Press.

Bacci, Pietro Giocomo. 1837. *Vita di San Filippo Neri*. Rome: Tip. Marini. First published Rome: per Giacomo Mascardi, 1622.

Bagley, C. H. 1967. "Litany of Loreto." In *New Catholic Encyclopedia*. New York: McGraw-Hill.

Baglione, Giovanni. *1995. Le vite de' pittori, scultori et architetti dal pontificato di Gregorio XIII del 1572 in fino a' tempi di Papa Urbano Ottavo nel 1642,* 3 vols. Ed. Jacob Hess and Herwarth Röttgen. Vatican City: Biblioteca apostolica vaticana.

Bailey, Gauvin Alexander. 1999a. *Art on the Jesuit Missions in Asia and Latin America, 1540–1773*. Toronto: University of Toronto Press.

1999b. " 'Le Style Jésuite N'existe Pas': Jesuit Corporate Culture and the Visual Arts." In O'Malley (1999b), 38–89.

1999c. "The Jesuits and Painting in Italy, 1550–1690: The Art of Catholic Reform." In Mormando (1999), 151–78.

2003. *Between Renaissance and Baroque: Jesuit Art in Rome, 1565–1610*. Toronto: University of Toronto Press.

Bakhtin, Mikhail. 1984. *Rabelais and His World*. Trans. Hélène Iswolsky. Bloomington: Indiana University Press.

Balde, Jacob, S.J. 1990. *Opera Poetica Omnia*, 8 vols. Ed. Wilhelm Kühlmann and Hermann Wiegand. Frankfurt: Keip.

Baldinucci, Filippo. 1974–75. *Notizie dei professori del disegno da Cimabue in qua*, vol. 3. Ed. Fernando Ranalli and Paola Barocchi. Florence: SPES.

Barasch, Moshe. 1975. "Character and Physiognomy: Bocchi on Donatello's *St George*, a Renaissance Text on Expression in Art." *Journal of the History of Ideas* 36: 413–30.

Barbieri, Costanza. 1995. " '*Invisibilia per visibilia*': S. Filippo Neri, le immagini e la contemplazione." In Strinati and Costamagna (1995), 32–67.

Barbieri, Costanza, Sofia Barchiesi, and Daniele Ferrara. 1995. *Santa Maria in Vallicella. Chiesa Nuova*. Rome: Palombi.

Barchiesi, Sofia. 1995. "S. Filippo Neri e l'iconografia mariana della Chiesa Nuova." In Strinati and Costamagna (1995), 130–49.

Barnes, Bernardine. 1997. "Aretino, the Public, and the Censorship of Michelangelo's *Last Judgment*." In *Suspended License: Censorship and the Visual*

Arts. Ed. Elizabeth C. Childs, 59–84. Seattle: University of Washington Press, 1997.

1998. *Michelangelo's Last Judgment: The Renaissance Response*. Berkeley: University of California Press.

Barocchi, Paola, ed. 1960–62. *Trattati d'Arte del Cinquecento, fra manierismo e Controriforma*, 3 vols. Bari: Laterza.

Baronio, Cesare. 1968. *Documenti per la storia dell'Architettura a Milano nel Rinascimento e nel Barocco*, vol. 2. Rome: Accademia Nazionale dei Lincei.

Baronius, Cesare. 1588–1607. *Annales Ecclesiastici*, 12 vols. Rome: Ex Typographia Congregationis Oratorij apud S. Mariam in Vallicella.

Barzman, Karen-Edis. 2000. *The Florentine Academy and the Early Modern State: The Discipline of Disegno*. Cambridge: Cambridge University Press.

Bascapé, Giacomo Carlo. 1983. *Vita e opere di Carlo arcivescovo di Milano Cardinale di S. Prassede*. Ed. Angelo Majo. Milan: NED.

Bätschmann, Oskar. 1992. "De Lumine et Colore. Der Maler Nicolas Poussin in seinen Bildern." In *Der Künstler über sich in seinem Werk. Internationales Symposium der Bibliotheca Hertziana, Rom 1998*. Ed. Matthias Winner, 463–83. Weinheim: VCH, Acta Humaniora.

Battaglia, Salvatore. 1964. *Grande Dizionario della lingua italiana*, vol. 3. Turin: UTET.

Bauer, George. 1987. "Experimental Shadow Casting and the Early History of Perspective." *Art Bulletin* 69.2: 211–19.

Baumstark, Reinhold, ed. 1997. *Rom in Bayern. Kunst und Spiritualität der ersten Jesuiten*. Exh. cat., Bayerisches Nationalmuseum, Munich. Munich: Hirmer.

Baxandall, Michael. 1971. *Giotto and the Orators: Humanist Observers of Painting in Italy and the Discovery of Pictorial Composition, 1350–1450*. Oxford: Clarendon Press.

1972. *Painting and Experience in Fifteenth Century Italy: A Primer in the Social History of Pictorial Style*. Oxford: Clarendon Press.

1995. *Shadows and Enlightenment*. New Haven, CT: Yale University Press.

Beggiao, Diego 1978. *La visita pastorale di Clemente VIII (1592–1600). Aspetti di riforma post-tridentina a Roma*. Rome: Libreria Editrice della Pontificia Università Lateranense.

Begheyn, Paul. 2001. "The Collection of Copperplates by Members of the Wierix Family in the Jesuit Church 'De Krijtberg' in Amsterdam." *Quaerendo* 31: 192–204.

Beissel, Stephan. 1910. *Die Geschichte der Verehung Marias in Deutschland während des Mittelalters*. Freiburg: Herder.

Bell, Janis. 1995. "Light and Color in Caravaggio's *Supper at Emmaus*." *Artibus et Historiae* 16.31: 139–70.

2003. "Zaccolini's Unpublished Perspective Treatise: Why Should We Care?" In *The Treatise on Perspective: Published and Unpublished*. Ed. Lyle Massey, 79–103. Studies in the History of Art 59, Center for Advanced Study in the Visual Arts. Washington, DC: National Gallery of Art / New Haven, CT: Yale University Press.

Bellori, Giovanni Pietro. 2005. *The Lives of the Modern Painters, Sculptors and Architects* [1672]. Trans. Alice Sedgwick Wohl. Cambridge: Cambridge University Press.

Belting, Hans. 1994. *Likeness and Presence: A History of the Image before the Era of Art.* Trans. Edmund Jephcott. Chicago: University of Chicago Press. Originially published as *Bild und Kult. Eine Geschichte des Bildes vor dem Zeitalter der Kunst.* Munich: C. H. Beck, 1990.

1998. "In Search of Christ's Body: Image or Imprint?" In *The Holy Face and the Paradox of Representation.* Ed. Herbert L. Kessler and Gerhard Wolf, 1–11. Villa Spelman Colloquia, vol. 6. Bologna: Nuova Alfa.

Benjamin, Walter. 1998. *The Origin of German Tragic Drama.* Trans. John Osborne. London: Verso. Originally published as *Ursprung des deutschen Trauerspiels.* Berlin: Ernst Rowohlt, 1928.

Bente, Martin, et al. 1989. *Kataloge Bayerischer Musiksammlungen* 5.1. Bayerische Staatsbibliothek: Chorbücher und Handschriften in chorbuchartiger Notierung. Munich: Henle.

Berliner, Rudolf. 1955. *Die Weihnachtskrippe.* Munich: Prestel.

Besch, Ulrike. 1983. *Studien zur Ausstattung von St. Kajetan in München. Ein Beitrag zur Funktion ephemerer Systemelemente in der Kunst des Barock.* Munich: Starnberg.

Beumer, Johannes. 1971. "Die Geschäftsordnung des Trienter Konzils." *Franziskanische Studien* 53: 289–306.

Biancani, Stefania. 1997. "La censura del nudo nel discorso di Paleotti e nella trattistica post-tridentina a Bologna." In *Bartolomeo Cesi e l'affresco dei canonici lateranesi,* ed. Vera Fortunati and Vincenzo Musumeci, 204–15. Fiesole: Nardini.

Bianchi, Ilaria. 2008. *La politica delle immagini nell'età della Controriforma. Gabriele Paleotti teorico e committente.* Bologna: Compositori.

Bireley, Robert. 1999. *The Refashioning of Catholicism, 1450–1700.* Washington, DC: Catholic University of America Press.

Bjurström, Per. 1972. "Baroque Theater and the Jesuits." In Wittkower and Jaffe (1972), 99–110.

Bloch, Ariel, and Chana Bloch. 1998. *The Song of Songs: A New Translation.* Berkeley: University of California Press.

Blue Letter Bible, The. 1996–2012. www.blueletterbible.org/.

Blunt, Anthony. 1978. *Artistic Theory in Italy, 1450–1600,* 2d ed. Oxford: Oxford University Press. (Originally published 1940, Clarendon Press; pbk. ed. 1962).

Bocchi, Francesco. 1592. *Opera di M. Francesco Bocchi sopra l'imagine miracolosa della Santissima Nunziata di Fiorenza …* Florence: Sermatelli.

1971. *Le Bellezze della Città di Fiorenza.* Facsimile of 1591 ed. (Florence: Sermatelli). Farnborough: Gregg International.

Bocchi, Francesco, and Giovanni Cinelli. 2004. *Le Bellezze della Città di Firenze.* Bologna: Forni.

Bohlmann, Carolin, et al. 2002. "Die Grenzen des Sichtbaren. Gespräch mit Victor Stoichita über Licht und Schatten in Tintorettos Abendmahl in San Giorgio Maggiore." *Kritische Berichte. Mitteilungsorgan des Ulmer Vereins Verband für Kunst- und Kulturwissenschaften* 30.4: 14–21.

Bonomelli, Marina, ed. 2008. *Milano e la corte di Spagna. Un carteggio inedito di Carlo Borromeo.* Milan: Bulzoni.

Borghini, Raffaello. 1584. *Il Riposo.* Florence: Giorgio Marescotti. 1967 facsimile of 1584 ed., with bibliography and index, 2 vols. Ed. Mario Rosci. Milan: Edizioni Labor.

2007. *Raffaello Borghini's "Il Riposo."* Trans. and ed. Lloyd H. Ellis, Jr. Toronto: University of Toronto Press.

Borromeo, Agostino. 1997. "I vescovi italiani e l'applicazione del Concilio di Trento." In *I tempi del Concilio. Religione, cultura e società nell'Europa tridentina.* Ed. Cesare Mozzarelli and Danilo Zardin, 27–105. Rome: Bulzoni.

Borromeo, Carlo. 1577. *Instructiones fabricae et supellectilis ecclesiasticae.* In Barocchi (1960–62), 3: 1–113.

1962. "Instructiones fabricae et supellectilis ecclesiasticae." In Barocchi (1960–62), 3: 3–113.

1977. "Charles Borromeo's *Instructiones fabricae et supellectilis ecclesiasticae*, 1577, Book I: A Translation with Commentary and Analysis." Trans. Evelyn Carole Voelker, Ph.D. diss., Syracuse University.

2000. *Instructionum fabricae et supellectilis ecclesiasticae, libri II Caroli Borromei (1577).* Ed. M. Marinelli with F. Adorni. Vatican City: Libreria editrice vaticana; Axios Group.

Borromeo, Carlo, and Pietro Galesio. 1582. *Acta Ecclesiae Mediolanensis Tribus Partibus Distincta. Quibus concilia provincialia, conciones, synodales, synodi dioecesanae, instructiones, liteare pastorales, edicta, regualae confratriarum, formuale, et alia denique continentur, quae Carolus S.R.E Cardinali tit. S. Praxedis Arciepiscopus egit.* Milan: Apud Pacificum Pontium.

Borromeo, Federico. 1932. *De pictura sacra* [1624]. Sora: Camastro.

1994. *Della Pittura Sacra. Libri Due.* Ed. Barbara Agosti. Pisa: Scuola normale superiore di Pisa.

2010. *Sacred Painting: Museum.* Ed. and trans. K. S. Rockwell. The i Tatti Renaissance Library 44. Cambridge, MA: Harvard University Press.

Boschloo, Anton W. A. 1974. *Annibale Carracci in Bologna: Visible Reality in Art after the Council of Trent.* Trans. R. R. Symonds. The Hague: Government Publishing Office.

Bottari, Giovanni, ed. 1822. *Raccolta di lettere sulla pittura, scultura ed architettura scritte da' più celebri personaggi del secolo XV, XVI, e XVII,* vol. 3. Milan.

Bouwsma, William. 1990. "The Two Faces of Humanism: Stoicism and Augustinianism in Renaissance Thought." In *Itinerarium Italicum: The Profile of the Italian Renaissance in the Mirror of Its European Transformations*, Ed. Heiko. A. Oberman with Thomas A. Brady, Jr. Leiden: E. J. Brill, 1975. Rpt. in William J. Bouwsma, *A Usable Past: Essays in European Cultural History.* Berkeley: University of California Press.

Braider, Christopher. 1998. "The Fountain of Narcissus: The Invention of Subjectivity and the Pauline Ontology of Art in Caravaggio and Rembrandt." *Comparative Literature* 50.4: 286–315.

Brock, Maurice. 2002. *Bronzino.* Trans. David Poole Radzinowicz and Christine Schultz-Touge. Paris: Flammarion.

Brodrick, James, S.J. 1935. *Saint Peter Canisius, S.J., 1521–1597.* London: Sheed and Ward.

Brooks, Julian. 2007. *Taddeo and Federico Zuccaro: Artist-Brothers in Renaissance Rome.* Exh. cat. Los Angeles: J. Paul Getty Museum, 2007.

Brooks, Neil C. 1921. *The Sepulchre of Christ in Art and Liturgy with Special Reference to the Liturgical Drama.* University of Illinois Studies in Language and Literature, vol. 7.2. Urbana: University of Illinois.

1928. "The *Sepulchrum Christi* and Its Ceremonies in Late Mediaeval and Modern Times." *Journal of English and Germanic Philology* 27: 147–61.

Brossette, Ursula. 2002. *Die Inszenierung des Sakralen. Das theatralische Raum- und Ausstattungsprogramm süddeutscher Barockkirchen in seinem liturgischen und zeremoniellen Kontext.* Weimer: VDG.

Brusatin, Manlio. 1987. "Colori e Passioni: La Luce Oscurata." *Eidos* 1: 26–33.

Bury, Michael. 1987. "The Senarega Chapel in San Lorenzo, Genoa; New Document about Barocci and Francavilla." *Mitteilungen des Kunsthistorischen Institutes in Florenz* 31.2/3: 327–56.

Cabaniss, James Allen. 1954. *Amalarius of Metz.* Amsterdam: North-Holland.

Caciali, Mario. 1997. *Milano, le chiese scomparse*, vol. 1. Milan: Castello sforzesco.

Caglioti, Francesco. 2000. *Donatello e i Medici. Storia del David e della Giuditta.* Florence: L. S. Olschki.

Cameron, Euan. 2004. "Dissent and Heresy." In Hsia (2004), 3–21.

Camille, Michael. 1992. *Images on the Edge: The Margins of Medieval Art.* Cambridge, MA: Harvard University Press.

Campbell, Stephen. 2004. "Bronzino's Martyrdom of Saint Lawrence: Counter Reformation Polemic and Mannerist Counter Aesthetics." *RES* 46 (Polemical Objects, Autumn): 99–121.

2005. "Eros in the Flesh: Petrarchism, the Embodied Eros Male Beauty in Italian Art, 1500–1540." *Journal of Medieval and Early Modern Studies* 35: 629–62.

2006. *The Cabinet of Eros: Renaissance Mythological Painting and the Studiolo of Isabella d'Este.* New Haven, CT: Yale University Press.

Campo, Pedro F., and Peter M. Daly. 2010. *Emblematic Images and Religious Texts: Studies in Honor of G. Richard Dimler, S.J.* Philadelphia: Saint Joseph's University Press.

Canisius, Peter. 1933. *Maria. Die unvergleichliche Jungfrau und hochheilige Gottesgebärerin.* Trans. Karl Telch. Warnsdorf: Opitz.

Canons and Decrees of the Council of Trent. 1978. Trans. Henry Joseph Schroeder, O.P. London: Herder, 1941. 2d ed. 1950. Rpt. Rockford, IL: Tan Books.

Canons and Decrees of the Sacred and Oecumenical Council of Trent. 1848. Ed. and trans. J. Waterworth. London: Dolman.

Cantimori, Delio. 1992. *Eretici Italiani del Cinquecento. Ricerche storiche.* Florence: G. C. Sansoni Editore, 1939; new edition by Adriano Prosperi, issued by Turin: Einaudi.

Capello, Paolo. 1880. *Della vita di Gaetano da Tiene.* Turin.

Cardella, Lorenzo. 1792–97. *Memorie storiche de' cardinali della Santa Romana Chiesa*, 9 vols. Rome: Typis Vaticanis.

Carroll, Stuart. 2003. "The Compromise of Charles Cardinal of Lorraine: New Evidence." *Journal of Ecclesiastical History* 54: 469–83.

Casale, Vittorio. 1976. "Trattato della pittura e scultura, opera stampata ad istanza del S.r Pietro da Cortona." *Paragone* 313: 67–99.

Casati, Roberto. 2004. "Methodological Issues in the Study of the Depiction of Cast Shadows: A Case Study in the Relationships Between Art and Cognition." *Journal of Aesthetics and Art Criticism* 62.2: 163–74.

Caterino, Ambrogio. 1552. "Disputatio de cultu et adoratione imaginum." In *Enarrationes.* Rome.

Cattaneo, Enrico. 1983. "La singulare fortuna degli Acta ecclesiae Mediolanensis." *La scuola cattolica*, no. 111: 191–217.

Celant, Germano. 1995. *Witkin.* Zürich: Scalo.

Chambers, David, and Brian Pullan, with Jennifer Fletcher, eds. 1992. *Venice: A Documentary History, 1450–1630.* Oxford: Blackwell.

Chambers, Edmund Kercherel, Sir. 1903. *The Mediaeval Stage.* Oxford: Oxford University Press.

Chappell, Miles L., and W. Chandler Kirwin. 1974. "A Petrine Triumph: The Decoration of the Navi Piccole in Sant Pietro under Clement VIII." *Storia dell'arte* 21: 119–70.

Chastel, André. 1984. *A Chronicle of Italian Renaissance Painting.* Trans. Linda Murray and Peter Murray. Ithaca, NY: Cornell University Press.

Châtellier, Louis. 1989. *The Europe of the Devout: The Catholic Reformation and the Formation of a New Society.* Trans. Jean Birrell. Cambridge: Cambridge University Press.

Cherubini, Laertio, and Angelo Maria Cherubino. 1638. *Bullarium Romanum Novissimum. A Clemente VIII usque ad Gregorium XV. Opus absolutissimum.* Rome: Ex Typographia Rev. Camera Apostolicae.

Chomarat, Jacques. 1981. *Grammaire et rhetorique chez Erasme.* Paris: Belles Lettres.

Chorpenning, Joseph. 1987. "Another Look at Caravaggio and Religion." *Artibus et Historiae* 8: 149–58.

Christiansen, Keith, ed. 2003. *Orazio and Artemisia: Father and Daughter Painters in Baroque Italy.* New York: Metropolitan Museum of Art.

Cistellini, Antonio. 1981. "Il Cardinale Federico Borromeo, S. Filippo e La Vallicella." *Atti dell'Accademia Di San Carlo* IV: 91–134.

1989. San Filippo Neri. *L'Oratorio e la Congregazione Oratoriana. Storia e Spiritualità,* 3 vols. Brescia: Morcelliana.

1994. *San Filippo Neri. Gli scritti e le massime.* Brescia: La Scuola.

Clark, Stuart. 2009. *Vanities of the Eye: Vision in Early Modern European Culture.* Oxford: Oxford University Press.

Clifton, James. 1999. "Gender and Shame in Masaccio's *Expulsion from the Garden of Eden.*" *Art History* 22.5: 637–55.

Cochrane, Eric. 1981. *Historians and Historiography in the Italian Renaissance.* Chicago: University of Chicago Press.

Coetzee, J. M. [John Maxwell]. 1996. *Giving Offense: Essays on Censorship.* Chicago: University of Chicago Press.

Cole, Michael W., ed. 2006. *Sixteenth-Century Italian Art.* Oxford: Blackwell.

Comanini, Gregorio. 2001. *The Figino, or on the Purpose of Painting: Art Theory in the Late Renaissance.* Ed. Ann Doyle-Anderson and Giancarlo Maiorino. Toronto: University of Toronto Press.

Concilium Tridentinum. Diariorum, actorum, epistularum, tractatuum nova collectio. 1901–2001. 13 vols. Ed. Societas Goerresiana Promovendis inter Germanos Catholicos Litterarum Studiis. Freiburg: Herder.

Condivi, Ascanio. 1976. *The Life of Michelangelo.* Ed and trans. Helmut Wohl and Alice Sedgwick Wohl. Baton Rouge: Louisiana State University Press.

Connors, Joseph. 1980. *Borromini and the Roman Oratory.* New York: Architectural History Foundation / Cambridge, MA: MIT Press, 1980.

Cooper, Tracy E. 1990. "The History and Decoration of the Church of San Giorgio Maggiore in Venice." Ph.D. diss., Princeton University.

1991. "Paolo Veronese–fa un modo per 'la riforma cattolica'?" In *Crisi e rinnovamenti nell'autunno del rinascimento.* Ed. Vittore Branca and Carlo Ossola, 271–92. Florence: Leo S. Olschki Editore.

1998. "Rhetorical Likeness." Review essay of Luba Freedman, *Titian's Portraits Through Aretino's Lens. International Journal of the Classical Tradition* 4: 567–71.

2006. *Palladio's Venice: Architecture and Society in a Renaissance Republic.* New Haven, CT: Yale University Press.

Costamagna, Alba. 1995. "'*La più bella et superba occasione di tutta Roma* . . .': Rubens per l'altar maggiore di S. Maria Vallicella." In Strinati and Costamagna (1995), 150–73.

Coster, Franciscus. 1588. *Libellus Sodalitatis*, rev. ed. Ingolstadt: David Sartorius.

Courtright, Nicola. 2003. *The Papacy and the Art of Reform in Sixteenth-Century Rome: Gregory XIII's Tower of the Winds.* Cambridge: Cambridge University Press.

2006. "Innovation, Imitation, and Renovation." In Cole (2006), 135–52.

Cox, Virginia. 1992. *The Renaissance Dialogue: Literary Dialogue in Its Social and Political Contexts, Castiglione to Galileo.* New York: Cambridge University Press.

Croce, Benedetto. 1969. *Aesthetic as Science of Expression and General Linguistic*, rev. ed. Trans. Ainslie Douglas. London: Peter Owen-Vision Press.

Crook, David. 1994. *Orlando di Lasso's Imitation Magnificats for Counter-Reformation.* Princeton, NJ: Princeton University Press.

Cropper, Elizabeth. 1995. "The Place of Beauty in the High Renaissance and Its Displacement in the History of Art." In *Place and Displacement in the Renaissance.* Ed. Alvin Vos, 159–205. Binghamton, NY: Center for Medieval and Early Renaissance Studies.

2010. "The *Fortuna Critica* of Agnolo Bronzino." In Falciani and Natali (2010), 23–33.

Cunningham, Andrew. 2010. *The Anatomist Anatomis'd: An Experimental Discipline in Enlightenment Europe.* Farnham: Ashgate.

D'Addario, Arnaldo. 1972. *Aspetti della controriforma a Firenze.* Rome: Ministero dell'interno.

Dante [Alighieri]. 1968. *De vulgari eloquentia.* Ed. A. Marigo and P. G. Ricci. Florence: Le Monnier.

Da Varagine, Jacopo [Jacobus de Voragine]. 1990. *Legenda Aurea*, 2 vols. Trans. Cecilia Lisi. Florence: Libreria editrice fiorentina.

Davidson, Bernice F. 1967. "Daniele da Volterra and the Orsini Chapel – II." *Burlington Magazine* 109: 553–61.

Davril, Anselme, and Timothy Thibodeau, eds. 1995–2000. *Guillelmi Duranti Rationale divinorum officiorum.* Turnhout: Brepols.

De Backer, Augustin, and Carlos Sommervogel. 1960. *Bibliothèque de la compagnie de Jésus*, 11 vols. Brussels, 1890–1932; rpt. and vol. 12, Louvain-Héverlée: Editions de la Bibliothèque S.J., Collège philosophique et théologique.

De Boer, Wietse. 1991. "Ad audiendi non videndi commoditatem. Note sull'introduzione del confessionale soprattutto in Italia." *Quaderni Storici* 77: 543–72.

1997. "Penitenza e moralità pubblica; le "Avvertenza" per i confessori di Carlo Borromeo." In *Carlo Borromeo e l'opera della "Grande riforma." Cultura, religione e arti del governo nella Milano del pieno Cinquecento.* Ed. F. Buzzi and D. Zardin, 105–14. Milan: Silvana.

2001. *The Conquest of the Soul: Confession, Discipline, and Public Order in Counter-Reformation Milan.* Leiden: Brill.

De Boor, Helmut. 1967. *Die Textgeschichte der lateinischen Osterfeiern.* Tübingen: Max Niemeyer.

De Courcelles, Dominique. 2004. "La ténèbre lumineuse dans l'oeuvre de Jean de la Croix." In *Du visible à l'intelligible. Lumière et ténèbres de L'Antiquité à la Renaissance*. Ed. Christian Trottmann and Anca Vasiliu, 373–87. Paris: Honoré Champion Éditeur.

Decreta authentica Congregationis Sacrorum Rituum ex actis eiusdem collecta eiusque auctoritate promulgata sub auspiciis ss. domini nostri Leonis Papae XII. 1898–1901. Rome: Ex Typographia Ployglotta.

De Filippi, Claudia. 2006. "Le donne nella chiesa ambrosiana." *Studia borromaica* 20: 155–184.

De Frachet, Gerard. 1896. *Vitae fratrum Ordinis Praedicatorum*, vol. 1 *of Monumenta Ordinis Fratrum Praedictorum historica*. Ed. Benedict Maria Reichert. Leuven: Charpentier & Schoonjans.

De Hollanda, Francisco. 1903. *Three Dialogues on Painting.* Trans. Charles Holroyd. In *Michael Angelo Buonarroti … with Translations of the Life of the Master by his Scholar, Ascanio Condivi, and Three Dialogues from the Portuguese by Francisco Hollanda.* London: Duckworth.

Dejob, Charles. 1884. *De l'influence du Concile de Trente sur la littérature et les beaux-arts chez les peuples catholiques.* Paris: Thorin.

Dekoninck, Ralph. 2005. *Ad Imaginem. Statuts, fonctions et usages de l'image dans la littérature spirituelle jésuite du XVIIe siècle.* Geneva: Droz.

Del Bravo, Carlo. 1983. "Sul Significato della Luce nel Caravaggio e in Gianlorenzo Bernini." *Artibus et Historiae* 4.7: 69–77.

Deleuze, Gilles, and Felix Guattari. 1994. In *What Is Philosophy?* Trans. Hugh Tomlinson and Graham Burchell. New York: Columbia University Press.

Della Torre, Stefano, and Richard Vaugh Schofield. 1994. *Pellegrino Tibaldi architetto e il S. Fedele di Milano. Invenzione e costruzione di una chiesa esemplare.* Milan-Como: Nodo.

Del Re, Niccolò. 1976. *Il vicegerente del Vicariato di Roma.* Rome: Istituto di studi romani.

1998. *La Curia romano. Lineamenti storico-giuridici.* Vatican City: Libreria editrice vaticana.

De Maio, Romeo. 1978. *Michelangelo e la Controriforma.* Rome: Laterza.

De Maio, Romeo, Agostino Borromeo, Luigi Gulia, Georg Lutz, and Aldo Mazzacane, eds. 1985. *Baronio e l'arte. Atti del Convegno internazionale di studi.* Sora: Centro di Studi Sorani "Vincenzo Patriarca."

Dempsey, Charles. 1982. "Mythic Inventions in Counter-Reformation Painting." In *Rome in the Renaissance: The City and the Myth.* Medieval and Renaissance Texts and Studies, no. 18. Binghamton, NY: Center for Medieval and Early Renaissance Studies.

2000. *Inventing the Renaissance Putto.* Chapel Hill, NC: University of North Carolina Press.

2006. "The Carracci and the Devout Style in Emilia." In Cole (2006), 388–402. Originally published in *Emilian Painting of the 16th and 17th Centuries.* Ed. Henry Millon, 75–87. Bologna: Nuova Alfa.

De Renzi, Silvia. 1999. "The Hospital of Santo Spirito in Rome." In *Health Care and Poor Relief in Counter-Reformation Europe.* Ed. Ole Peter Grell, Andrew Cunningham, and Jon Arrizabalaga, 102–31. London: Routledge.

Dern, Alexandra. 2003. *Scipione Pulzone (ca. 1546–1598).* Weimar: VDG.

De Vecchi, Pierluigi. 1984. *Michelangelo pittore.* Milan: Jaca.

1986. "Michelangelo's Last Judgment." In *The Sistine Chapel: The Art, the History, and the Restoration*, 176–207. New York: Harmony Books.

Di Bello, Patrizia, and Gabriel Koureas. 2010. *Art, History and the Senses: 1830 to the Present*. Aldershot: Ashgate.

Diez, Karlheinz. 1987. *Christus und seine Kirche. Zum Kirchenverständnis des Petrus Canisius*. Paderborn: Bonifatius-Druckerei.

Dimler, G. Richard. 1974. "A Geographic and Genetic Survey of Jesuit Drama in German-speaking Territories from 1555–1602." *Archivum Historicum Societatis Jesu* 43: 133–46.

2007. *Studies in the Jesuit Emblem*. New York: AMS Press.

Ditchfield, Simon. 2004. "Of Dancing Cardinals and Mestizo Madonnas: Reconfiguring the History of Roman Catholicism in the Early Modern Period." *Journal of Early Modern History* 8: 386–408.

2007. "Tridentine Worship and the Cult of Saints." In *The Cambridge History of Christianity*, vol. 6: *Reform and Expansion 1500–1660*. Ed. R. Po-chia Hsia, 201–24. Cambridge: Cambridge University Press.

Dizionario biografico degli italiani. 1964. "Baronio." Rome, Istituto dell'Enciclopedia Italiana, 6: 470–78.

Dolce, Lodovico. 1960. *Dialogo della pittura intitolato l'Aretino* (1557). In Barocchi (1960–62), 1: 141–206.

1969. *Dolce's "Aretino" and Venetian Art Theory of the Cinquecento*. Trans. Mark W. Roskill. New York: New York University Press. 2d. ed., 2000. Toronto: University of Toronto Press.

Donnelly, John Patrick. 1981. "Peter Canisius, 1521–1597." In *Shapers of Religious Traditions in Germany, Switzerland, and Poland, 1560–1600*. Ed. Jill Raitt, 141–56. New Haven, CT: Yale University Press.

Du Cange, Charles du Fresne, sieur. 1938. *Glossarium mediae et infimae latinitatis*, vol. 4. Paris: Librairie des sciences et des arts.

Duchesne, Louis, ed. 1886–1892. *Liber pontificalis*, 3 vols. Paris: Thorin, 1886–1892. Rpt. Paris: De Boccard, 1955.

Duhr, Bernhard. 1907–28. *Geschichte der Jesuiten in den Ländern deutscher Zunge*, 4 vols. in 6 parts. Freiburg-im-Breisgau: Herder.

Dupeux, Cécile, Peter Jezler, and Jean Wirth. 2000. *Bildersturm: Wahnsinn oder Gottes Wille?* Munich: Fink.

Durand, Guillaume. 2007. *The "Rationale Divinorum Officiorum" of William Durand of Mende*. Ed. Timothy M. Thibodeau. New York: Columbia University Press.

Dyer, Joseph. n.d. "Roman Catholic Church Music. II. The 16th Century in Europe." *Grove Music Online*, Oxford Music Online, ed. L. Macy, www.grovemusic.com (accessed 15 April 2008).

Eire, Carlos M. N. 1986. *War Against the Idols: The Reformation of Worship from Erasmus to Calvin*. Cambridge: Cambridge University Press.

Eisenberg, Marvin. 2002. "The Stoning of St. Stephen in an Altarpiece by Mariotto di Nardo: Again the Cast Shadow." In *Reading Medieval Images: The Art Historian and the Object*, Ed. Elizabeth Sears and Thelma K. Thomas, 231–38. Ann Arbor: University of Michigan Press.

Ekserdjian, David. 1997. *Correggio*. New Haven, CT: Yale University Press.

2006. *Parmigianino*. New Haven, CT: Yale University Press.

Elias, Norbert. 1983. *The Court Society*. Trans. Edmund Jephcott. Oxford: Blackwell.

Emiliani, Andrea. 1985. *Federico Barocci Urbino, 1535–1612*, 2 vols. Bologna: Nuova Alfa.

Erasmus of Rotterdam. 1963. *The Enchiridion of Erasmus*. Trans. Raymond Himelick. Bloomington: Indiana University Press.

1991. *Ecclesiastes*, bks. I and II. Ed. Jacques Chomarat. Amsterdam: North Holland.

1994. *Ecclesiastes*, bks. III and IV. Ed. Jacques Chomarat. Amsterdam: North Holland.

Erb, James. 1990. *Orlando di Lasso: A Guide to Research*. New York: Garland.

Ettelt, Beatrix, ed. 1991. *Die Jesuiten in Ingolstadt*. Exh. Cat. Ingolstadt: Stadtarchiv.

Evennett, H. Outram. 1930. *The Cardinal of Lorraine and the Council of Trent: A Study in the Counter-Reformation*. Cambridge: Cambridge University Press.

Falciani, Carlo, and Antonio Natali, eds. 2010. *Bronzino: Artist and Poet at the Court of the Medici*. Florence: Mandragora.

Farago, Claire. 1991. "Leonardo's Color and Chiaroscuro Reconsidered: The Visual Force of Painted Images." *Art Bulletin* 73.1: 63–88.

Fehl, Philipp P. 1961. "Veronese and the Inquisition: A Study of the Subject Matter of the So-called 'Feast in the House of Levi.'" *Gazette des Beaux-Arts*, ser. 6, 58 (1961): 325–54.

1992. *Decorum and Wit: The Poetry of Venetian Painting*. Essays in the History of the Classical Tradition. Vienna: Irsa.

Fehleison, Jill R. 2005. "Appealing to the Senses: The Forty Hours Celebrations in the Duchy of Chablais, 1597–98." *Sixteenth Century Journal* 36: 375–96.

Fehrenbach, Frank. 2005a. "Bernini's Light." *Art History* 28.1: 1–42.

2005b. "Veli sopra veli: Leonardo und die Schleier." In *Ikonologie des Zwischenraums: Der Schleier als Medium und Metapher*. Ed. Johannes Endres et al., 121–47. Munich: Wilhelm Fink.

Ferrari, Daniele, ed. 1992. *Giulio Romano, Repertorio di fonti documentarie*, vol. 2. Rome: Ministero per i beni culturali.

1995. "Artisti e committenze alla Chiesa Nuova." In Strinati and Costamagna (1995), 108–29.

Feuchtmayr, Andrea. 1989. *Kulissenheiliggräber im Barock. Entstehungsgeschichte und Typologie*. Munich: Tuduv.

Filippi, Bruna. 2001. *Il teatro degli argomenti. Gli scenari seicenteschi del teatro gesuitico romano*. Rome: Institutum Historicum S.I.

2006. "The Orator's Performance: Gesture, Word, and Image in Theatre at the Collegio Romano." In O'Malley (2006c).

Findlen, Paula. 1993. "Humanism, Politics and Pornography in Renaissance Italy." In *The Invention of Pornography*. Ed. Lynn Hunt. 49–108. New York: Zone Books.

Fiorani, Francesca. 2008. "The Colors of Leonardo's Shadows." *Leonardo* 41.3: 271–78.

Fiorani, Luigi. 1980. "Le visite apostoliche del Cinque-Seicento e la società religiosa romana." *Ricerche per la storia religiosa di Roma* 4: 53–148.

Fiorio, Maria Teresa, ed. 1985. *Le chiese di Milano*. Milan: Electa.

Firpo, Massimo. 2004. "The Italian Reformation." In Hsia (2004), 169–84.

Fisher, Alexander. 2004. *Music and Religious Identity in Counter-Reformation Augsburg, 1580–1630*. Aldershot: Ashgate.

2007. "'Per mia particolare devotione': Orlando di Lasso's *Lagrime di San Pietro* and Catholic Spirituality in Counter-Reformation Munich." *Journal of the Royal Musical Association* 132: 167–220.

Fisher, Philip. 2002. "Darkness and the Demand for Time in Art." In *Art History, Aesthetics, Visual Studies*. Ed. Michael Ann Holly and Keith Moxey, 87–104. Williamstown, MA: Sterling and Francine Clark Art Institute / New Haven, CT: Yale University Press.

Flacius, Matthias, et al. 1559–1574. *Ecclesiastica Historia*, vol. 13. Basel: J. Oporinus.

Formentini, Marco. 1881. *La dominazione spagnuola in Lombardia*. Milan: Giuseppe Ottino.

Foschi, Paola. 1988. "La chiesa di S. Lucia e i collegi dei Jesuiti. Vicende costruttive." In *Dall'Isola alla città. I Jesuiti a Bologna*. Ed. G. P. Brizzi and A. M. Matteucci. Bologna: Nuova Alfa.

Foucault, Michel. 1980. *History of Sexuality*, vol. 1: *An Introduction*. Trans. Robert Hurley. New York: Random House.

Fragnito, Gigliola. 1997. "Vescovi e ordini religiosi in Italia all'indomani del Concilio." In *I tempi del Concilio. Religione, cultura e società nell'Europa tridentina*. Ed. Cesare Mozzarelli and Danilo Zardin, 13–25. Rome: Bulzoni.

Fragnito, Gigliola, and Ugo Rozzo. 1997. "La censura libraria tra Congregazione dell'Indice, Congregazione dell'Inquisizione e Maestro del Sacro Palazzo (1571–1596)." In *La censura libraria nell'Europa del secolo XVI. Atti del Convegno internazionale di studi Cividale del Friuli, 9–10 novembre 1995*, 163–76. Udine: Forum.

Franca Mellano, Maria. 1986. "La donna nell'opera riformatrice di S. Carlo." In *S. Carlo e il suo tempo*, 2 vols., 1073–1134. Rome: Edizioni di storia e letteratura.

Franck, Sebastian. 1534. *Weltbüch: Spiegel und Bildtnisz des gantzen Erdtbodens*. Tübingen: Vlrich Morhart.

Frangenberg, Thomas. 1990. *Der Betrachter. Studien zur florentinischen Kunstliterature des 16. Jahrhunderts*. Berlin: Mann.

Freedberg, David. 1971. "Johannes Molanus on Provocative Paintings: *De Historia Sanctarum Imaginum et Picturarum*, Book II, Chapter 42." *Journal of the Warburg and Courtauld Institute* 34: 229–45.

1988. "Molanus and Theological Recommendations about Imagery in the Netherlands after the Iconoclasm." In *Iconoclasm and Painting in the Revolt of the Netherlands (1566–1609)*, 134–66. New York: Garland.

1989. *The Power of Images: Studies in the History and Theory of Response*. Chicago: University of Chicago Press.

2011. "Memory in Art: History and the Neuroscience of Response." In *The Memory Process: Neuroscientific and Humanistic Perspectives*. Ed. Susan Nalbantian, Paul M. Matthews, and James L. McClelland, 337–58. Cambridge, MA: MIT Press.

Freedberg, Sydney J. 1961. *Painting of the High Renaissance in Rome and Florence*, 2 vols. Cambridge, MA: Harvard University Press.

1965. "Observations on the Painting of the Maniera." *Art Bulletin* 47: 187–97.

1993. *Painting in Italy, 1500–1600* [1971], 3d ed. New Haven, CT: Yale University Press.

Freedman, Luba. 1990. "Masaccio's *St. Peter Healing with His Shadow*: A Study in Iconography." *Notizie da Palazzo Albani* 19.2: 13–30.

Freiberg, Jack. 1995. *The Lateran in 1600: Christian Concord in Counter-Reformation Rome*. Cambridge: Cambridge University Press.

Frere, Walter Howard, ed. 1898. *The Use of Sarum: The Original Texts*. Cambridge: Cambridge University Press.

Friedlaender, Walter. 1957. "The Anticlassical Style." In *Mannerism and Anti-Mannerism in Italian Painting*, 3–43. New York: Columbia University Press. Originally published as "Die Entstehung des antiklassischen Stiles in der italienischen Malerei um 1520" (1925).

Frommel, Christoph L., and Gerhard Wolf, eds. 2006. *L'immagine di Cristo. Dall'Acheropita alla mano d'artista; dal tardo medioevo all'età barocca*. Vatican City: Biblioteca apostolica vaticana.

Fubini, Riccardo. 1990. *Umanesimo e secolarizzazione da Petrarca a Valla*. Rome: Bulzoni.

Gabrieli, G. 1933–34. "Federico Borromeo a Roma." *Archivio della Società Romana di Storia Patria* 56/57: 157–217.

Galassi Paluzzi, Carlo. 1951. *Storia segreta dello stile dei gesuiti*. Rome: F. Mondini.

Gallonio, Antonio. 1600. *Vitae B. P. Philippi Nerii Florentini*. Rome.

Ganss, George E., S.J., ed. 1991. *Ignatius of Loyola: The Spiritual Exercises and Selected Works*. New York: Paulist Press.

Gaston, Robert W. 1995. "Sacred Erotica: The Classical *Figura* in Religious Painting of the Early Cinquecento." *International Journal of the Classical Tradition* 2.2: 238–64.

1996. "Decorum." In *The Dictionary of Art*. Ed. Jane Turner, 8: 612–14. London: Macmillan.

1996–97. "Pictorial Representation and Ekphrasis in *Elogio de la madrastra*." *Antipodas: Journal of Hispanic Studies* 18/19: 216–29.

1998a. "Erwin Panofsky and the Classical Tradition." *International Journal of the Classical Tradition* 4.4: 613–23.

1998b. "The Renaissance Artist as *Dantista*: A Reassessment." *Lectura Dantis* 22/23: 5–44.

2001. "Attention in Court: Visual Decorum in Medieval Prayer Theory and Early Italian Art." In *Visions of Holiness: Art and Devotion in Renaissance Italy*. Ed. Andrew Ladis and Shelley E. Zuraw, 136–62. Athens: Georgia Museum of Art.

2003. Review of Gregorio Comanini, *The Figino, or On the Purpose of Painting: Art Theory in the Late Renaissance*, ed. Ann Doyle-Anderson and Giancarlo Maiorino (Toronto, Buffalo, and London: University of Toronto Press, 2001). *International Journal of the Classical Tradition* 10.2: 316–19.

Geissler, Heinrich. 1960. "Christoph Schwarz, ca. 1548–1592." Diss., Albert-Ludwig-Universität, Freiburg im Breisgau.

n.d. "Schwarz, Christoph." *Grove Art Online*. Oxford University Press, www.groveart.com (accessed 15 April 2008).

Gentili, Augusto, with Marco Lattanzi and Flavia Polignano. 1985. *I giardini di contemplazione: Lorenzo Lotto, 1503/1512*. Rome: Bulzoni.

Gerken, Claudia. 2004. "Vom Porträt zum Heiligenbild: Filippo Neri als 'Vivum Exemplar' und die Legitimation seines Bildkultes." In *Ästhetik des Unsichtbaren. Bildtheorie und Bildgebrauch in der Vormodern*. KultBild: Visualität und Religion in der Vormodern, 1. Ed. David Ganz and Thomas Lentes, 220–49. Berlin: Dietrich Reimer.

Gigli, Giacinto. 1958. *Diario romano*. Ed. Giuseppe Ricciotti. Rome: Tumminelli.

Gilio, Giovanni Andrea. 1961. *Dialogo nel quale si ragiona degli errori e degli abusi de' pittori circa l'istorie [1564]*. In Barocchi (1960–62) 2: 1–116.

1986. *Due dialogi*. Ed. Paola Barocchi. Florence: Studio per edizioni scelte.

Gilio da Fabriano, Giovanni Andrea. 1580. *Topica poetica*. Venice: De' Gobbi.

Gill, Meredith. 2005. *Augustine in the Italian Renaissance: Art and Philosophy from Petrarch to Michelangelo.* Cambridge: Cambridge University Press.

Gilmore, Myron P. 1969. "Erasmus and Alberto Pio, Prince of Carpi." In *Action and Conviction in Early Modern Europe, Essays in Honor of E. H. Harbison.* Ed. Theodore Rabb and J. E. Seigel, 299–318. Princeton, NJ: Princeton University Press.

Ginzburg, Carlo. 1976. *Il formaggio e vermi: il cosmo di un mugnaio del'500.* Turin: Einaudi.

Giustiniani, Vincenzo. 1981. *Discorsi Sulle Arti e Sui Mestieri.* Ed. Anna Banti. Florence: Sansoni.

Glaser, Hubert, ed. 1980. *Wittelsbach und Bayern. Um Glauben und Reich: Kurfürst Maximilian I.* Exh. cat. Munich: Hirmer.

Goldberg, Rose Lee. 1988. *Performance Art: From Futurism to the Present*, rev. ed. New York: Abrams.

Gombrich, Ernst Hans. 1972. *Symbolic Images: Studies in the Art of the Renaissance.* London: Phaidon.

1995. *Shadows: The Depiction of Cast Shadows in Western Art.* London: National Gallery Publications / New Haven, CT: Yale University Press.

Göttler, Christine, Wietse de Boer, and Herman Roodenburg, eds. Forthcoming. *Religion and the Senses in Early Modern Europe.* Leiden: Brill.

Graeve, Mary A. 1958. "The Stone of Unction in Caravaggio's Painting for the Chiesa Nuova." *Art Bulletin* 40: 223–37.

Gramberg, Werner. 1984. "Guglielmo della Portas Grabmal fur Paul III Farnese in San Pietro in Vaticano." *Romisches Jahrbuch fur Kunstgeschichte* 24: 253–364.

Grass, Nikolaus. 1957. "Barock-Heiliggräber: Ein Beitrag zur Kultur- und Kunstgeschichte Tirols." In *Ostern in Tirol.* Ed. Nikolaus Grass, 221–69. Innsburck: Wagner.

Grazzini, Anton Francesco. 1882. "Capitolo in lode della statua di San Giorgio." In *Le rime burlesche edite e inedite.* Florence: Sansoni.

Greenblatt, Stephen. 1980. *Renaissance Self-Fashioning: From More to Shakespeare.* Chicago: University of Chicago Press.

1988. *Shakespearean Negotiations: The Circulation of Social Energy in Renaissance England.* Berkeley: University of California Press.

Gregori, Mina, and Rodolfo Maffeis, eds. 2007. *Un'altra bellezza: Francesco Furini.* Florence: Mandragora.

Gregory I, Pope. 1984. *Commentaire sur le Cantique des cantiques.* Trans. Rodrigue Bélanger. Paris: Éditions du Cerf.

Grendler, Paul F. 1969. *Critics of the Italian World, 1530–1560: Anton Francesco Doni, Nicolò Franco & Ortensio Lando.* Madison: University of Wisconsin Press.

Grimaldi, Giacomo. 1972. *Descrizione della Basilica Antica di S. Pietro in Vaticano. Codice Barberini Latin 2733.* 1622. Codices e Vaticanis selecti, vol. 32. Ed. Reto Niggl. Vatican City: Biblioteca apostolica vaticana.

Gschwend, Kolumban. 1965. *Die Depositio und Elevatio Crucis im Raum der alten Diözese Brixen: Ein Beitrag zur Geschichte der Grablegung am Karfreitag und der Auferstehungsfeier am Ostermorgen.* Sarnen: Ehrli.

Gualdo Priorato, Galeazzo. 1666. *Relatione della città e stato di Milano.* Milan: L. Monza.

Guarinonius, Hippolytus. 1610. *Die Grewel der Verwüstung menschlichen Geschlects.* Ingolstadt.

Haastrup, Ulla. 1987. "Medieval Props in the Liturgical Drama." *Hafnia: Copenhagen Papers in the History of Art* 11: 133–70.

Hall, Marcia B. 1979. *Renovation and Counter-Reformation: Vasari and Duke Cosimo in Sta. Maria Novella and Sta. Croce, 1565–1577.* Oxford: Oxford University Press.

1999. *After Raphael: Painting in Central Italy in the Sixteenth Century.* Cambridge: Cambridge University Press.

ed. 2005a. *Michelangelo's "Last Judgment."* Cambridge: Cambridge University Press.

ed. 2005b. *Rome.* Cambridge: Cambridge University Press.

2011. *The Sacred Image in the Age of Art: Titian, Tintoretto, Barocci, El Greco, Caravaggio.* New Haven, CT: Yale University Press.

Hallman, Barbara. 1985. *Italian Cardinals, Reform and the Church as Property, 1492–1563.* Berkeley: University of California Press.

Hamberg, Per Gustaf. 2002. *Temples for Protestants: Studies in the Architectural Milieu of the Early Reformed Church and of the Lutheran Church.* Gothenberg: Acta Universitatis Gothoburgensis.

Hamburger, Jeffrey. 2000. "Seeing and Believing : The Suspicion of Sight and the Authentication of Vision in Late Medieval Art And Devotion." In *Imagination and Wirklichkeit: zum Verhältnis von mentalen und realen Bildern in der Kunst der frühen Neuzeit.* Ed. Klaus Krüger and Alessandro Nova, 47–69. Mainz: von Zabern.

Hardison, O. B. [Ostome Bennet]. 1965. *Christian Rite and Christian Drama in the Middle Ages: Essays in the Origin and Early History of Modern Drama.* Baltimore: Johns Hopkins Press.

Harper, John. 1991. *The Forms and Orders of the Western Liturgy from the Tenth to the Eighteenth Century: A Historical Introduction and Guide for Students and Musicians.* Oxford: Clarendon Press.

Harvey, Elizabeth, D., ed. 2003. *Sensible Flesh: On Touch in Early Modern Culture.* Philadelphia: University of Pennsylvania Press.

Haskell, Francis, and Nicholas Penny. 1981. *Taste and the Antique: The Lure of Classical Sculpture, 1500–1900.* New Haven, CT: Yale University Press.

Haub, Rita. 1996. "Petrus Canisius as Schriftsteller." In Oswald and Rummel (1996), 151–77.

Haussherr, Reiner. 1984. *Convenevolezza.* Weisbaden: Franz Steiner.

Heal, Bridget. 2007. *The Cult of the Virgin Mary in Early Modern Germany.* Cambridge: Cambridge University Press.

Hecht, Christian. 1997. *Katholische Bildertheologie im Zeitalter von Gegenreformation und Barock. Studien zu Traktaten von Johannes Molanus, Gabriele Paleotti und anderen Autoren.* Berlin: Gebr. Mann.

2003. *Die Glorie. Begriff, Thema, Bildelement in der europäischen Sakralkunst vom Mittelalter bis zum Ausgang des Barock.* Regensburg: Schnell & Steiner.

Heideman, Johanna Elfriede Louise. 1982. *The Cinquecento Chapel Decorations in S. Maria in Aracoeli in Rome.* Amsterdam: Academische pers B.V.

Hell, Helmut, and Horst Leuchtmann. 1982. *Orlando di Lasso: Musik der Renaissance am Münchner Fürstenhof.* Exh. cat., Bayerische Staatsbibliothek, Munich. Wiesbaden: Reichert.

Hellegouarc'h, Joseph. 1963. *Le vocabulaire latin des relations et des partis politiques sous la République.* Paris: Belles Lettres.

Helmholz, Richard H. 1996. *The Spirit of Classical Canon Law.* Athens: University of Georgia Press.

Heming, Carol Piper. 2003. *Protestants and the Cult of the Saints in German-Speaking Europe, 1517–1531*. Kirksville, MO: Truman State University Press.

Herklotz, Ingo. 2000. Review of Hecht (1997). *Journal für Kunstgeschichte* 4.1: 43–49.

Herrmann-Schneider, Hildegard. 1985. *Die Musikhandschriften der St. Michaelskirche in München*, 16: 179–86. Munich: Henle.

Hess, Daniel, and Dagmar Hirschfelder, eds. 2010. *Renaissance, Barock, Aufklärung: Kunst und Kultur vom 16. bis zum 18. Jahrhundert* [Germanisches Nationalmuseum]. Nuremberg: Germanischen Nationalmuseums.

Hess, Günter, Sabine M. Schneider, and Claudia Wiener, eds. 1997. *Trophaea Bavarica-Bayerisches Siegeszeichen*. Regensburg: Schnell & Steiner.

Hirst, Michael. 1967. "Daniele da Volterra and the Orsini Chapel – I: The Chronology and the Altar-piece." *Burlington Magazine* 109: 498–509.

Hollingsworth, Mary, and Carol M. Richardson, eds. 2010. *The Possessions of a Cardinal: Politics, Piety, and Art, 1450–1700*. University Park: Pennsylvania State University Press.

Hollstein, F. W. H. [Friedrich Wilhelm], gen. ed. 1949–. *Dutch and Flemish Etchings, Engravings, and Woodcuts 1450–1700*. Amsterdam: M. Hertzberger.

Höltgen, Karl Josef. 1999. "Henry Hawkins: A Jesuit Writer and Emblematist in Stuart England." In O'Malley (1999b), 600–26.

Honig, Elizabeth Alice. 1998. "Making Sense of Things: On the Motive of Dutch Still Life." *RES: Anthropology and Aesthetics* 34: 166–83.

Horn-Oncken, Alste. 1967. *Über das Schickliche. Studien zur Geschichte der Architekturtheorie*. Göttingen: Vandenhoeck & Ruprecht.

Hospinianus, Rodolphus. 1603. *De templis*. Zürich: Wolfiana.

Howes, David, ed. 2005. *Empire of the Senses: The Sensual Culture Reader*. Oxford: Oxford University Press.

2008. "Can These Dry Bones Live? An Anthropological Approach to the History of the Senses." *Journal of American History* 95: 442–51.

ed. 2009. *The Sixth Sense Reader*. Oxford: Berg.

Hsia, Adrian, et al., eds. 2005. *Mission und Theater: Japan und China auf den Bühnen der Gesellschaft Jesu*. Regensburg: Schnell & Steiner.

Hsia, R. Po-chia, ed. 1997. *The World of Catholic Renewal, 1540–1770* (2d ed., 2005). Cambridge: Cambridge University Press.

ed. 2004. *A Companion to the Reformation World*. Oxford: Blackwell.

Hub, Berthold. 2005. "... e fa dolce la morte: Love, Death, and Salvation in Michelangelo's *Last Judgement*." *Artibus et Historiae* 26: 103–30.

Ignatius of Loyola. 1970. *The Constitutions of the Society of Jesus*. Ed. and trans. George E. Ganss. St. Louis, MO: Institute of Jesuit Sources.

Imorde, Joseph. 1999. "'Allegoricus semper interpres, & historiae fugiens veritatem': Zur Bildervalenz der Eucharistie." In *Barocke Inszenierung*. Ed. Joseph Imorde, Fritz Neumeyer, and Tristan Weddigen, 104–15. Emsdetten: Edition Imorde.

Incisa della Rocchetta, Giovanni. 1972. "La Sala Rossa e la cappella interna di San Filippo." In *Oratorium: archivium historicum Oratorii S. Philippi Nerii* 3: 87–92.

Irving, D. R. M. [David]. 2010. *Colonial Counterpoint*. Oxford: Oxford University Press.

Jacob, Fredrika H. 2008. "Divine and Demonic Presence in Images of Exorcism." In *CASVA Center Report* 28: 113–15.

Jaffé, Michael. 1981. "'The Penitent Magdalene in a Landscape' by Annibale Carracci." *Burlington Magazine* 123.935: 88–91.

Jansen, Jeroen. 2001. *Decorum: Observaties over de literaire gepastheid in de renaissancitische poëtica.* Hilvershum: Verloren.

Javitch, Daniel, 1978. *Poetry and Courtliness in Renaissance England.* Princeton, NJ: Princeton University Press.

Jedin, Hubert. 1935. "Entstehung und Tragweite de Trienter Dekrets über die Bilderverherung." *Tübingen Teologische Quartalschrift* 116: 134–88, 277–91.

1948–75. *Geschichte des Konzils von Trient,* 4 vols. in 5. Freiburg: Herder. Italian trans., *Storia del Concilio di Trento,* 4 vols. Brescia: Morcelliana, 1949–81. *A History of the Council of Trent.* Trans. Ernest Graf, first 2 vols. only. London: Thomas Nelson, 1957–61.

1963. "Das Tridentinum und die bildenden Künste: Bemerkungen zu Paolo Prodi, Richerche [*sic*] sulla teorica delle arti figurative nella Riforma Cattolica (1962)." *Zeitschrift für Kirchengeschichte* 74: 321–39.

1966a. "Die Geschäftsordunungen der beiden letzten ökumenischen Konzilien in ekklesiologischer Sicht." In *Kirche des Glaubens: Kirche der Geschichte,* 2 vols. Freiburg: Herder, 2: 577–88.

1966b. "Entstehung und Tragweite des Trienter Dekrets über die Bilderverehrung." In *Kirche des Glaubens: Kirche der Geschichte. Ausgewälte Aufsätze und Vorträge,* 2 vols. Freiburg: Herder, 2: 460–98. Originally published in *Tübinger Theologische Quartalschrift* 116 (1935): 143–88.

1967. *Crisis and Closure of the Council of Trent.* Trans. N. D. Smith. London: Sheed and Ward.

1982. *Il Cardinale Cesare Baronio. L'inizio della storiografia cattolica nel sedicesimo secolo.* Brescia: Morcelliana.

Jedin, Hubert, and Paolo Prodi, eds. 1979. *Il Concilio di Trento come crocevia della politica europea.* Bologna: Il Mulino.

Jezler, Peter. 1983. "Bildwerke im Dienste der dramatischen Ausgestaltung der Osterliturgie – Befürworter und Gegner." In *Von der Macht der Bilder: Beiträge des C.I.H.A –Kolloquiums, "Kunst und Reformation."* Ed. Ernst Ullmann, 236–49. Leipzig: E. A. Seemann.

1989. "Das 'handelnde Christusbild' und seine Verwendung in der städtischen Zelebration der Herrenfeste im spätmittelalterlichen Deutschland." In *World Art: Themes of Unity in Diversity.* Ed. Irving Lavin, 619–22. University Park: Pennsylvania State University Press.

Jones, Amelia. 1998. *Body Art / Performing the Subject.* Minneapolis: University of Minnesota Press.

Jones, Caroline A. 2006. *Eyesight Alone: Clement Greenberg's Modernism and the Bureaucratization of the Senses.* Chicago: Chicago University Press.

Jones, Pamela M. 1993. *Federico Borromeo and the Ambrosiana: Art Patronage and Reform in Seventeenth-Century Milan.* Cambridge: Cambridge University Press.

1995. "Art Theory as Ideology: Gabriele Paleotti's Hierarchical Notion of Painting's Universality and Reception." In *Reframing the Renaissance: Visual Culture in Europe and Latin America, 1450–1650.* Ed. Claire Farago, 127–39. New Haven, CT: Yale University Press.

1997. "Art's Role in Personal Reform: Christian Optimism and Federico Borromeo's Pinacoteca Ambrosiana." In *I tempi del Concilio. Religione, cultura e società nell'Europa tridentina.* Ed. Cesare Mozzarelli and Danilo Zardin, 387–407. Rome: Bulzoni.

2006. "Landscapes and Still Lifes." In Cole (2006), 153–66. Previously published in Pamela M. Jones, *Federico Borromeo and the Ambrosiana*, 76–84. Cambridge: Cambridge University Press (1993).

2008. *Altarpieces and Their Viewers in the Churches of Rome from Caravaggio to Guido Reni*. Aldershot: Ashgate.

Judovitz, Dalia. 2006. "Georges de La Tour: The Enigma of the Visible." In *The Beholder: The Experience of Art in Early Modern Europe*. Ed. Thomas Frangenberg and Robert Williams, 143–63. Aldershot: Ashgate.

Julian, John. 1957. *A Dictionary of Hymnology* [1907]. Reprinted in 2 vols. New York: Dover.

Jung, Tanya A. 2006. "The Phenomenal Lives of Movable Christ Sculptures." Ph.D. Diss., University of Maryland.

Jütte, Robert. 2005. *A History of the Senses: From Antiquity to Cyberspace*. Cambridge: Polity.

Kallendorf, Craig, ed. and trans. 2002. *Humanist Educational Treatises*. Cambridge, MA: Harvard University Press.

Kanz, Roland. 2000. "Der Capriccio-Begriff bei Vasari und Gilio in der Kontroverse um Michelangelos *Jüngstes Gericht*." In *Künste und Natur in Diskursen der frühen Neuzeit*, 497–513. Wiesbaden: Harrasowitz.

Karant-Nunn, Susan. 2010. *The Reformation of Feeling: Shaping the Religious Emotions in Early Modern Germany*. Oxford: Oxford University Press.

Kauffman, Linda S. 1998. *Bad Girls and Sick Boys*. Berkeley: University of California Press.

Kaufmann, Thomas Da Costa. 1975. "The Perspective of Shadows: The History of the Theory of Shadow Projection." *Journal of the Warburg and Courtauld Institutes* 38: 258–87.

Kaulbach, Hans-Martin, with Guido Messling and Heinrich Geissler, 2007. *Deutsche Zeichnungen vom Mittelalter bis zum Barock. Bestandskatalog*. [Staatsgalerie Stuttgart, Graphische Sammlung]: Ostfildern.

Kemp, Martin. 1995. " 'Wrought by No Artist's Hand': The Natural, the Artificial, the Exotic and the Scientific in some Artifacts from the Renaissance." In *Reframing the Renaissance*. Ed. Claire Farago, 177–96. New Haven, CT: Yale University Press.

Kindermann, Udo, ed. 2002. *Kunstdenkmäler zwischen Antwerpen und Trient. Beschreibungen und Bewertungen des Jesuiten Daniel Papebroch aus dem Jahre 1660*. Cologne: Böhlau.

Klein, Robert, and Henri Zerner, ed. 1966. *Italian Art, 1500–1600: Sources and Documents*. Englewood Cliffs, NJ: Prentice Hall.

Knaap, Anna C. 2005. "Meditation, Ministry, and Visual Rhetoric in Peter Paul Rubens's Program for the Jesuit Church in Antwerp." In O'Malley and Bailey (2005), 157–81.

Knowles, John, ed. 1831. *The Life and Writings of Henry Fuseli*. London: Henry Colburn and Richard Bentley.

Knox, Dilwyn. 1991. "*Disciplina*: The Monastic and Clerical Origins of European Civility." In *Renaissance Society and Culture: Essays in Honor of Eugene F. Rice, Jr.* Ed. John Monfasani and Ronald G. Musto, 107–35. New York: Italica Press.

Körte, Werner. 1935. *Der Palazzo Zuccari in Rom. Sein Freskenschmuck und seine Geschichte*. Leipzig: Heinrich Keller.

Krause, Katharina, ed. 2007. *Geschichte der bildenden Kunst in Deutschland*, vol. 4: *Spätgotik und Renaissance*. Munich: Prestel.

Kristeller, Paul Oskar. 1992. "Thomism and the Italian Thought of the Renaissance." In *Medieval Aspects of Renaissance Learning: Three Essays by Paul Oskar Kristeller*. Ed. and trans. Edward P. Mahoney, 29–91. New York: Columbia University Press.

Kroesen, Justin. 2000. *The Sepulchrum Domini Through the Ages: Its Form and Function*. Leuven: Peeters.

Kroesen, Justin, and Regnerus Steensma. 2004. *The Interior of the Medieval Village Church*. Leuven: Peeters.

Kummer, Stefan. 1987. *Anfänge und Ausbreitung der Stuckdekoration im römischen Kirchenraum (1500–1600)*. Tübingen: Wasmuth.

LaMarche, Gara. 1991. "Some Thoughts on the Chilling Effect." *Art Journal* 50.4: 56–58.

Lanham, Richard A. 1991. *A Handlist of Rhetorical Terms*, 2d ed. Berkeley: University of California Press.

Lanzi, Luigi. 1809. *Storia pittorica dell'Italia dal risorgimento delle belle arti fin presso al fine del XVIII secolo*, 6 vols. Bassano: Remondino. Trans. Thomas Roscoe [1828], *History of Painting in Italy*. London: H. G. Bohn, 1847. (Original 1-vol. ed., 1792; 3-vol. 2d ed., 1795–96.)

Lassus, Orlando. 1982. *Alma Redemptoris Mater, Ave Regina Caelorum, Regina Caeli, and Salve Regina: Four Marian Antiphons for 6, 7, and 8 Voices*. Trans. and ed. Clive Wearing. London: Mapa Mundi Renaissance Performing Scores.

1989. *Missa Osculetur Me for Double Choir*. The Tallis Scholars directed by Peter Phillips. Oxford: Gimell CDGIM 018, 1989.

Laughran, Michelle. 2003. "Oltre la pelle. I cosmetici e il loro uso." In *Storia d'Italia. Annali 19*. Ed. C. M. Belfanti and F. Giusberti, 42–82. Torino: Einaudi.

Laun, Rainer. 1982. *Studien zur Altarbaukunst in Süddeutschland, 1560–1650*. Munich: Tuduv.

Lazar, Lance Gabriel. 2005. *Working in the Vineyard of the Lord: Jesuit Confraternities in Early Modern Italy*. Toronto: University of Toronto Press.

Lea, Henry Charles. 1911–1915. *Storia della confessione auricolare e delle indulgenze della chiesa latina*, 2 vols. Trans. P. Cremonini. Mendrisio: Cultura moderna.

Leclerq, Henri. 1910. *Dictionnaire d'archéologie chrétienne e de liturgie, s.v. Baptistère*, vol. 2.1 of 15 vols. (1907–53). Ed. Fernand Cabrol. Paris: Librairie Letouzey et Ane.

Lee, Rensselaer W. 1967. *Ut pictura poesis: The Humanistic Theory of Painting*. New York: Norton. Originally published in *Art Bulletin* 22.4 (1940): 197–269.

Le Gall, Yvon. 2000. "Le *Traité de peinture et de sculpture* de G. Domenico Ottonelli et Pietro da Cortona. La fin des imprécateurs?" *Études littéraires* 32.1–2: 71–93.

Leonard, Mark, Narayan Khandekar, and Dawson Carr. 2001. "'Amber Varnish' and Orazio Gentileschi's 'Lot and His Daughters.'" *Burlington Magazine* 143: 4–10.

Leproux, Guy-Michel. 1991. "La corporation romaine des peintres 'et autres' de 1548 à 1574." *Bibliothèque de l'École des chartes* 149.2: 293–348.

Leuchtmann, Horst. 1976. *Orlando di Lasso: Sein Leben*. Wiesbaden: Breitkopf and Härtel.

Leuchtmann, Horst, and Hartmut Schaefer. 1994. *Orlando di Lasso: Prachthandschriften und Quellenüberlieferung aus den Beständen der Bayerischen Staatsbibliothek München*. Tutzing: Schneider.

Leuppi, Heidi, ed. 1995. *Der liber ordinarius des Konrad von Mure. Die Gottesdienstordnung am Grossmünster in Zürich.* Freiburg: Universitätsverlag.

Leuschner, Eckhard. 1998. "The Papal Printing Privilege." *Print Quarterly* 15.4: 359–70.

Levy, Giuseppe di, ed. 1887. *La Legazione di Roma di Paolo Paruta (1592–1595).* Reale deputazione di storia patria per le Venezie. Monumenti storici, ser. 4. Miscellanea, vols. 7–9. Venice: a spese della Società.

Levy, Yvonne. 2004. *Propaganda and the Jesuit Baroque.* Berkeley: University of California Press.

Lewis, Charlton T., and Charles Short. 1969. *A Latin Dictionary.* Oxford: Clarendon Press.

Lieb, Norbert. 1980. *Octavian Secundus Fugger (1549–1600) und die Kunst.* Tübingen: J. C. B. Mohr.

Lincoln, Evelyn. 2000. *The Invention of the Italian Renaissance Printmaker.* New Haven, CT: Yale University Press.

Lingo, Stuart. 2001. "Retrospection and the Genesis of Federico Barocci's *Immaculate Conception.*" In *Coming About ... : A Festschrift for John Shearman.* Ed. Lars R. Jones, 215–21. Cambridge, MA: Harvard University Art Museums.

2008. *Federico Barocci: Allure and Devotion in Late Renaissance Painting.* New Haven, CT: Yale University Press.

Lipowsky, Felix Joseph. 1816. *Geschichte der Jesuiten in Baiern.* Munich: J. Giel.

1819. Geschichte der Jesuiten in Schwaben, 2 vols. Munich: J. Giel.

Lipphardt, Walther. 1975. *Lateinische Osterfeiern und Osterspiele.* Berlin: De Gruyter.

Lippomano, Luigi. 1553. *Confirmatione et stabilimento di tutti i dogmi catholici.* Venice: Per Domenico Zio.

Löcher, Kurt, and Carola Gries. 2007. *Germanisches Nationalmuseum Nürnberg. Die Gemälde des 16. Jahrhunderts.* Ostfildern-Ruit: Gerd Hatje.

Lönne, Karl Egon, ed. 2003. *Carteggio Croce-Schlosser.* Bologna: Il Mulino.

Loh, Maria H. 2007. *Titian Remade: Repetition and the Transformation of Early Modern Italian Art.* Los Angeles: J. Paul Getty Museum.

Lucantoni, Silvia. 2004. "Il Palazzo Cesarini a Roma." In *Le corti rinascimentali. Committenti e artisti.* Ed. Luciana Cassanelli, 183–224. Rome: Sinnos.

Lucianus. 1967. *Lucian.* Trans. M. D. Macleod, 8: 151–235. Cambridge, MA: Harvard University Press.

Luciani, Roberto. 1996. *Santa Maria Maggiore e Roma.* Fratelli Palombi: Patriarcale Basilica di Santa Maria Maggiore.

Luebke, David M., ed. 1999. *The Counter-Reformation: The Essential Readings.* Malden, MA: Blackwell.

Lukehart, Peter M. 2007. "Parallel Lives: The Example of Taddeo Zuccaro in Late Sixteenth-Century Rome." In *Taddeo and Federico Zuccaro: Artist-Brothers in Renaissance Rome.* Ed. Julian Brooks. 105–11. Exh. cat. Los Angeles: J. Paul Getty Museum.

2009a. *The Accademia Seminars: The Accademia di San Luca in Rome, c. 1590–1635.* Ed. Peter M. Lukehart. Washington, DC: Center for Advanced Study in the Visual Arts.

2009b. "Visions and Divisions in the Early History of the Accademia di San Luca." In Lukehart (2009a), 161–95.

ed. and director. 2010. "The History of the Accademia di San Luca, c. 1590–1635: Documents from the Archivio di Stato di Roma." National Gallery of Art, Center for Advanced Study in the Visual Arts, www.nga.gov/casva/accademia.

Macioce, Stefania. 1990. *Undique Splendente. Aspetti della Pittura Sacra nella Roma di Clemente VIII Aldobrandini (1592–1605).* Rome: De Luca.

Mack, Peter. 1993. *Renaissance Argument: Valla and Agricola in the Traditions of Rhetoric and Dialectic.* Leiden: Brill.

Madonna, Maria Luisa, ed. 1993. *Roma di Sisto V. Le arti e la cultura.* Exh. cat., Palazzo Venezia, Rome. Rome: Edizione De Luca.

Maggioni, Giovanni Paolo. 1998. *Iacopo da Varazzo: Legenda Aurea.* Florence: Sismel.

Maisel, Markus. 2002. *Sepulchrum Domini. Studien zur Ikonographie und Funktion großplastischer Grablegungsgruppen am Mittelrhein und im Rheinland.* Mainz: Gesellschaft für Mittelrheinische Kirchengeschichte.

Mâle, Émile. 1932. *Art religieux après le Concile de Trente. Étude sur l'iconographie de la fin du XVIe siècle, du XVIIe, du XVIIIe siècle – Italie, France, Espagne, Flandres.* Paris: Colin.

Mancinelli, Fabrizio. 1998. "Il Giudizio Universale: storia tecnica e restauro." In *La Cappella Sistina: Il* Giudizio *restaurato*, 155–86. Novara: De Agostini.

Mancinelli, Fabrizio, Gianluigi Colalucci, and Nazzareno Gabrieli. 1994. "The *Last Judgment*: Notes on Its Conservation History, Technique, and Restoration." In *The Sistine Chapel: A Glorious Restoration.* Ed. Pierluigi de Vecchi, 236–55. New York: Abrams.

Mancini, Giulio. 1956. *Considerazioni sulla Pittura.* Ed. Adriana Marucchi and Luigi Salerno. Rome: Accademia Nazionale dei Lincei.

Mandowsky, Erna. 1939. *Ricerche intorno all'Iconologia di Cesare Ripa.* Florence: Olschki.

Mangrum, Bryan D., and Scavizzi, Giuseppe, ed. 1998. *A Reformation Debate: Karlstadt, Emser, and Eck on Sacred Images – Three Treatises in Translation*, 2d ed. Toronto: Centre for Reformation and Renaissance Studies.

Maniura, Robert, and Rupert Sheperd, ed. 2006. *Presence: The Inherence of the Prototype Within Images and Other Objects.* Aldershot: Ashgate.

Manning, John, and Marc Van Vaeck, ed. 1999. *The Jesuits and the Emblem Tradition.* Turnhout: Brepols.

Mansi, Giovanni Domenico. 1759–98. *Sacrorum conciliorum nova et amplissima collectio.* Florence: Antonio Zatta.

Mansi, Joannes Dominicus. 1960–62. *Sacrorum Conciliorum nova et amplissima collectio*, 54 vols. in 59. Graz: Akademische Druck- und Verlagsanstalt.

Marcora, Carlo. 1962a. "Il processo diocesano informativo sulla vita di S. Carlo per la sua canonizzazione." *Memorie Storiche della Diocesi di Milano* 9: 76–735.

1962b. "Un tentativo di processo arcivescovile contro le nobildonne milanesi." *La Martinella* 16: 316–18.

1965. "Il diario di Giambattista Casale (1554–1598)." *Memorie Storiche della Diocesi di Milano* 12: 209–437.

1985. "Trattati d'arte sacre al tempo del Baronio." In Romeo De Maio et al. (1986), 189–246.

Marinelli, Sergio. 1974. "Lo spazio ideologico di Paolo Veronese." *Comunità* 173: 302–64.

Martin, John Jeffries. 2004. *Venice's Hidden Enemies: Italian Heretics in a Renaissance City* [1993]. Baltimore: Johns Hopkins University Press.

Mauquoy-Hendrickx, Marie. 1979–83. *Les Estampes des Wierix*, 4 vols. Brussels: Bibliothèque Royale de Belgique.

Mazzone, Umberto, and Angelo Turchini, eds. 1985. *Le visite pastorali. Analisi si una fonte.* Bologna: il Mulino.

McCabe, William H. 1983. *An Introduction to the Jesuit Theater.* Ed. Louis J. Oldani. St. Louis: Institute of Jesuit Sources.

Meijer, Bert W. 1999. "New Light on Christoph Schwarz in Venice and the Veneto." *Artibus et Historiae*, 20.39: 127–56.

Melasecchi, Olga. 1995. "Nascita e sviluppo dell'iconografia di S. Filippo Neri dal Cinquecento al Settecento." In Strinati and Costamagna (1995), 34–49.

Melasecchi, Olga, D., and Stephen Pepper. 1998. "Guido Reni, Luca Ciamberlano and the Oratorians: Their Relationship Clarified." *Burlington Magazine* 140: 596–603.

Melion, Walter S., and Lee Palmer Wandel, ed. 2009. *Early Modern Eyes.* Leiden: Brill.

Memorie storiche della diocesi di Milano. 1954–64. Vols. 1–16. Milan: Biblioteca Ambrosiana.

Merbeck, Mitchell. 1999. *The Thief, the Cross and the Wheel: Pain and the Spectacle of Punishment in Medieval and Renaissance Europe.* Chicago: Chicago University Press.

Merleau-Ponty, Maurice. 1964. *Sense and Non-Sense.* Trans. Hubert L. Dreyfus and Patricia Allen Dreyfus. Evanston, IL: Northwestern University Press. Originally published as *Sens et non-sens.* Paris: Nagel, 1948.

Michaud-Quantin, Pierre. 1970. *Études sur le vocabulaire philosophique du moyen âge.* Rome: Edizioni dell'Ateneo.

Migne, J.-P. [Jacques-Paul], ed. 1841–61. *Patrologiae cursus completus. Series latina.* Paris: J.-P. Migne.

Mildner, Ursula. 1994. "Decorum 2. Malerei, Architektur." *Historisches Wörterbuch der Rhetorik*, 2: 434–51. Tübingen: Max Niemeyer.

Mildner-Flesch, Ursula. 1983. *Das Decorum. Herkunft, Wesen, und Wirkung des Sujetstils am Beispiel Nicolas Poussins.* Sankt Augustin: Richarz.

Miles, Margaret R. 1985. *Image as Insight: Visual Understanding in Western Christianity and Secular Culture.* Boston: Beacon Press.

Millner, Matthew. 2011. *The Senses and the English Reformation.* Aldershot: Ashgate.

Minnich, Nelson H. 1988. "The Debate between Desiderius Erasmus of Rotterdam and Alberto Pio of Carpi on the Use of Sacred Images." *Annuarium historiae Conciliorum* 20: 1–2: 379–413. Rpt. with the original pagination in Minnich, *The Catholic Reformation: Council, Churchmen, Controversies.* Aldershot: Variorum, 1993.

1998. "The Voice of Theologians in General Councils from Pisa to Trent." *Theological Studies* 59: 420–41.

Miranda, Salvador. *The Cardinals of the Holy Roman Church.* www2.fiu.edu/~mirandas/bios1539.htm (modified 26 January 2012; accessed 23 February 2011).

Missirini, Melchiorre. 1823. *Memorie per servire alla storia della Romana Accademia di S. Luca fino alla morte di Antonio Canova.* Rome: De Romanis.

Molanus, Johannes. 1570. *De Picturis et Imaginibus Sacris, liber unus, tractans de vitandis circa eas abusibus ac de earundem significationibus.* Leuven: Walleus.

1996. *Traité Des Saintes Images*, 2 vols. Trans. François Boespflug, Olivier Christin, and Benoît Tassel. Paris: Cerf.
Monfasani, John. 1993. "Aristotelians, Platonists, and the Missing Ockhamists: Philosophical Liberty in Pre-Reformation Italy." *Renaissance Quarterly* 46: 247–76.
Monson, Craig. 2002. "The Council of Trent Revisited." *Journal of the American Musicological Society* 55: 1–37.
Montagu, Jennifer. 1992. "The Theory of the Musical Modes in the Académie Royale de Peinture et de Sculpture." *Journal of the Warburg and Courtauld Institutes* 55: 233–48.
Monticone, Alberto. 1953. "L'applicazione a Roma del Concilio di Trento. Le visite del 1565–66." *Rivista di storia della Chiesa in Italia* 7: 225–50.
Morelli, Arnaldo. 1991. *Il Tempio Armonico. Musica nell'Oratorio dei Filippini in Roma (1575–1705)*. Laaber: Laaber Verlag.
Mormando, Franco, ed. 1999. *Saints & Sinners: Caravaggio & the Baroque Image*. Chicago: University of Chicago Press.
Mouchel, Christian. 1990. *Cicéron et Sénèque dans la rhétorique de la Renaissance*. Marburg: Hitzeroth.
Müller, A. 1909. *Die Kölner Bürger-Sodalität, 1608–1908*. Paderborn: Junfermann.
Muir, Edward. 1997. *Ritual in Early Modern Europe*. Cambridge: Cambridge University Press.
Muraoka, Anne H. 2009. "Il Fine della Pittura: Canon Reformulation in the Age of Counter-Reformation – The Lombard–Roman Confluence." Ph.D. diss., Temple University.
Muzzarelli, Maria Giuseppina. 2003. "Le leggi suntuarie." In *Storia d'Italia. Annali 19*. Ed. C. M. Belfanti and F. Giusberti. Torino: Einaudi.
Nadal, Jerónimo. 2003–2007. *Annotations and Meditations on the Gospels*, 3 vols. Trans. Frederick A. Homann, intro. Walter S. Melion. Philadelphia: Saint Joseph's University Press.
Nagel, Alexander. 1993. "Leonardo and *sfumato*." *RES* 23 (Spring): 7–20.
2000. *Michelangelo and the Reform of Art*. Cambridge: Cambridge University Press.
2011. *The Controversy of Renaissance Art*. Chicago: Chicago University Press.
Nead, Lynda. 1992. *The Female Nude*. New York: Routledge.
Nelson, Robert S. 2000. *Visuality before and beyond the Renaissance: Seeing as Others Saw*. Cambridge: Cambridge University Press.
Nencioni, Giovanni, and Barocchi Paola, eds. "Vocabolario della Crusca (1612)." In *Vocabolario degli accademici della Crusca*, 2001–. vocabolario.signum.sns.it (accessed 23 February 2011).
Newhauser, Richard. 2010. "Foreword: The Senses in Medieval and Renaissance Intellectual History." *Senses and Society* 5: 1.
Nichols, Stephen G., Andreas Kablitz, and Alison Calhoun. 2008. *Rethinking the Medieval Senses: Heritage/Fascinations/Frames*. Baltimore: Johns Hopkins University Press.
Nicolson, Benedict. 1985. "Orazio Gentileschi and Giovanni Antonio Saulli." *Artibus et Historiae* 6.12: 9–25.
Nising, Horst. 2004. "... in keiner Weise prächtig." *Die Jesuitenkollegien der süddeutschen Provinz des Ordens und ihre städtebauliche Lage im 16–18.* Jahrhundert. Petersberg: Imhof.
Norberg-Schulz, Christian. 1971. *Baroque Architecture*. New York: Abrams.

Nordenfalk, Carl. 1985a. "The Five Senses in Flemish Art before 1600." In *Netherlandish Mannerism*. Ed. Görel Cavalli-Björkman, 135–54. Stockholm: Nationalmuseum.

1985b. "The Five Senses in Late Medieval and Renaissance Art." *Journal of the Warburg and Courtauld Institutes* 48: 1–22. Originally published as "Les Cinq Sens dans l'art du Moyen-âge." *Revue de l'art* 34 (1976): 17–28.

Nubola, Cecilia. 1996. "Visite Pastorali fra Chiesa e Stato nei secoli XVI e XVII." In *Il Concilio di Trento e il Moderno*. Ed. Paolo Prodi and Wolfgang Reinhard, 383–414. Bologna: Il Mulino.

Nubola, Cecilia, and Angelo Turchini. 1993. *Visite pastorali ed elaborazione dei dati*. Bologna: Il Mulino.

Nugent, Donald. 1974. *Ecumenism in the Age of the Reformation: The Colloquy of Poissy*. Cambridge, MA: Harvard University Press.

Nussdorfer, Laurie. 1987. "The Vacant See: Ritual and Protest in Early Modern Rome." *Sixteenth Century Journal* 18.2: 173–89.

2009. "Notaries and the Accademia di San Luca, 1590–1630." In Lukehart (2009a), 54–67.

Ogden, Dunbar H. 2002. *The Staging of Drama in the Medieval Church*. Newark: University of Delaware Press.

O'Malley, John W. 1979. *Praise and Blame in Renaissance Rome: Rhetoric, Doctrine, and Reform in the Sacred Orators of the Papal Court, c. 1450–1521*. Durham, NC: Duke University Press.

1981. "The Feast of Thomas Aquinas in Renaissance Rome: A Neglected Document and Its Import." *Rivista di Storia della Chiesa in Italia* 35: 1–27.

1985. "Erasmus and the History of Sacred Rhetoric: The *Ecclesiastes* of 1535." *Erasmus of Rotterdam Society Yearbook* 5 (1985): 1–29.

ed. 1988. *Collected Works of Erasmus*, vol. 66: *Spiritualia*. Toronto: University of Toronto Press.

1993. *The First Jesuits*. Cambridge, MA: Harvard University Press.

1999a. "A Historiographical Frame for the Paintings: Recent Interpretations of Early Modern Catholicism." In Mormando (1999), 19–27.

ed. 1999b. *The Jesuits: Cultures, Sciences, and the Arts, 1, 1540–1773*. Toronto: University of Toronto Press.

ed. 1999c. *Collected Works of Erasmus*, vol. 69: *Spiritualia and Pastoralia*. Toronto: University of Toronto Press.

2000. *Trent and All That: Renaming Catholicism in the Early Modern Era*. Cambridge, MA: Harvard University Press.

2002. "The Council of Trent: Myths, Misunderstandings, and Misinformation." In *Spirit, Style, Story: Essays Honoring John W. Padberg, S.J.* Ed. Thomas M. Lucas, 205–26. Chicago: Loyola Press.

2004a. *Four Cultures of the West*. Cambridge, MA: Harvard University Press.

2004b. "The Society of Jesus." In Hsia (2004), 223–36.

2006a. "Celibacy: Decisive Moments in Its History." In *Sexuality and the U.S. Catholic Church: Crisis and Renewal*. Ed. Lisa Sowle Cahill et al., 94–106. New York: Crossroad.

2006b. "Ignatius, Saint of a Middle Way." *America* (31 July 2006), 10–14.

ed. 2006c. *The Jesuits II: Cultures, Sciences, and the Arts, 1540–1773*. Toronto: Toronto University Press.

ed. 2008. *Constructing a Saint Through Images: The 1609 Illustrated Biography of Ignatius of Loyola*. Philadelphia: Saint Joseph's University Press.

O'Malley, John W., and Gauvin Alexander Bailey, eds. 2005. *The Jesuits and the Arts, 1540–1773*. Philadelphia: Saint Joseph's University Press.

Ong, Walter J., S.J. 2004. *Ramus, Method, and the Decay of Dialogue: From the Art of Discourse to the Art of Reason [1958]*. Chicago: Chicago University Press.

Onians, John. 2007. *Neuroarthistory: From Aristotle and Pliny to Baxandall and Zeki*. New Haven, CT: Yale University Press.

Onida, Nicoletta. 2002. "Il problema dei 'luoghi per confessionali' nelle chiese dei barnabiti. Il contributo di Lorenzo Binago." *Arte lombarda*, n.s. 134: 150–60.

Osborne, Peter, ed. 2000. *From an Aesthetic Point of View: Philosophy, Art and the Senses*. London: Serpent's Tail.

Ostrow, Steven F. 1996. *Art and Spirituality in Counter-Reformation Rome: The Sistine and Pauline Chapels in S. Maria Maggiore*. Cambridge: Cambridge University Press.

Oswald, John, and Peter Rummel, eds. 1996. *Petrus Canisius: Reformer der Kirche*. Augsburg: Sankt Ulrich.

Ottonelli, Giovan Domenico, and Pietro Berrettini [da Cortona]. 1652. *Trattato della pittura, e scultura, uso, et abuso loro*. Florence: Giovanni Antonio Bonardi. Rpt. Treviso: Canova, 1973.

Ozment, Steven. 1980. *The Age of Reform 1250–1550: An Intellectual and Religious History of Late Medieval and Reformation Europe*. New Haven, CT: Yale University Press.

Padberg, John W., Martin D. O'Keefe, and John L. McCarthy, eds. 1994. *For Matters of Great Moment, the First Thirty Jesuit General Congregations: A Brief History and a Translation of the Decrees*. St. Louis: Institute of Jesuit Sources.

Pagano, Sergio. 1980. "Le visite apostoliche a Roma nei secoli XVI–XIX. Repertorio delle fonti." *Ricerche per la storia religiosa di Roma* 4: 317–464.

1984. *Ricerca sulla Teorica delle arti figurative nella Riforma Cattolica*. Bologna: Nuova Alfa.

Paleotti, Gabriele. 1582. *Discorso intorno alle imagini sacre e profane*. In Barocchi (1960–62), 2: 117–503.

2002. *Discorso intorno alle immagini sacre e profane (1582)*. Vatican City: Libreria editrice vaticana.

Palestra, Anselme. 1977. "Le visite pastorali del Card. Carlo Borromeo al Duomo e alla veneranda fabbrica del Duomo di Milano." In AA.VV., *Duomo di Milano. Cuore e simbolo di Milano. IV Centenario della Dedicazione (1577–1977)*, 156–230. Milan: Centro ambrosiano di documentazione e studi religiosi.

Pampalone, Antonella. 2000. "La Pentecoste di San Filippo Neri: iconografia e iconologia." In Russo and Del Re (2000), 145–78.

Panofsky, Erwin. 1955. *Meaning in the Visual Arts: Papers in and on Art History*. Garden City, NY: Doubleday.

1969. "Erasmus and the Visual Arts." *Journal of the Warburg and Courtauld Institutes* 32: 200–27.

Parks, George Bruner, ed. 1969. *Roma sancta (1581)*. Rome: Edizioni di storia e letteratura.

Parma Armani, Elena. 1986. *Perin del Vaga. L'anello mancante*. Genoa: Sagep.

Paruta, Paolo. 1887. *La legazione di Roma di Paolo Paruta (1592–1595)*. Ed. Giuseppe di Levy. Reale deputazione di storia patria per le Venezie. Monumenti storici, ser. 4. Miscellanea, vols. 7–9. Venice: a spese della Società.

Paschini, Pio. 1926. *S. Gaetano Thiene, Gian Pietro Carafa e le origini dei chierici regolari teatini.* Rome: Scuola tip. Pio X.

Paterson, Mark. 2007. *The Senses of Touch: Haptics, Affects and Technologies.* Oxford: Berg.

Patrologia Latina: The Full-Text Database. 1996. Alexandria, VA: Chadwyck-Healey.

Paulus, Nikolaus. 1902. "Die Einführung der lauretanischen Litanei in Deutschland durch den seligen Canisius." *Zeitschrift für katholische Theologie* 26: 574–83.

Perella, Nicolas James. 1969. *The Kiss Sacred and Profane.* Berkeley: University of California Press.

Pieters, Jürgen. 2001. *Moments of Negotiation: The New Historicism of Stephen Greenblatt.* Amsterdam: Amsterdam University Press.

Pigozzi, Marinella. 1989. "Domenico Tibaldi, architetto e teorico. Architettura come metafora." In *L'Architettura a Roma e in Italia (1580–1621).* Ed. G. Spagnesi, 315–33. Rome: Centro di Studi per la Storia dell'Architettura.

Pina Polo, Francisco. 2004. "Die nützliche Erinnerung: Geschichtsschreibung, *mos maiorum* und die römische Identität." *Historia* 53: 147–72.

Pirri, Pietro. 1955. *Giovanni Tristano e i primordi della architettura jesuitica.* Rome: Institutum Historicum Societatis Iesu.

Ponnelle, Louis, and Louis Bordet. 1928. *Saint Philippe Neri et la société romaine de son temps.* Paris: Bloud & Gay.

Possevino, Antonio. 1595. *Tractatio De Poesi Et Pictura Ethnica, Humana Et Fabulosa Collata Cum Vera, Honesta Et Sacra: Adjectus Est in Hac Editione Novus Index Qui Omnia Notatu Digna Complectitur.* Lyon: apud J. Pillehotte.

Possevino, Giovanni Battista. 1591. *Discorsi della vita et ationi di Carlo Borromeo prete cardinale di santa chiesa del titolo di S. Prassede, arcivescovo di Milano.* Rome: Giacomo Tornieri.

Pozzi, Mario. 1967. "*L'ut pictura poesis* in un dialogo di L. Dolce." *Giornale Storico della Letteratura Italiana* 144: 234–60.

Pracchi, Attilio. 1996. *La cattedrale antica di Milano.* Rome: Einaudi.

Praz, Mario. 1964. *Studies in Seventeenth-Century Imagery*, 2d ed. Rome: Edizioni di storia e letteratura.

Preti, Girolamo. 2002. "Discorso intorno all'onestà della poesia." In *Edizioni Res.* www.edres.it/preti.pdf (accessed 22 February 2011).

Processo. 1957–63. *Il primo Processo per la canonizzazione di San Filippo Neri*, 4 vols. Ed. Giovanni Incisa della Rocchetta and Niccolò Vian. Vatican.

Prodi, Paolo. 1959–67. *Il Cardinale Gabriele Paleotti (1522–1597)*, 2 vols. Rome: Edizioni di storia e letteratura.

1962. "Ricerca sulla teorica delle arti figurative nella Riforma Cattolica." Archivio Italiano per la Storia della Pietà 4 (1965): 121–212. Rome: Edizioni di storia e letteratura.

1984. *Ricerca sulla teorica delle arti figurative nella Riforma Cattolica.* Rome: Edizioni di storia e letteratura. Rpt. Bologna: Nuova Alfa.

Prodi, Paolo, ed. 1995. *Filippo Neri nella Roma della Controriforma.* Florence La Nuova Italia Ed. (special issue of *Storia dell'arte* 85).

Prodi, Paolo, and Elisabeth Möller-Luckner, eds. 1993. *Glaube und Eid. Treuformeln, Glaubensbekenntnisse und Sozialdisziplinierung zwischen Mittelalter und Neuzeit.* Munich: Oldenbourg.

Prodi, Paolo, and Carla Penuti, eds. 1994. *Disciplina dell'anima, disciplina del corpo e disciplina della società tra medioevo ed età moderna.* Bologna: Il Mulino.

Prosperi, Adriano. 1996. *Il tribunale della coscienza. Inquisitori, confessori, missionari.* Turin: Einaudi.

Pullapilly, Cyriac K. 1992. "Agostino Valier and the Conceptual Basis of the Catholic Reformation." *Harvard Theological Review* 85.3: 307–33.

Puttenham, George. 1970. *The Arte of English Poesie* [1936]. Ed. Gladys Doidge Willock and Alice Walker. Cambridge: Cambridge University Press.

2007. *The Arte of English Poesie.* Ed. Frank Whigham and Wayne Rebhorn. Ithaca, NY: Cornell University Press.

Quiviger, François. 2010. *The Sensory World of Italian Renaissance Art.* London: Reaktion Books.

Rabus, Johann Jakob. 1925. *Rom, eine Münchner Pilgerfahrt im Jubeljahr 1575.* Ed. Karl Schottenloher. Munich: Münchner Drucke.

Rainey, Ronald. 1991. "Dressing Down the Dressed-up: Reproving Feminine Attire in Renaissance Florence." In *Renaissance Society and Culture: Essays in Honor of Eugene Rice.* Ed. John Monfasano and Ron G. Musto, 217–37. New York: Italic Press.

Randolph, Adrian. 1997. "Regarding Women in Sacred Space." In *Picturing Women in Renaissance and Baroque Italy.* Ed. Geraldine A. Johnson and Sara F. Matthews Greco, 17–41. Cambridge: Cambridge University Press.

2002. *Engaging Symbols: Gender, Politics, and Public Art in Fifteenth-Century Florence.* New Haven, CT: Yale University Press.

Rasmussen, Jörg. 1974. *Die Nürnberger Altarbau-Kunst der Dürerzeit.* Hamburg: Author.

1980–81. "Bildersturm und Restauatio." In *Welt im Umbruch. Augsburg zwischen Renaissance und Barock.* Exh. cat., Stadt Augsburg, 3 vols. Augsburg: Augsberger Druck- und Verlagshaus.

Rebhorn, Wayne. 2000. "Outlandish Fears: Defining Decorum in Renaissance Rhetoric." *Intertexts* 4:1. www.intertexts.org.

Repishti, Francesco. 2006. "I disegni per il pulpito dell'antico testamento del Duomo di Milano." In *Arte e storia di Lombardi. Scritti in memoria di Grazioso Sironi* in *Biblioteca della nuova rivista storica* 40: 265–72. Rome: Società Editrice Dante Alighieri.

Repishti, Francesco, and Richard Vaughn Schofield. 2004. *Architettura e controriforma. I dibattiti per la facciata del Duomo di Milano, 1582–1682.* Milan: Electa.

Rice, Eugene F. 1985. *Saint Jerome in the Renaissance.* Baltimore: Johns Hopkins University Press.

Rice, Louise. 1997. *The Altars and Altarpieces of New St. Peter's: Outfitting the Basilica, 1621–1666.* Cambridge: Cambridge University Press.

Richeôme, Louis. 1604. *Le pelerin de Lorete.* Bordeaux: Impr. de S. Millange.

1611. *La peinture spirituelle.* Lyon: Chez Pierre Rigaud.

Rietbergen, Peter. 2006. *Power and Religion in Baroque Rome: Barbarini Cultural Policies.* Leiden: Koninklijke Brill NV.

Ringbom, Sixten. 1984. *Icon to Narrative: The Rise of the Dramatic Close-Up in Fifteenth-Century Devotional Painting,* 2d ed. Doornspijk: Davaco.

Ripa, Cesare. 1611. *Iconologia.* Padua: Pietro Paolo Tozzi.

Ristori, Renato. 1986. "L'Aretino, Il David di Michelangelo e la 'Modestia Fiorentina.'" *Rinascimento* 26: 77–97.

Rittershausen, Joseph Sebastian. 1788. *Die vornehmste Merkwürdigkeiten der Residenz-Stadt München für Liebhaber der bildenden Künste.* Munich: Lentner.

Robertson, Clare. 1992. *'Il gran cardinale': Alessandro Farnese, Patron of the Arts.* New Haven, CT: Yale University Press.

Roccasecca, Pietro. 2009. "Teaching in the Studio of the Accademia del Disegno dei pittori, scultori e architetti di Roma (1594–1636)." In Lukehart (2009a), 122–59.

Rock, Judith. 1996. *Terpsichore at Louis-le-Grand: Baroque Dance on the Jesuit Stage in Paris.* St. Louis: Institute of Jesuit Sources.

Rocke, Michael. 1996. *Forbidden Friendships: Homosexuality and Male Culture in Renaissance Florence.* Oxford: Oxford University Press.

Rodaway, Paul. 1994. *Sensuous Geographies: Body, Sense, and Place.* London: Routledge.

Rolle, Theodor. 1989. "Die Anfänge der Marianischen Kongregationen in Augsburg." *Jahrbuch des Vereins für Augsburger Bistumsgeschichte* 23: 27–68.

Rosignoli, C. Gregorio. 1696. *La Pittura in Giudicio.* Bologna: Il Longhi.

Rotelle, John E., ed. 2000. *Soliloquies: Augustine's Inner Dialogue.* Trans. Kim Paffenroth, O.S.A. Hyde Park, NY: New City Press.

Röttgen, Herwarth. 2002. *Il Cavalier Giuseppe Cesari d'Arpino. Un Grande Pittore nello Splendore della Fama e nell'incostanza della Fortuna.* Rome: Ugo Bozzi.

Rovetta, Alessandro. 1999. "Tra un 'paragone' e un 'abbozzo' di Giacomo Valeri. Milano città d'arte ai tempi di Federico Borromeo e Cesare Monti." In *Studi di storia dell'arte in onore di Maria Luisa Gatti Perer.* Ed. M. Rossi and A. Rovetta, 307–15. Milan: Università Cattolica del Sacro Cuore.

Rudolph, Conrad. 2000. *The Things of Greater Importance: Bernard of Clairvaux's Apologia and the Medieval Attitude Toward Art.* Philadelphia: University of Pennslyvania Press.

Rummel, Erika. 1995. "Monachatus Non Est Pietas: Interpretations and Misinterpretations of a Dictum." In *Erasmus' Vision of the Church.* Ed. Hilmar M. Pabel, 41–55. Kirksville, MO: Sixteenth Century Journal Publishers.

Rurale, Flavio. 1992. *I Jesuiti a Milano. Religione e politica nel secondo Cinquecento.* Rome: Bulzoni.

Russo, Maria Teresa Bonadonna, and Niccolò del Re, eds. 2000. *San Filippo Neri nella realtà romana del XVI secoli.* Atti del convegno di studio in occasione del IV centenario della morte di San Filippo Neri (1595–1995), 11–13 May, Rome. Rome: Società Romana di Storia Patria.

Rzepińska, Maria. 1986. "Tenebrism in Baroque Painting and Its Ideological Background." *Artibus et Historiae* 7.13: 91–112.

Saba, Agostino. 1936. *La biblioteca di S. Carlo Borromeo.* Florence: Sansoni.

Sacrosancti et Oecumenici Concilii Tridentini … Canones et Decreta. 1824. Paris: Méquignon / Lyon: Périsse.

Sailer, Sebastian. 1997. *Geistliche Schaubühne des Leidens Jesu Christi, in gesungenen Oratorien aufgeführt.* Weißenhorn: Konrad.

Salvagni, Isabella. 2009. "The Università dei Pittori and the Accademia di San Luca: From the Installation in San Luca sull'Esquilino to the Reconstruction of Santa Martina al Foro Romano." In Lukehart (2009a), 68–121.

Salviucci Insolera, Lydia. 2004. *L'Imago primi saeculi (1640) e il significato dell'imagine allegorica nella Compagnia di Gesù.* Rome: Editrice Pontificia Università Gregoriana.

Sandrart, Joachim von. 1994. *Teutsche Academie der edlen Bau-, Bild- und Malerei-Künste* [1675–80], 3 vols. Nördlingen: Uhl.

Sanger, Alice, and Siv Tove Kulbrandstad Walker, eds. 2012. *Sense and the Senses in Early Modern Art and Cultural Practice.* Aldershot: Ashgate.

Sassi, Giovanni Antonio. 1747–48. *S. Caroli Borromei … Homiliae,* 5 vols. Milan: Biblioteca Ambrosiano.

Sattler, Maximilian Vinzenz. 1864. *Geschichte der Marianischen Congregationen in Bayern*. Munich: J. J. Lentner.

Sauter, Marion. 2004. *Die oberdeutschen Jesuitenkirchen (1550–1650). Bauten, Kontext und Bautypologie.* Petersberg: Imhof.

Scavizzi, Giuseppe. 1974. "La teologia cattolica e le immagini durante il XVI secolo." *Storia dell'arte* 21: 171–213.

1981. *Arte e architettura sacra. Cronache e documenti sulla controversia tra riformati e cattolici (1500–1550).* Rome: Casa del Libro.

1987. "Storia ecclesiastica e arte nel secondo Cinquecento." *Storia dell'arte* 59: 29–46.

1992. *The Controversy on Images from Calvin to Baronius.* Toronto Studies in Religion, no. 14. New York: Peter Lang.

Schade, Herbert. 1960. "Die Berufung der Jesuiten nach München und der Bau von St. Michael." In *Der Mönch im Wappen. Das Geschichte und Gegenwort des katholischen München*, 209–57. Munich: Schnell & Steiner.

Schlitt, Melinda. 2005. "Painting, Criticism, and Michelangelo's Last Judgment in the Age of the Counter-Reformation." In Hall (2005b), 113–49.

Schlosser, Julius von. 1924. *Die Kunstliteratur. Ein Handbuch zur Quellenkunde der neueren Kunstgeschichte.* Vienna: A. Schroll.

1956. *Die Kunstliteratur. Ein Handbuch zur Quellenkunde der neueren Kunstgeschichte [1924].* Ed. Otto Kurz. Florence: La Nuova Italia.

1996. *La letteratura artistica. Manuale delle fonti della storia dell'arte moderna.* Trans. Filippo Rossi. Florence: La Nuova Italia.

1997. *La letteratura artistica. Manuale delle fonti della storia dell'arte moderna.* Paperbacks classici, 6. Trans. Filippo Rossi. Florence: La Nuova Italia.

Schmidt, Anja. 2000. *Augsburger Ansichten. Die Darstellung der Stadt in der Druckgraphik des 15. bis 18. Jahrhunderts.* Augsburg: Wissner.

Schneider, Bernhard. 1991. "Die Sodalitäten und Bruderschaften am Trierer Jesuitenkollege." In *Für Gott und die Menschen. Die Gesellschaft Jesu und ihr Wirken im Erzbistum Trier*, 273–81. Mainz: Verlag der Gesellschaft für mittelrheinische Kirchengeschichte.

Schneider, Rebecca. 1997. *The Explicit Body in Performance.* London: Routledge.

Schnusenberg, Christine. 1988. *The Relationship Between the Church and the Theatre: Exemplified by Selected Writings of the Church Fathers and by Liturgical Texts Until Amalarius of Metz, 775–852 A.D.* Lanham, MD: University Press of America.

Schofield, Richard Vaughn. 2001. Review of C. Borromeo (2000). *Annali di architettura* 13: 206–10.

2004. "Architecture and the Assertion of the Cult of Relics in Milan's Public Spaces." *Annali di architettura* 16: 79–120.

2006. "Tu es porta Diaboli; Carlo Borromeo, misoginia e l'architettura." In Stabenow (2006), 282–352.

Schroeder, Henry Joseph, O.P., trans. 1950. *Canons and Decrees of the Council of Trent* [1941]. St. Louis: Herder. Rpt. Rockford, IL: Tan Books, 1978.

Schwarzweber, Annemarie. 1940. *Das heilige Grab in der deutschen Bildnerei des Mittelalters.* Freiburg: Eberhard Albert Universitätsbuchhandlung.

Scribner, Robert W. 1987. *Popular Culture and Popular Movements in Reformation Germany.* London: Hambledon Press.

Senie, Harriet, and Sally Webster, eds. 1992. *Critical Issues in Public Art: Content, Context, and Controversy.* New York: Icon Editions.

Sgarbi, Vittorio, ed. 2006. *Luce e ombra nella pittura italiana tra Rinascimento e Barocco. Da Tiziano a Bernini*. Geneva: Skira.

Shearman, John. 1962. "Leonardo's Color and Chiaroscuro." *Zeitschrift für Kunstgeschichte* 25: 13–47.

1967. *Mannerism*. Harmondsworth: Penguin.

1992. *Only Connect . . . :Art and the Spectator in the Italian Renaissance*. A.W. Mellon Lectures in the Fine Arts (1988), National Gallery of Art, Washington, DC. Princeton: Princeton University Press.

Sheingorn, Pamela. 1978. "The *Sepulchrum Domini*: A Study in Art and Liturgy." *Studies in Iconography* 4: 37–60.

Sherman, Claire Richter, and Peter M. Lukehart, eds. 2000. *Writing on Hands: Memory and Knowledge in Early Modern Europe*. Exh. cat. Carlisle: Trout Gallery.

Silos, Giuseppe. 1672. *Vita di S. Gaetano Thiene*. Milan: Ludovico Monza.

Smith, Jeffrey Chipps. 1994. *German Sculpture of the Later Renaissance, c. 1520–1580: Art in an Age of Uncertainty*. Princeton, NJ: Princeton University Press.

2002. *Sensuous Worship: Jesuits and the Art of the Early Catholic Reformation in Germany*. Princeton, NJ: Princeton University Press.

2006. *The Art of the Goldsmith in Late Fifteenth-Century Germany: The Kimbell Virgin and Her Bishop*. New Haven, CT: Yale University Press.

2008. "A Tale of Two Cities: Nuremberg and Munich." In *Embodiments of Power: Building Baroque Cities in Europe*. Ed. Gary B. Cohen and Franz A. J. Szabo, 164–90. New York: Berghahn.

Smith, Mark M. 2008. *Sensing the Past: Seeing, Hearing, Smelling, Tasting, and Touching in History*. Berkeley: University of California Press.

2010. "Looking Back: the Explosion of Sensory History." *Psychologist* 23.10: 860–63.

Smyth, Craig Hugh. 1992. *Mannerism and Maniera* [1963]. Intro. Elizabeth Cropper. Vienna: IRSA.

Snyder, Jon R. 1989. *Writing the Scene of Speaking: Theories of Dialogue in the Late Italian Renaissance*. Stanford, CA: Stanford University Press.

Spagnolo, Maddalena. 2005. *Correggio. Geografia e storia della fortuna (1528–1657)*. Milan: Silvana Editoriale.

Stabenow, Jörg. 2006. "Il duplice pulpito di Carlo Borromeo nel Duomo di Milano." In Stabenow (2006), 227–80.

ed. 2006. *Lo spazio e il culto. Relazioni tra edificio ecclesiale e uso liturgico dal XV al XVI secolo*. Venice: Marsilio.

Stafford, Barbara Maria, and Frances Terpak, eds. 2001. *Devices of Wonder: From the World in a Box to Images on a Screen*. Los Angeles: Getty Research Institute.

Stefaniak, Regina. 2008. *Mysterium Magnum: Michelangelo's Doni Tondo*. Leiden: Brill.

Steinberg, Leo. 1983. "The Sexuality of Christ in Renaissance Art and in Modern Oblivion." *October* 25: 1–198, 204–22.

1997. *The Sexuality of Christ in Renaissance Art and in Modern Oblivion*, rev. ed. Chicago: University of Chicago Press.

Steinberg, Ronald. 1977. *Fra Girolamo Savonarola, Florentine Arts, and Renaissance Historiography*. Athens, GA: Ohio University Press.

Stenhouse, William. 2005. *Reading Inscriptions and Writing Ancient History: Historical Scholarship in the Late Renaissance*. London: Institute of Classical Studies.

Sterling, Charles. 1958. "Gentileschi in France." *Burlington Magazine* 100.661: 112–21.

Stoichita, Victor I. 1997. *A Short History of the Shadow*. London: Reaktion Books.

Stortoni, Laura Anna, ed. 1997. *Women Poets of the Italian Renaissance*. New York: Italica Press.

Strecker, Freya. 1998. *Augsburger Altäre zwischen Reformation (1537) und 1635*. Münster: Lit.

Strieder, Peter. 1951. "Entwürfe zu 'Heiligen Gräbern' in Münchner Kirchen." *Das Münster* 4: 281–87.

Strinati, Claudio. 1980. "Roma nell'anno 1600. Studio di pittura." *Ricerche di storia dell'arte* 10: 15–48.

Strinati, Claudio, and Alba Costamagna, eds. 1995. *La Regola e la Fama. San Filippo Neri e l'arte*. Exh. cat., Museo Nazionale del Palazzo Venezia, Rome. Milan: Electa.

Strunck, Christina. 2007. "The Original Setting of the Early Life of Taddeo Series: A New Reading of the Pictorial Program in the Palazzo Zuccari, Rome." In *Taddeo and Federico Zuccaro: Artist-Brothers in Renaissance Rome*. Ed. Julian Brooks, 113–25. Exh. cat. Los Angeles: J. Paul Getty Museum.

Summers, David. 1972. "Maniera and Movement: The *Figura Serpentinata*." *Art Quarterly* 35: 269–301.

1987. *The Judgment of Sense: Renaissance Naturalism and the Rise of Aesthetics*. New York: Cambridge University Press.

2007. *Vision, Reflection and Desire in Western Painting*. Chapel Hill, NC: University of North Carolina Press.

Summers, William J. 1999. "The Jesuits in Manila, 1581–1621: The Role of Music in Rite, Ritual, and Spectacle." In O'Malley (1999b), 659–79.

Surius, Laurentius. 1567. *In quatuor tomos conciliorum omnium tum generalium tum provincialium … index*, 4 vols. Cologne: Gervinus Calenius.

Symonds, John Addington. 1914. *Sketches in Italy and Greece*. Ed. Horatio R. F. Brown. London: John Murray.

Symons, Thomas. 1953. *The Monastic Agreement of the Monks and Nuns of the English Nation*. Trans. Thomas Symons. New York: Oxford University Press.

Tacchella, Lorenzo. 1972. *S. Carlo Borromeo ed il card. Agostino Valier (carteggio)*. Verona: Istituto per gli studi veronesi.

1974. *Il card. A. Valier e la riforma Tridentina nelle diocesi di Trieste*. Udine: Editrice Arti Grafiche Friuliane.

Tadlock, Stephanie L. 2005. "Fra Bartolommeo and the Vision of Saint Bernard: An Examination of Savonarolan Influence." Ph.D. diss., University of Maryland.

Tallon, Alain. 1997. *La France et le Concile de Trente (1518–1563)*. Rome. École Française de Rome.

Talvacchia, Bette. 2010. "The Double Life of St. Sebastian in Renaissance Art." In *The Body in Early Modern Italy*. Ed. Julia Hairston and Walter Stephens, 226–48. Baltimore: Johns Hopkins University Press.

Tanner, Norman, ed. 1990. *Decrees of the Ecumenical Councils*, 2 vols. Washington, DC: Georgetown University Press.

Tarchi, Rossella, Cecilia Nubola, and Angelo Turchini. 1993. "Per un'indicazione computerizzata degli atti della visite pastorali della diocesi di Firenze. La visita di Alessandro de' Medici del 1589." In *Visite Pastorali ed elaborazione dei dati. Esperienze e metodi*. Ed. Cecilia Nubola and Angelo Turchini, 81–140. Annali dell'Istituto storico italo-germanico in Trento. Bologna: Il Mulino.

Taubert, Gesine, and Johannes Taubert. 1969. "Mittelalterliche Kruzifixe mit schwenkbaren Armen: Ein Beitrag zur Verwendung von Bildwerken in der Liturgie." *Zeitschrift des deutschen Vereins für Kunstwissenschaft* 23: 79–121.

Taviani, Ferdinando. 1969. *La commedia dell'arte e la societa barocca*. Rome: Bulzoni.

Taylor, John Hammond, trans. 1982. *The Literal Meaning of Genesis*, vol. 2. New York: Newman Press.

Thayer, Joseph Henry. 1996. *Thayer's Greek–English Lexicon of the New Testament: Coded with the Numbering System from Strong's Exhaustive Concordance of the Bible*. Peabody, MA: Hendrickson.

Thiers, Jean-Baptiste. 1777. *Traité de l'exposition du s. sacrement de l'autel*. Avignon: L. Chambeau.

Thro, E. Broydrick. 1966. "Leonardo's Early Work on the Pinhole Camera: The Astronomical Heritage of Levi ben Gerson." *Achademia Leonardi Vinci* 9: 20–54.

Tischendorf, Konstantin von. 1872. *Novum Testamentum Graece*, 2 vols. Leipzig: H. Mendelssohn.

Tongiorgi Tomasi, Lucia, and Tony Willis, eds. 2009. *An Oak Spring Herbaria: Herbs and Herbals from the Fourteenth to the Nineteenth Centuries*. Upperville, VA: Oak Spring Garden Library.

Toscano, Gennaro. 1985. "Baronio e le immagini." In De Maio et al. (1985), 409–23.

Tosini, Patrizia, ed. 2009. *Arte e committenza nel Lazio nell'età di Cesare Baronio. Atti del convegno internazionale di studi Frosinone, 2007*. Rome: Gangemi.

Traube, Ludwig. ed. 1881. *Poetae Latini aevi Carolini*. Berlin: Apud Weidmann.

Trinkaus, Charles. 1970. *"In Our Image and Likeness": Humanity and Divinity in Italian Humanist Thought*, 2 vols. Chicago: University of Chicago Press.

Tripps, Johannes. 1998. *Das handelnde Bildwerk in der Gotik. Forschungen zu den Bedeutungsschichten und der Funktion des Kirchengebäudes und seiner Ausstattung in der Hoch- und Spätgotik*. Berlin: Gebr. Mann.

Tüchle, Hermann. 1977. "Die Münsteraltäre des Spätmittelalters. Stifter, Heilige, Patrone und Kapläne." In *600 Jahre Ulmer Münster – Festschrift*. Ed. Hans Engen Specker and Reinhard Wörtmann, 126–82. Ulm: Stadtarchiv.

Turchini, Angelo. 1996. "La visita come strumento di governo del territorio." In *Il concilio di Trento ed il moderno*. Ed. Paolo Prodi and Wolfgang Reinhard. Bologna: Il Mulino.

Turks, Paul. 1995. *Philip Neri: The Fire and Joy*. New York: Alba House.

Tuve, Rosemond. 1947. *Elizabethan and Metaphysical Imagery*. Chicago: University of Chicago Press.

Ughelli, Ferdinando. 1717. *Italia Sacra*. Venice: apud Sebastianum Coleti.

Ugolnik, Anthony. 1989. "The *Libri Carolini*: Antecedents of Reformation Iconoclasm." In *Iconoclasm vs. Art and Drama*. Ed. Clifford Davidson and Ann Eljenholm Nichols, 1–32. Kalamazoo: Western Michigan University, Medieval Institute Publications.

Ussia, Salvatore. 1988. "Il tema letterario della Maddalena nell'età della Controriforma." *Rivista di storia e letteratura religiosa* 24: 386–424.

1975. *Il dialogo della gioia cristiana* [1591]. Ed. Antonio Cistellini, D.O. Brescia: La scuola.

Valla, Lorenzo. 1540. *Laurentii Vallae Opera*. Basel: Henricum Petrum.

Van Eikema Hommes, Margriet. 2000. "Discoloration or Chiaroscuro? An Interpretation of the Dark Areas in Raphael's *Transfiguration of Christ*." *Simiolus* 28.1–2: 4–43.

Vannini, Phillip, Dennis Waskul, and Simon Gottschalk. 2011. *The Senses in Self, Society, and Culture: A Sociology of the Senses*. London: Routledge.

Varriano, John L. 1999. "Caravaggio and Religion." In O'Malley (1999b), 206.

2006. *Caravaggio: The Art of Realism*. University Park, Pa: Pennsylvania State University Press.

Vasari, Giorgio. 1881. *Le vite de' più eccellenti pittori, scultori ed architettori*, vol. 7. Ed. Gaetano Milanesi. Florence: G. C. Sansoni.

1966–87. *Le vite de più eccellenti pittori, scultori e architettori. Nelle redazioni del 1550 e 1568*. Ed. Rosanna Bettarini and Paola Barrocchi. Florence: Sansoni and Studio per edizioni scelte.

1996. *Lives of the Painters, Sculptors and Architects*. Trans. Gaston du C. de Vere, intro. David Ekserdjian. New York: Alfred Knopf.

1997. *Le vite de' piu eccellenti pittori, scultori e architettori. Nelle redazioni del 1550 e 1568*, vol. 6. Ed. Rosanna Bettarini and Paola Barrocchi. Florence: Studio per edizioni scelte.

Venatorius, Thomas. 1529. *Thomae Venatorii de Virtute Christiana Libri III*. Nuremberg: Foedericus Peypus.

Venturelli, Paola. 1999. *Vestire e apparire. Il sistema vestimentario femminile nella Milano spagnola (1539–1679)*. Rome: Bulzoni.

Venturoli, Alberto. 1988. *San Filippo Neri. Vita, contesto storico e dimensione mariana*. Casale Monferrato: Piemme.

Verstegen, Ian. 2003a. "Federico Barocci: The Art of Painting and the Rhetoric of Persuasion." Ph.D. diss., Temple University. Ann Arbor, MI: UMI Dissertation Services.

2003b. "Federico Barocci, Borromeo and the Oratorian Orbit." *Renaissance Quarterly* 56: 56–87.

Vetter, Ewald M. 1994. *Speculum salutis. Arbeiten zur christlichen Kunst*. Münsterschwarzach: Vier-Türme.

Vignau-Wilberg, Thea, ed. 2005. *In Europa zu Hause. Niederländer in München um 1600*. Exh. cat., Neue Pinakothek, Munich. Munich: Hirmer.

Villaret, Émile. 1947. *Les Congrégations mariales*, vol. 1: *Des origines à la suppression de la compagnie de Jésus, 1540–1773*. Paris: Beau Chesne.

Villari, Pasquale. 1888. *Life and Times of Girolamo Savanarola*, vol. 1. London: T. Fisher Unwin.

Voelker, Evelyn C. 1977. "Charles Borromeo's 'Instructiones fabricae et supellectilis ecclesiasticae,' 1577: A Translation with Commentary and Analysis." PhD. Diss., Syracuse University. Ann Arbor, Michigan: University Microfilms International, 1981.

Volk-Knüttel, Brigitte. 1988. "Candid nach Schwarz." *Münchner Jahrbuch der bildenden Kunst* 39: 113–32.

2010. *Peter Candid (um 1548–1628): Gemälde, Zeichnungen, Druckgraphik*. Berlin: Kunstwissenschaft.

Von Pastor, Ludwig. 1923–53. *The History of the Popes from the Close of the Middle Ages*, 40 vols. Trans. and ed. Ralph Francis Kerr. London: Kegan Paul.

1938–61. *The History of the Popes from the Close of the Middle Ages*, 40 vols. Trans. and ed. Ralph Francis Kerr. London: Routledge & Kegan Paul.

Von Posse, Hans. 1931. "Die Rekonstruktion der Venus mit dem Cupido von Giorgione." *Jahrbuch der Preußischen Kunstsammulgen* 52: 29–35.

Voragine, Jacobus de. 1969. *The Golden Legend of Jacobus de Voragine*. Trans. Granger Ryan and Helmut Ripperger. New York: Arno.

Wagner, Karl, and Albert Keller, eds. 1983. *St. Michael in München*. Munich: Schnell & Steiner.

Warner, Marina. 1976. *Alone of All Her Sex: The Myth and the Cult of the Virgin Mary*. New York: Knopf.

Warning, Rainer. 2001. *The Ambivalences of Medieval Religious Drama*. Trans. Steven Rendall. Stanford, CA: Stanford University Press.

Wazbinski, Zygmut. 1977. "Artisti e pubblico a Firenze nel '500." *Paragone* 28: 3–24.

1986. "Lo studio: la scuola fiorentina di Federico Zuccari." *Mitteilungen des Kunsthistorischen Institutes in Florenz* 25: 275–346.

1987. "Il *modus* semplice: un dibattito sull'*ars sacra* fiorentina intorno al 1600." In *Studi su Raffaello*, 2 vols. Ed. Micaela Sambucco Hamoud and Maria Letizia Strocchi, 1: 625–48. Urbino: Quattro Venti.

Wegmann, Peter. 1985. " 'Öfters mehr ein Theater': Bemerkungen zu barocken Heiligen Gräbern." In *Grenzbereiche der Architektur*. Ed. Thomas Bolt et al., 243–58. Basel: Birkhäuser.

Welt im Umbruch. Augsburg zwischen Renaissance und Barock. 1980–81. Exh. cat., Stadt Augsburg, 3 vols. Augsburg: Augsburger Druck- und Verlagshaus.

Wheeler, Jo. 2007. "Stench in Sixteenth-Century Venice." In *The City and the Senses: Urban Culture Since 1500*. Ed. Alexander Cowan and Jill Stewart, 25–38. Burlington, VT: Ashgate.

Williams, Robert. 1989. "A Treatise by Francesco Bocchi in Praise of Andrea del Sarto." *Journal of the Warburg and Courtauld Institutes* 52: 111–39.

1997. *Art, Theory, and Culture in Sixteenth-Century Italy: From Techne to Metatechne*. Cambridge: Cambridge University Press.

Wimböck, Gabriele. 1998. *Der Ingolstädter Münsteraltar*. Munich: Lipp.

Winston-Allen, Anne. 1997. *Stories of the Rose: The Making of the Rosary in the Middle Ages*. University Park: Pennsylvania State University Press.

Witcombe, Christopher L. C. E. 2004. *Copyright in the Renaissance: Prints and the Privilegio in Sixteenth-Century Venice and Rome*. Studies in Medieval and Reformation Traditions. Leiden: Brill.

Wittkower, Rudolf, and Irma B. Jaffe, eds. 1972. *Baroque Art: The Jesuit Contribution*. New York: Fordham University Press.

Woeckel, Gerhard P. 1992. *Pietas Bavaricae*. Weissenhorn: Anton Konrad.

Wohl, Helmut. 1999. *The Aesthetics of Italian Renaissance Art: A Reconsideration of Style*. New York: Cambridge University Press.

Wölfflin, Heinrich. 1953. *Classic Art* [1899]. Trans. Peter Murray and Linda Murray. London: Phaidon.

Woolgar, C. M. [Christopher Michael]. 2006. *The Senses in Late Medieval England*. New Haven, CT: Yale University Press.

Young, Karl. 1920. *The Dramatic Associations of the Easter Sepulchre*. University of Wisconsin Studies in Language and Literature, vol. 10. Madison: University of Wisconsin.

1962. *The Drama of the Medieval Church*. Oxford: Clarendon Press.

Zager, Daniel. 1995. "Liturgical Rite and Musical Repertory: The Polyphonic Latin Hymn Cycle of Lasso in Munich and Augsburg." In *Orlandus Lassus and His Time*. Ed. Ignace Bossuyt, Eugeen Schreurs, and Annelies Wouters, 215–31. Peer: Alamire Foundation.

Zampelli, Michael. 2002. "Giovan Battista Andreini's *Maddalena* of 1617: Staging the Redemption of the Theatrical Profession." In *From Rome to Eternity. Catholicism and the Arts in Italy, ca. 1550–1650*. Ed. Pamela Jones and Thomas Worcester, 63–83. Leiden: Brill.

2006. " 'Lascivi Spettacoli': Jesuits and Theater (from the Underside)." In O'Malley (2006c), 550–72.

Zanlonghi, Giovanna. 2002. *Teatri di formazione. Actio, parola e immagine nella scena gesuitica del Sei-Settecento a Milano.* Milan: Vita e Pensiero.

Zapperi, Roberto. 1994. *Eros e Controriforma. Preistoria della Galleria Farnese.* Turin: Bollati Boringhieri.

1998. *La leggenda del papa Paolo III. Arte e censura nella Roma pontificia.* Turin: Bollati Boringhieri.

Zeri, Federico. 1957. *Pittura e Controriforma. L'arte senza tempo di Scipione da Gaeta.* Turin: Einaudi.

Zini, Pietro Francesco. 1556. *Boni pastoris exemplum.* Venice: Giovanni Battista Sessa.

Zuccari, Alessandro. 1981. "La politica culturale dell'Oratorio romano nella seconda metà del Cinquecento." *Storia dell'arte* 41: 77–112.

1983. "La politica culturale dell'Oratorio Romano nelle imprese artistiche promosse da Cesare Baronio." *Storia dell'arte* 43: 171–93.

1984. *Arte e committenza nella Roma di Caravaggio.* Turin: Edizioni Rai.

1992. *I pittori di Sisto V.* Rome: Fratelli Palombi.

1995a. "Cesare Baronio: le immagini, gli artisti." In Strinati and Costamagna (1995), 80–97.

1995b. "Cultura e predicazione nelle immagini dell'oratorio." In Prodi (1995), 340–54.

1996. "Immagini e sermoni dell'Oratorio nei dipinti della Chiesa Nuova." In *La Congregazione dell'Oratorio di San Filippo Neri nelle Marche del '600.* Ed. Flavia Emanuelli, 173–93. Fiesole: Nardini.

Zuccaro, Federico. 1607. *L'Idea de' pittori, scultori, et architetti*, 2 vols. Turin: Disserolio.

INDEX